CLINICAL HYPNOSIS IN PAIN THERAPY AND PALLIATIVE CARE

ABOUT THE AUTHOR

Dr. Paola Brugnoli, M.D., with Specialization in Anesthesia and Critical Care and master's in Pain Therapy and Palliative Care, Pediatric Anesthesiology and Psychogerontology and Psychogeriatric. She is a Palliativist and Pain Therapist in Medical Staff of Pain Therapy, at University Department of Anesthesiology, Critical Care and Pain Therapy, University of Verona, Italy.

She is internationally recognized for her work in clinical hypnosis, pain therapy and palliative care, routinely teaching to professional audiences in Europe, United States, and all over the world and in schools of specialization in psychotherapy.

She is the author of seven books, in Italian and English. She is AIST President, the Italian Association for the study of Pain Therapy and Clinical Hypnosis (www.aist-pain.it).

E-mail: paola.brugnoli@libero.it

CLINICAL HYPNOSIS IN PAIN THERAPY AND PALLIATIVE CARE

A Handbook of Techniques for Improving the Patient's Physical and Psychological Well-Being

By

MARIA PAOLA BRUGNOLI, M.D.

Department of Anesthesiology
Critical Care and Pain Therapy
University of Verona
Verona, Italy

Foreword by Julie H. Linden and Consuelo C. Casula

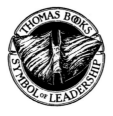

CHARLES C THOMAS • PUBLISHER, LTD.
Springfield • Illinois • U.S.A.

Published and Distributed Throughout the World by

CHARLES C THOMAS • PUBLISHER, LTD.
2600 South First Street
Springfield, Illinois 62704

© 2014 by CHARLES C THOMAS • PUBLISHER, LTD.

ISBN 978-0-398-08765-4 (hard)
ISBN 978-0-398-08766-1 (paper)
ISBN 978-0-398-08767-8 (ebook)

Library of Congress Catalog Card Number: 2013023179

With THOMAS BOOKS *careful attention is given to all details of manufacturing and design. It is the Publisher's desire to present books that are satisfactory as to their physical qualities and artistic possibilities and appropriate for their particular use.* THOMAS BOOKS *will be true to those laws of quality that assure a good name and good will.*

Printed in the United States of America
MM-R-3

Library of Congress Cataloging-in-Publication Data

Brugnoli, Maria Paola, author.
 Clinical hyponosis in pain therapy and palliative care : a handbook of techniques for improving the patient's physical and psychological well-being / by Maria Paola Brugnoli ; foreword by Julie H. Linden and Consuelo C. Casula.
 p. ; cm.
 Includes bibliographical references and index.
 ISBN 978-0-398-08765-4 (hard) -- ISBN 978-0-398-08766-1 (pbk.) --
ISBN 978-0-398-08767-8 (ebook)
 1. Title.
 [DNLM: 1. Hypnosis—methods. 2. Hypnosis, Anesthetic. 3. Pain Management—methods. 4. Palliative Care,methods. 5. Spiritual Therapies. WM 415]

 RC499.A8
 615.8'5122—dc23
                                        2013023179

FOREWORD

Anesthetist and pain specialist, Paola Brugnoli, brings together her experience, knowledge and emotional intelligence in this integrative work on clinical hypnosis and pain management. Unlike many other books that address the topic of pain treatments, this one is expansive. Conceptually, Brugnoli explores the links between ancient philosophy and quantum physics, reviews consciousness and modified states of consciousness, and updates our understanding of neurophysiology and neuropsychology as they each influence our understanding of how to relieve pain and suffering.

A clinical hypnotherapist, she considers the shared roots of clinical hypnosis and mindfulness and provides a spiritual overview of the universal contributions to healing that come from the practices of many meditative states in different philosophies and religions. Finally, she is able to frame this in a life-span perspective noting the diverse approaches with children and adults.

Her deep sensitivity is most notable in her attention to the dignity of the person in pain. She gathers together the techniques for distracting them from the painful present and transporting them to another dimension. One can imagine her psychological hand-holding and support as she moves her patients from suffering to relief.

Practically, Brugnoli is generous in providing the reader the scripts for many inductions. The handbook is enriched by medical and hypnotic techniques for pain analgesia as well as hypnotic deepening techniques to activate spiritual awareness. It also indicates when and how to use them with children and adults.

With extensive references, this book offers accessible concepts and practical suggestions to the reader. It highlights the relational and the creative process, encouraging each clinician to find his or her own way of facilitating the mechanisms in the patient to alleviate pain and suffering. The book demonstrates the vast experience Brugnoli accumulated in her work as anesthesiologist, palliative care specialist and Pain Therapist at University Department of Anesthesiology.

JULIE H. LINDEN, PH.D.
CONSUELO C. CASULA, PSY.D.

INTRODUCTION

And a man said, speak to us of self knowledge.
And he answered saying:
Your hearts know in silence the secrets of the days and of the nights.
But your ears thirst for the sound of your heart's knowledge.
You would know in words that which you have always known in thought.
You would touch with your fingers the naked body of your dreams.
And it is well you should.
The hidden well-spring of your soul must rise and run murmuring to the sea;
And the treasure of your infinite depths would be revealed to your eyes.

Kahlil Gibran

Yesterday I thought myself a fragment quivering
without rhythm in the sphere of life.
Now I know that I am the sphere,
and all life in rhythmic fragments moves within me.

Kahlil Gibran

*C*linical Hypnosis in Pain Therapy and Palliative Care refers to the conscious, calm awareness of cognitions, sensations, emotions, and experiences. This state can be achieved through mindfulness and meditative states, which are practices that cultivate nonjudgmental awareness of the present moment. Mindfulness (from Pāli; *sati;* and Sanskrit; *smṛti;* furthermore, translated as awareness) is a spiritual or psychological faculty (indriya) that is considered to be important in the path to enlightenment according to the teaching of the Buddha. It is one of the seven factors of enlightenment. "Correct" or "right" mindfulness is the seventh element of the noble eightfold path. Mindfulness meditation can also be traced back to the earlier Upanishads, part of Hindu scripture.

The Abhidhammattha Sangaha, a key Abhidharma text from the Theravada tradition, defines sati as follows: "The word *sati* derives from a root meaning 'to remember,' but as a mental factor it signifies the presence of mind, attentiveness to the present, rather than the faculty of memory regarding the past. It has the characteristic of not wobbling, not floating away from the object. Its function is the absence of confusion or nonforgetfulness. It is manifested as guardianship, or as the state of confronting an objective field. Its proximate cause is strong perception (*thirasanna*) or the four foundations of mindfulness."

Mindfulness practice, inherited from the Buddhist tradition, is increasingly being employed in Western psychology to alleviate a variety of mental and physical conditions. Scientific research into mindfulness, generally falls under the umbrella of positive psychology. Research has been ongoing over the last twenty or thirty years, with a surge of interest over the last decade in particular.

In 2011, the National Institutes of Health's (NIH) National Center for Complementary and Alternative Medicine (NCCAM) released the findings of a study in which magnetic resonance images of the brains of 16 participants, two weeks before and after mindfulness meditation practitioners joined the meditation program, were taken by researchers from Massachusetts General Hospital, Bender Institute of Neuroimaging in Germany, and the University of Massachusetts Medical School. It concluded that "these findings may represent an underlying brain mechanism associated with mindfulness-based improvements in mental health" (National Center, 2011).

The high likelihood of recurrence in depression is linked to a progressive increase in emotional reactivity to stress (stress sensitization). Mindfulness-based therapies teach mindfulness skills, designed to decrease emotional reactivity in the face of negative affect-producing stressors. Given that emotional reactivity to stress is an important psychopathological process underlying the chronic and recurrent nature of depression, mindfulness skills are important in adaptive emotion regulation when coping with stress (Britton, Shahar, Szepsenwol, & Jacobs, 2012).

In this model, self-regulated attention (an important component of consciousness) involves conscious awareness of one's current thoughts, feelings, and surroundings. Consciousness is extremely elusive from the empirical point of view. Scientists of consciousness usually proceed as if such a definition were already available. In clinical hypnosis, mindfulness, and meditative states, we assume a priori that consciousness is an object and exists in an observer-independent way.

A primary point of contention among the major theories of consciousness is whether attention is generally necessary for consciousness. The global workspace theory (Deahene et al., 2006) holds that an inability to accurately report supraliminal stimuli that are unattended indicates that they are processed unconsciously (inattentional blindness).

The neurogenetics of consciousness has three main components:

1. The neurophysiological neurogenesis, brain morphogenesis, and neuron maturation, which are all under the guidance of genes
2. The neuron-based continuum of consciousness that involves neurological and epigenetic factors, microtubules and neuroplasticity
3. The end of life processes that involves neurodegeneration

This suggests that it is important to go beyond the mask of brain anatomy to explore the fine spatiotemporal patterns and the underlying mechanisms of consciousness. The human brain consists of about one billion neurons, and each neuron has synapses on the order of 1000. Thus, the capability of the human brain is 1016 operations per second. We know that each neuron in the human brain consists of large number of microtubules. Penrose and Hameroff (2007) proposed that consciousness involves sequences of quantum computation in microtubules inside brain neurons.

Recent studies (Demertzi et al., 2009) show that awareness is an emergent property of the collective behavior of frontoparietal top-down connectivity. With this network, external (sensory) awareness depends on lateral prefrontal parietal cortices, and internal (self) awareness correlates with precuneal mesiofrontal midline activity. Both functional magnetic resonance imaging (MRI) and electrophysiology suggest that attention and consciousness share neural correlates. The fields of pain and palliative care have undergone a great revolution, and this volume reflects these exciting advances.

We are so accustomed to viewing pain as a sensory phenomenon that we have long ignored the fact that injury does more than produce pain; it also disrupts the brain's homeostatic regulation system, thereby producing "stress" and initiating complex programs to reinstate homeostasis. Stress can be defined as an activation of the limbic system of the central nervous system (CNS) that then activates neurohumoral mechanisms of arousal. Stress produced by painful experiences initiates a cascade of neurophysiological, humoral, and phenomenological events that challenge our understanding but also provide valuable clues in dealing with chronic pain (Melzack, 1998, 1999).

I wrote this textbook as a contribution to pain and suffering therapy in palliative care. Advances in pain and suffering therapy have tremendously influenced the development of new nonpharmacological and noninvasive pain management. Psychological therapies that were generally used when drugs or anesthesiology or neurosurgery failed are now integrated into mainstream pain management strategies.

The stress associated with advancing and incurable illness inevitably causes distress for patients, families, and caregivers. A palliative approach to care aims to improve the quality of life for patients with a life-limiting illness by reducing suffering through early identification; assessment; and optimal management of pain and physical, cultural, psychological, social, and spiritual needs.

This book is quite different from others in its unique focus on the assessment of pain and suffering therapy through clinical hypnosis and mindfulness, rather than through conventional pharmacological, anesthesiological, and invasive techniques that have previously been dealt with in many other texts. The book explores the fields of clinical hypnosis and mindfulness as applied to the therapy of suffering and various type of acute and chronic pain and in dying patients. We were conscious of how much there is to learn in these areas, we believe that the dissemination of this rapidly growing body of knowledge will stimulate further research and exploration into the use of specific consciousness states for healing and wellness work.

This book is organized in order to show all scientific neuropsychological theories currently in use regarding various types of pain and suffering. Recent advances in the understanding of fundamental neurobiological mechanisms of nociception have provided insights into the evaluation and treatment of clinical pain (Melzack, 2002). Acute pain serves the purpose of alerting the organism to the presence of harmful stimuli in the internal or external environment. Acute pain may be repetitive in circumstances in which recurrent and/or progressive tissue injury is experienced.

The chronic "pain state" term is usually used in the context of patients who report pain on a long-term basis with no apparent tissue injury component or at least no apparent evidence of persistent nociceptor activation. The psychological counterparts to the chronic pain state include depression, anxiety, and other affective states and are key to understanding the disability associated with this condition (Cleeland & Syrjala, 1992). The different aspects of pathophysiological pain (neurophysiology and psychology), are described followed by a classification of anatomiconeurophysiological and neuropsychological pain.

Scientific literature distinguishes the philosophy of neuroscience and neurophilosophy. The former concerns foundational issues within the neurosciences. The latter concerns application of neuroscientific concepts, to traditional philosophical questions. Exploring various neurological concepts of representation employed in neuroscientific theories is an example of the former.

Examining implications of neurological syndromes for the concept of a unified self and in different states of consciousness, as in clinical hypnosis and mindfulness, is an example of the latter. I will discuss examples of both in the therapy of pain and suffering and will describe hypnosis techniques useful for the management of physical pain and mental suffering.

Therefore, I have chosen to describe many different techniques of clinical hypnosis and mindfulness. This book has been carefully studied, edited, and strongly desired by the author, who has a vast experience in the specific field of physical, mental, and spiritual suffering therapy in subjects afflicted by various types of pain, acute and chronic; disability; and cancer illness in order to relieve, within limits their anxiety and worry regarding a better quality of life.

If we look at the Contents, we can see that the arguments are dealt with in a scientific way but also from a psychological and spiritual point of view. The book highlights the importance the author gives to the study of clinical hypnosis and interior awareness, consolidating the studies carried out by psychologists at first and then by scientists through neurosciences. The World Health Organization (WHO) defines palliative care as "The active total care of patients whose disease is not responsive to curative treatment." One of the primary issues of palliative care for patients with advanced cancer is symptom control and quality-of-life issues.

This book presents a hypnotic model for improving the patient's physical and psychological well-being. There exists a need for a broad and inclusive model of mind-body interventions for pain therapy and palliative care. This is supported by the observation that symptoms related to psychological distress and existential concerns are even more prevalent than are pain and other physical symptoms among those with life-limiting conditions.

The hypnotic trance is a consciousness state of heightened awareness and focused concentration that can be used to manipulate the perception of pain and has been effective in the treatment of cancer-related pain. Our ordinary state of consciousness is not something natural or given but is a highly complex construction, a specialized tool for coping with our environment (Tart, 1972).

The last change comes from the new techniques of brain imaging, for which we must know the traditional separation of sensory and motor mechanisms of consciousness. The chapter titles of this book show how the author has incorporated this fundamentally new thinking about the origins of pain and suffering and the direction of new therapies. The conscious mind is one of the most unresolved problems of neuroscience. What are the conscious sensations that accompany neural activities of the brain? What is the bridge between pain perception and the experience of anxiety and suffering? Moreover, how can we cure suffering and pain in all their aspects, not only physical but also mental? How does a neurochemical phenomenon like pain, which starts from a biological state, transform into a psychological sensation?

Even if our neurophysiological knowledge should one day enable us to identify the exact neurochemical correlation of a psychic phenomenon, we must not forget that neurochemical knowledge is not sufficient to explain all the subjective experiences in people. The conscious mental properties interact in causal and lawlike ways with other fundamental properties such as those of physics; however, their existence is neither ontologically dependent upon nor derivative from any other properties (Chalmers, 1996).

A major turning point in philosophers' interest in neuroscience came with the publication of Patricia Churchland's *Neurophilosophy* (1986). The Churchlands (Pat and husband Paul) were already notorious for advocating eliminative materialism. In her book, Churchland distilled eliminativist arguments of the past decade, unified the pieces of the philosophy of science underlying them, and sandwiched the philosophy between a five-chapter introduction to neuroscience and a seventy-page chapter on three then-current theories of brain function (1986). She was unapologetic about her intent. She was introducing philosophy of science to neuroscientists and neuroscience to philosophers (Bickle, 2003).

Science still does not know the mechanisms that produced awareness experiences, however, and does not have a clear definition of them. Consciousness then is more than the sum of its constituent neurophysiological events and substrates. The physician and mathematician John Taylor recently observed "the study of consciousness is like a black hole for those that study it. Once the scientific study is done they lose sight of their normal scientific activity and give an explanation of the phenomena that does not correspond to a scientific explanation" (Taylor, 2000).

In cancer patients and in palliative care, pain is neurophysiological, psychological, social, and spiritual. As David Chalmers wrote, "even if we explained all the physical events inside and around the brain and how all the neural functions operate something would be missing: consciousness" (1996). The question then naturally arises: Is it possible to incorporate both science and mysticism into a single, coherent worldview? Quantum mechanics shows that the materialistic common sense notion of reality is an illusion. The appearance of an objective world distinguishable from a subjective self is but the imaginary form in which consciousness perfectly realizes itself (McFarlane, 1995). How can one approach consciousness in a scientific manner? There are many forms of consciousness, such as those associated with seeing, thinking, emotions, pain, suffering and so on.

Clinical hypnosis can help the patients to improve their self-consciousness and self-awareness. The techniques of relaxation, hypnosis, and mindfulness in meditative states are open gates on the self in pain and suffering therapy. Psychological interventions are an important part of a multimodal approach to pain and suffering management. Such interventions frequently are used in conjunction with appropriate analgesics for the management of pain.

One goal is to help the patients gain a sense of control over pain and suffering. Changing how they think about pain, we can change their sensitivity to it and their feelings and reactions toward it. In *Analysis Terminable and Interminable* (1937) Freud wrote, "Only the simultaneous working together and against each other of both primordial drives, of Eros and death drive, can explain the colourfulness of life, never the one or the other all by itself." Erickson, like Freud, suffered all his life. His basic attitude toward his patients also reflected this basic dialectic of the life and death drive: "I think that you should take a patient as he is. He is only going to live today, tomorrow, next week, next month, next year. His living conditions are those of today" (Erickson, Rossi, & Rossi, 1976).

There is therefore a permanent task for the beginner and for the experienced practitioner as well: through symbolization, through clinical and experimental researches and theorizing, we have to convert the mirage of hypnosis into a disciplined analysis of our condition as human subjects made of body, mind, and spirit. Several techniques can be used to achieve a mental and physical state of relaxation. Muscular tension, and mental distress exacerbate pain (Benson, 1975; Brugnoli, Brugnoli, & Norsa, 2006; Cleeland, 1987; Loscalzo & Jacobsen, 1990).

Hypnosis can be a useful adjunct in the management of pain and clinical trials (Erickson, 1959; Jensen & Patterson, 2005; Levitan, 1992; Spiegel, 1985). The hypnotic trance is a essentially a state of heightened and focused concentration, and thus it can be used to manipulate the perception of pain. The use of hypnosis involves control over the focus of attention and can be used to make the patient less aware of the noxious stimuli (Bates, Broome, Lillis, & McGahe, 1992)

The use of clinical hypnosis and mindfulness in pain therapy and palliative care, makes us give to the patients empathy and listening skills; empathic listening sometimes leads to good therapy, relationships, and emotional intimacy. Their use may also lead to a conversation partner feeling like she or he is receiving a hug, a "psychological hug." The consciousness approach through clinical hypnosis and meditative states can be used not only in a verbal channel, but also in patients with cognitive disorders through feelings and perceiving sensations. The realm of emotional responses constitutes the personal sphere wherein one interacts with the environment, past, thoughts, and one's and others immediate and ultimate values.

Components of emotional events include liminal-subliminal perception of real, or imaging of imaginary, objects, representations of those objects, reflexive motor responses, and a range of unattended higher and higher-order emotional experiences. The problem faced by both sciences and psychology is dualism: The apparent duality between subjective and objective or consciousness and matter. The solution is in clinical hypnosis and mindfulness: It is not to side either with brain but somehow–whether through neuroscience, psychology, philosophy, or spiritual practice–to attain nonduality.

Consciousness study has been the focus of an extensive practice in spiritual traditions since ancient times. Many spiritual meditations have provided detailed revelations of different states of consciousness. It is enlightening to study clinical hypnosis, mindfulness and the modified states of consciousness in different traditions, to achieve the primary objective of self-realization and higher consciousness. Generally, we know various "states of consciousness," in particular, wakefulness; dreams; and sleep, which the physiologists divide into "slow sleep" and "paradoxical sleep." Methods of relaxation allow us to describe a "modified state," a particular state of consciousness to which we can give a special value. This state comprises peace, serenity, "absorption," even "presence," and ineffability.

In this book, I present a new system approach to study the neurophysiological states of consciousness to improve the use of clinical hypnosis and mindfulness in pain therapy and palliative care. The contents of the book cover:

- What consciousness is
- Neurophysiology and neuropsychology of pain
- The modified states of consciousness in pain therapy and palliative care
- A new system approach and classification of clinical hypnosis and mindfulness in consciousness states
- The hypnosis techniques, the meditative states, and mindfulness techniques to relieve pain in palliative care
- Relaxation and hypnosis in pediatric patients: techniques for pain and suffering relief
- Music therapy to achieve deep hypnosis and mindfulness
- Metaphor's techniques in pain therapy and palliative care
- Modified states of consciousness and quantum physics: the mind beyond matter

Our ordinary state of consciousness is not something natural or given but a highly complex construction, a specialized tool for coping with our environment and the people in it. In this book, I propose a new approach, using neurophysiologic and neuropsychological explanations that help to formulate empirically testable hypotheses about the nature of consciousness states. Because we are creatures with a certain kind of body and nervous system, a large number of human potentials are, in principle, available to use, but each of us is born into a particular culture that selects and develops a small number of these potentials, rejects others, and is ignorant of many.

The small number of experiential abilities selected by our culture, plus some unplanned factors, constitutes the structural elements from which our ordinary state of consciousness is constructed. After all, we are the victims of our culture's particular selection. The power and the possibility of tapping and developing latent potentials that lie outside the cultural norm by entering a modified state of consciousness, by temporarily restructuring consciousness, are the basis of the great interest in such states (Tart, 1990). As we look at consciousness closely, we see that it can be analyzed into many parts: neurophysiology of the brain, neuropsychology of the mind, spirituality, and awareness. These parts function together in a pattern, however: they form a system. Although the components of consciousness can be studied in isolation, they exist as parts of a complex system, consciousness, and can be fully understood only when we see this function in the overall system.

In this book, I carefully examine the role and use of specific states of consciousness, clinical hypnosis techniques, and meditative states for the best management of pain and relief of suffering in adults and children. This book is intended for all the professionals working every day with pain and suffering. Every day, because the mind reflects habitual thoughts, it is therefore our responsibility to influence our brain with positive emotions, thoughts, and energy as the dominating factors in our mind and in our life.

After experiencing many levels of consciousness and the higher consciousness, we become able to live in its energy continuously. Then, with further practice and development, we become permanently awakened and live in uninterrupted higher consciousness. We can direct our inner strength to move and express itself in our own life and the lives of our loved ones.

REFERENCES

Benson, H. (1975). *The Relaxation Response.* New York: William Morrow.

Bickle, J. (2003). *Philosophy and Neuroscience: A Ruthlessly Reductive Account.* Norwell, MA: Kluwer Academic Press.

Britton, W. B., Shahar, B., Szepsenwol, O., & Jacobs, W. J. (2012). Mindfulness-based cognitive therapy improves emotional reactivity to social stress: Results from a randomized controlled trial. *Behavioral Therapy, 43*(2), 365–380.

Broome, M., Lillis, P., McGahe, T., & Bates, T. (1992). The use of distraction and imagery with children during painful procedures. *Oncology Nursing Forum 19,* 499–502.

Brugnoli, M. P., Brugnoli, A., & Norsa, A. (2009). *Nonpharmacological and noninvasive management in pain.* Verona, Italy: La Grafica Editrice.

Chalmers, D. (1996). *The conscious mind.* Oxford, UK: Oxford University Press.

Churchland, P. (1986). *Neurophilosophy.* Cambridge, MA: MIT Press.

Cleeland, C.S. (1987). Nonpharmacologic management of cancer pain. *Journal of Pain and Symptom Control, 2,* 523–528.

Cleeland, C. S., & Syrjala, K. L. (1992). How to assess cancer pain. In D .C. Turk & R. Melzack (Eds.), *Handbook of pain assessment* (pp. 360–387). New York: Guilford Press.

Erickson, M. H. (1959). Hypnosis in painful terminal illness. *American Journal of Clinical Hypnosis, 1,* 1117–1121.

Erickson, M.H., Rossi, E.L., & Rossi, S.I. (1976). Hypnotic Realities: The Induction of Clinical Hypnosis and Forms of Indirect Suggestion. New York: Irvingtone.

Farthing, G. W. (1992). *The psychology of consciousness.* Englewood Cliffs, NJ: Prentice-Hall.

Freud, S. (1937). *Analysis terminable and interminable. The standard edition of the complete psychological works of Sigmund Freud* (Vol. 23 [1937–1939], pp. 209–254). London: Hogart Press, 1964.

Gibran, K. (1992). *Sabbia e Spuma e Il Vagabondo* [*Sand and foam and the wanderer*]. Rome, Italy: Newton Compton Editori.

Gibran, K. (1993). *Il Profeta* [*The prophet*]. Verona, Italy: Editrice Demetra.

Jensen, M. P., & Patterson, D. R. (2005, April). Control conditions in hypnotic analgesia clinical trials: challenges and recommendations. *International Journal of Clinical and Experimental Hypnosis, 53*(2), 170–197.

Levitan, A. (1992). The use of hypnosis with cancer patients. *Psychiatry and Medicine, 10,* 119–131.

Loscalzo, M., & Jacobsen, P. B. (1990). Practical behavioural approaches to the effective management of pain and distress. *Journal of Psychosocial Oncology, 8,* 139–169.

McFarlane, T. J. (1995). Quantum mechanics and reality [Online]. Available at www.integralscience.org

Melzack, R. (1998). Pain and stress: Clues toward understanding chronic pain. In M. Sabourin, F. Craik & M. Robert (Eds.), *Advances in psychological science* (Vol. 2, Biological and Cognitive Aspects, pp. 63–85). London: Psychology Press.

Melzack, R. (1999). Pain and stress: A new perspective. In R.J. Gatchel & D.C. Turk (Eds.), *Psychosocial factors in pain* (pp. 89–106). New York: Guilford Press.

Melzack, R. (2002). *Evolution of Pain Theories.* Program and Abstracts of the 21st Annual Scientific Meeting of the American Pain Society, March 14–17, Baltimore, Maryland. Abstract 102.

National Center for Complementary and Alternative Medicine (NCCAM). (2011, January 30). Research Spotlight: Mindfulness meditation is associated with structural changes in the brain [Online]. Available at http://nccam.nih.gov/research/results/spotlight/012311.htm

Spiegel, D. (1985). The use of hypnosis in controlled cancer pain. *CA: A Cancer Journal for Clinicians, 4,* 221–231.

Tart, C. T. (1972). States of consciousness and state-specific sciences. *Science, 176,* 1203–1210.

Taylor, J. (2000, February). The enchanting subject of consciousness (or is it a black hole?). *PSYCHE, 6*(2).

SUGGESTED READINGS

Armstrong, D. M. (1978). Naturalism, Materialism and First Philosophy. *Philosophia, 8,* 261–276.

Boccio, F. J. (2004). *Mindfulness yoga: The awakened union of breath, body and mind.* Somerville, MA: Wisdom Publishers.

Bonica, J. J. (Ed.). (1990). *The management of pain* (2nd ed.). Philadelphia: Lea & Febiger.

Brahm, A. (2005). *Mindfulness, bliss, and beyond: A meditator's handbook.* Somerville, MA: Wisdom Publications.

Brugnoli, A. (2005). *Stati di coscienza modificati neurofisiologici.* Verona, Italy: La Grafica Editrice.

Brugnoli, M. P. (2009). *Clinical hypnosis, spirituality and palliation: The way of inner peace.* Verona, Italy: Del Miglio Editore.

Carruthers, P. (2000). *Phenomenal consciousness.* Cambridge: Cambridge University Press.

Chalmers, D. J. (1995). Facing up to the problem of consciousness. *Journal of Consciousness Studies, 2*(3), 200–219.

Chochinov, H. M., Krisjanson, L. J., Hack, T. F., Hassard, T., McClement, S., & Harlos, M. (2006, June). Dignity in the terminally ill: Revisited. *Journal of Palliative Medicine, 9*(3), 666–672.

Crick, F., & Koch, C. (1995a). Are we aware of neural activity in primary visual cortex? *Nature, 375,* 121–123

Crick, F., & Koch, C. (1995b). Cortical areas in visual awareness [Reply]. *Nature, 377,* 294–295.

Dalai Lama. (1999). *The Dalai Lama's book of wisdom.* London: Thorsons.

Damasio, A. (1994). *Descartes' error: Emotions, reason, and the human brain.* New York: Avon Books.

Graffam, S., & Johnson, A. (1987). A comparison of two relaxation strategies for the relief of pain and its distress. *Journal of Pain and Symptom Management, 2*(4), 229–231.

Guenther, H. V., & Kawamura, L. S. (1975). *Mind in Buddhist psychology: The necklace of clear understanding by Ye-shes rGyal-mtshan* [Tibetan Translation Series] [Kindle edition]. Berkeley, CA: Dharma Publishing.

Gunaratana, B. H. (2002). *Mindfulness in plain English.* Somerville, MA: Wisdom Publications.

Handel, D. L. (2001, February). Complementary therapies for cancer patients: What works, what doesn't, and how to know the difference. *Texas Medicine, 97*(2), 68–73.

Hendler, C. S., & Redd, W. H. (1986). Fear of hypnosis: The role of labeling in patients' acceptance of behavioral interventions. *Behavior Therapy, 17*(1), 2–13.

His Divine Grace A. C. Bhaktivedanta Swami Prabhupada. (1972). *Bhagavad-Gita.* Krishna Store.

Hoopes, A. (2007). *Zen yoga: A path to enlightenment through breathing, movement and meditation.* Tokyo: Kodansha International.

Huai-chin, N. (1993). *Working toward enlightenment: The cultivation of practice.* York Beach, ME: Samuel Weiser.

Kallio, S., & Revonsuo, A. (2003). Hypnotic phenomena and altered states of consciousness: A multilevel framework of description and explanation. *Contemporary Hypnosis, 20*(3), 111–164.

Kihlstrom, J. F. (1997). Convergence in understanding hypnosis? Perhaps, but perhaps not quite so fast. *International Journal of Clinical and Experimental Hypnosis, 45,* 324–332.

Kolcaba, K. Y., & Fisher, E. M. (1996, February). A holistic perspective on comfort care as an advance directive. *Critical Care Nursing Quarterly, 18*(4), 66–76.

Levine, J. (1983). Materialism and qualia: The explanatory gap. *Pacific Philosophical Quarterly, 64,* 354–361.

Manzotti, R., & Gozzano, S. (2004). Verso una scienza della coscienza. *Networks 3–4:* i-iii. Available at http://www.swif.uniba.it/lei/ai/networks/

Masters, E. L. (1988). *Antologia di Spoon River* [*Spoon River anthology*]. Rome, Italy: Newton Compton Editori.

Mathieu, V. (1969). *Storia della filosofia e del pensiero scientifico.* Brescia, Italy: Editrice La Scuola.

McCaffery, M., & Beebe, A. (1989). *Pain: Clinical manual for nursing practice.* St. Louis: Mosby.

McCaul, K. D., & Malott, J. M. (1984). Distraction and coping with pain. *Psychology Bulletin, 95*(3), 516–533.

McGrath, P. A. (Ed.). (1990). *Pain in children: Nature, assessment, and treatment.* New York: The Guilford Press.

Melzack, R. (2001). Pain and the neuromatrix in the brain. *Journal of Dental Education, 65,* 1378–1382.

Melzack, R., & Wall, P. D. (1965). Pain mechanisms: A new theory. *Science, 150,* 971–979.

Mosca, A. (2000). A review essay on Antonio Damasio's The Feeling of What Happens: Body and Emotion in the Making of Consciousness. *PSYCHE, 6*(10).

Munro, S., & Mount, B. (1978). Music therapy in palliative care. *Canadian Medical Association Journal, 119*(9), 1029–1034.

Nagel, T. (1974). What is it like to be a bat? *Philosophical Review, 4,* 435–450.

Nhat Hanh, T. (1996). *The miracle of mindfulness: A manual on meditation.* Boston: Beacon Press.

Reeves, J. L., Redd, W. H., Storm, F. K., & Minagawa, R. Y. (1983). Hypnosis in the control of pain during hyperthermia treatment of cancer. In J.J. Bonica, U. Lindblom & A. Iggo (Eds.), *Proceedings of the Third World Congress on Pain,* Edinburgh. (Vol. 5, Advances in Pain Research and Therapy, pp. 857–861). New York: Raven Press.

Rinpoche, S. (2002). *The Tibetan book of living and dying* (2nd ed.). San Francisco: HarperCollins.

Russel, R. (1961). *Brain, memory, learning.* Oxford, UK: Oxford University Press.

Searle, J. (1992). *The rediscovery of the mind.* Cambridge, MA: MIT Press.

Searle, J. R. (1990). Consciousness, explanatory inversion and cognitive science. *Behavioral and Brain Sciences, 13,* 585–642.

Shapiro, D. (1977). A biofeedback strategy in the study of consciousness. In N.E. Zinberg (Ed.), *Alternate states of consciousness* (pp. 145–37). New York: The Free Press.

Siegel, R. D. (2010). *The mindfulness solution: Everyday practices for everyday problems.* The Guilford Press.

Syrjala, K. L. (1990). Relaxation techniques. In J. J. Bonica (Ed.), *The management of pain* (2nd ed., pp. 1742–1750). Philadelphia: Lea & Febiger.

Travis, C. (2004). The silence of the senses. *Mind, 113,* 57–94.

Van Gulick, R. (2004). Higher-order global states (HOGS): An alternative higher-order model of consciousness. In R. J. Gennaro (Ed.), *Higher-order theories of consciousness: An anthology* (pp. 67–92). Amsterdam: John Benjamins B.V.

Weiss, A. (2004). *Beginning mindfulness: Learning the way of awareness.* Novato, CA: New World Library.

ACKNOWLEDGMENTS

I would like to thank my family for the support, strength, and encouragement they gave me throughout my life. Particularly, I appreciate the love of my husband Andrea, my two sons Luca and Alessandro, my parents Angelico and Elda, my brother Marco, and my sister Angelica.

I would like to express my immense gratitude to my master and father Dr. Angelico Brugnoli, M.D., for improving my knowledge and studies in clinical hypnosis and stages of consciousness. I appreciate his vast knowledge and skills in many areas: in 1965, he and Dr. Gualtiero Guantieri, M.D., founded in Verona, Italy, the Italian Institute for the Study of Psychotherapy and Clinical Hypnosis "H. Bernheim."

I especially thank my colleagues and friends: Dr. Daniel Handel (past president of American Society of Clinical Hypnosis [ASCH]), and professors Sylvain Néron, Alladin Assen, Dabney Ewin, Donald Moss, Camillo Loriedo, Giovanni Gocci; Dr. Michael Yapko, Dr. Alessandro Norsa, Dr. Consuelo Casula (president elect of European Society of Hypnosis [ESH]), Professors Éva Bányai and Katalin Varga, Dr. Nicole Ruysschaert (president of ESH), and Dr. Julie Linden (past president of ASCH and president of International Society of Hypnosis [ISH]) for sharing with me workshops and studies in the United States, in Europe, and in Italy about clinical hypnosis.

I thank my friends Dr. Mike Flynn, psychologist and Christian priest, and Giampaolo Mortaro, theologist, anthropologist and Catholic Comboni priest, for improving my studies about the Christian religion.

The information and Eastern religious studies contained in this book are obtained by following several practice periods and studies with the following teachers: Pandit Kanta Prashad Mishra, Brahmin and Hindu monk, and Pandit Marco Shivchandra Parolini, Brahmin and Hindu monk, from Varanasi Benares, India. In conclusion, I recognize that the Eastern religious knowledge would not have been possible without their assistance.

I greatly thank my colleagues and friends of Agra University in India, Dr. Anirudh Kumar Satsangi, director of the Dayalbagh Educational Institute, and Dr. Siddharth Agarwal, M.D., for willingly sharing our researches about meditative stages and clinical hypnosis.

I am very grateful to all the Professors of Nanjing University of Traditional Chinese Medicine (NJUCM); I attended NJUCM in China in 2007 to improve my knowledge in traditional Chinese medicine (TCM) and my spiritual life in my practice of Chinese medicine, receiving TAO in Italy, 2013.

Very special thanks go out to my friends and English teachers Gary Judge, Vlatka Kalecak, Ricci Gementiza, Letizia Fenzi Stephenson, and Dr. Stefania Dodoni for helping me in translations; it was a pleasure to collaborate with you.

Furthermore, I would like to extend my gratitude to Professor Harvey Max Chochinov. He is internationally recognized as a leader in palliative care research; he is professor of psychiatry at the University of Manitoba and Director of the Manitoba Palliative Care Research Unit, Canada. Thank you, Harvey, for your enthusiasm in sharing your vast knowledge and, then, our conversations about dignity therapy in palliative care.

It is a great pleasure to thank my colleagues and friends: Professor Enrico Polati, director of the Unit Anesthesiology, Critical Care and Pain Therapy at Verona University, and Dr. Vittorio Schweiger, chief of the pain therapy team, for having offered me the opportunity of working with the university team of pain therapy in Verona and developing exciting research projects.

I would also like to thank my publisher, Michael Thomas, and all those who helped this book to become a reality. There are no words that can express the gratitude I feel toward these special people.

Finally, thanks to all my angels who have left this world but are close to me every day (especially my brother Michele) and the One, who perfectly manifests creative excellence and love. Thank you God, for giving me another day, another chance to give and experience love and awareness. Thank you for the energy that feeds my soul. Stay connected to me today and always. God, make me a channel of your energy and help me understand suffering people. Keep us all close to you.

CONTENTS

CLINICAL HYPNOSIS IN PAIN THERAPY AND PALLIATIVE CARE

Chapter I

CONSCIOUSNESS IN CLINICAL HYPNOSIS AND MINDFULNESS

1. PHILOSOPHY, NEUROPHYSIOLOGY AND NEUROPSYCHOLOGY OF CONSCIOUSNESS

A. What is Consciousness?

Consciousness poses the most enigmatic problems in the science of the mind. Consciousness is a term concerning the ability to perceive; to feel; or to be conscious of events, objects, or patterns, which does not necessarily imply understanding. "I see nothing but Becoming. It is the fault of your limited outlook and not the fault of the essence of things if you believe that you see firm land anywhere in the ocean of Becoming and Passing" (Heraclitus, 500 B.C.).

I find the unification of ancient metaphysics and philosophy with modern physics and cosmology very fascinating and inspiring. Certainly, it is now clear that matter interacts with all other matter in the universe. The wave structure of matter provides a very simple sensible explanation of why this is so. "There is nothing that we know more intimately than conscious experience, but there is nothing that is harder to explain. All sorts of mental phenomena have yielded to the scientific investigation in recent years, but consciousness has stubbornly resisted" (Chalmers, 1995).

Although in general speech, we tend to use the terms awareness and consciousness to represent basically the same thing, I use them here with somewhat different meanings.

In medicine, consciousness is assessed by observing a patient's arousal and responsiveness and can be seen as a continuum of states ranging from full alertness and comprehension; through disorientation, delirium, loss of meaningful communication; and finally to loss of movement in response to painful stimuli.

In recent years, consciousness has become a significant topic of research in psychology and neuroscience. The primary focus is on understanding what it means biologically and psychologically for information to be present in consciousness, that is, on determining the neural and psychological correlates of consciousness. Consciousness is the quality or state of being aware of external neurophysiological stimuli or object or something within oneself.

The philosophy of the mind has given rise to many stances regarding consciousness. In this book, I analyze how we can use the modified states of consciousness in clinical hypnosis, meditative states, and mindfulness to relief pain and suffering.

Awareness is much more than consciousness; it is the state or ability to perceive; to feel; or to be conscious of events, objects, or sensory patterns. In this higher level of consciousness, sense data can be confirmed by an observer without necessarily implying understanding. More broadly, it is the state or quality of being aware of something.

Through the different modified states of consciousness, we can reach higher consciousness and awareness: it refers to the awareness or knowledge of an ultimate reality that traditional theistic religions have named God and Gautama Buddha referred to as the unconditioned element and knowledge.

B. The Philosophy of Consciousness: The "Hard" and the "Easy" Problems

According to the philosopher David Chalmers (1995), there is not just one problem of consciousness. Consciousness is an ambiguous term, referring to many different phenomena. Each of these phenomena needs to be explained, but some are easier to explain than others. Chalmers divides the associated problems of consciousness into "hard" and "easy" problems. The easy problems of consciousness are those that seem directly susceptible to the standard methods of cognitive science, whereby a phenomenon is explained in terms of calculative or neural mechanisms. The easy problems of consciousness include those of explaining the following phenomena:

- the ability to be discriminate, categorize, and react to environmental stimuli
- the integration of knowledge by a neurocognitive system
- the different mental states
- the capacity of a system to access its own internal states
- the focus of attention

- the control of behavior
- the difference between wakefulness, hypnosis and sleep

The hard problems are those that seem to resist those methods: the really hard problem of consciousness is the problem of experience and knowledge.

There is no real matter about whether these phenomena can be explained scientifically. All of them are straightforwardly vulnerable to an explanation in terms of computational or neural mechanisms. Consciousness generally refers to awareness in a much more complex way; consciousness is awareness as modulated by the structure of the mind. Mind refers to the totality of both inferable and potentially experienced phenomena, of which awareness and consciousness are components.

I agree with Charles Tart (1972) that awareness refers to the basic knowledge that something is happening, to perceiving or feeling or cognizing in its simplest form. What are the conscious sensations that accompany neural activities of the brain? Can we share the problem of consciousness only biologically or should we develop other methods?

This book is organized in order to show the scientific neurophysiological theories currently in use regarding the many modalities of consciousness states. Consequently, I have chosen to describe many different states of concentration, relaxation, hypnosis, mindfulness, and meditative states to help patients in pain and suffering relief. I will purposefully not examine the pathological modified states of consciousness, such as coma states or states of modified consciousness through drugs or medicines.

Popular ideas about consciousness suggest the phenomenon describes a condition of being aware of one's awareness, or self-awareness. Efforts to explain consciousness in neurological terms have focused on describing networks in the brain that increase awareness of the qualia, developed by other networks.

C. Qualia

"Qualia" (singular "quale," from the Latin for "sort of" or "what kind") is a term used in philosophy, to describe the subjective quality of conscious experience. Examples of qualia are the pain of a headache, the taste of wine, or the redness of an evening sky. Daniel Dennett (1991) writes that qualia is "an unfamiliar term for something that could not be more familiar to each of us: the ways things seem to us."

Balduzzi and Tononi (2009) studied a new theory of consciousness explained by qualia at the Department of Psychiatry, University of Wisconsin,

Madison, WI, USA. According to their integrated information theory, the quantity of consciousness is the amount of integrated information generated by a complex of elements, and the quality of the experience is specified by the informational relationships it generates.

Their study outlines a structure for characterizing the informational relationships generated by such systems. They think that qualia space (Q) is a space having an axis for each possible state (activity pattern) of a complex. Within Q, each submechanism specifies a point corresponding to a repertoire of system states. Arrows between repertoires in Q define informational relationships. Together, these arrows specify a quale: a shape that completely and univocally characterizes the quality of a conscious experience. Qualia is the quantity of consciousness associated with the experience and knowledge.

There are several conclusions from these premises: the quale is determined by both the mechanism and the state of the system. Thus, two distinct systems having identical activity patterns may generate different qualia. Conversely, the same quale may be generated by two systems that differ in both activity and connectivity. Both active and inactive elements specify a quale, but elements that are inactivated do not. Furthermore, the activation of an element affects the experience by changing the shape of the quale. The present framework may offer a good way for translating qualitative properties of experience into mathematics and biophysics.

Basic awareness of one's and external world depends on the brainstem. "Higher" forms of consciousness and awareness, including self-awareness, require cortical inputs. The "primary consciousness" or "basic awareness" as an ability to integrate sensations from the background of one's immediate goals and feelings in order to guide behavior springs from the brainstem, which human beings share with most of the vertebrates.

Psychologist Carroll Izard emphasizes that this form of primary consciousness consists of capacity to generate emotions and an awareness of a one's not an ability to talk about what one has experienced. In the same way, people can become conscious of a feeling that they cannot describe, a phenomenon that is especially common in infants.

Daniel Dennett (1991) identifies four properties that are commonly ascribed to qualia.

According to Dennet, qualia are

- *ineffable;* that is, they cannot be communicated or apprehended by any other means than direct experience
- *intrinsic;* that is, they are nonrelational properties that do not change depending on the experience's relation to other things

- *private;* that is, all interpersonal comparisons of qualia are systematically impossible
- *directly;* or immediately apprehensible in consciousness; that is, to experience a quale is to know one experiences a quale and to know all there is to know about that quale.

D. Neurophysiology of Consciousness and Quantum Consciousness

Consciousness depends on spontaneously emitted pulses from brainstem neurons that ascend in a complex mesh of activating circuits to awaken neurons in the limbic system, thalamus, and cerebral cortex. Without this ascending activation, humans lapse into a coma. Damasio (1994) has suggested that whereas the senses of vision, hearing, touch, taste, and smell function by nerve activation patterns that correspond to the state of the external world, emotions are nerve-activation patterns that correspond to the state of the internal world. If we experience a state of fear, our brains subsequently will record this body state in nerve cell-activation patterns obtained from neural and hormonal feedback, and this information may, then be used to adapt behavior appropriately.

Four neurotransmitters appear to be most important in creating consciousness: norepinephrine, serotonin, dopamine, and acetylcholine. Drugs such as anesthetics, which interrupt consciousness, interfere with cortical activation (Vertes, 2002). In their review of ten years of studying the connections of thalamic nuclei in rats, Van der Werf, Witter, and Groenewegen (2002) stated, "The thalamic midline and intralaminar nuclei, long thought to be a non-specific arousing system in the brain, have been shown to be involved functions seems to be a role in awareness." They proposed that the midline and intralaminar nuclei mediate awareness.

Each of the groups has a distinct role in a different aspect of awareness: there are separate and definite brain functions, such as specific cognitive, sensory and motor functions. They ar fundamental to the participation of the midline and intralaminar nuclei:

1. a dorsal group, consisting of the paraventricular, paratenial, and intermediodorsal nuclei, involved in visceral-limbic functions
2. a lateral group comprising the central lateral and paracentral nuclei and the anterior part of the central medial nucleus, involved in cognitive functions

3. a ventral group made up of the reuniens and rhomboial nuclei and the posterior part of the central medial nucleus, involved in multimodal sensory processing
4. a posterior group consisting of the central medial and parafascicular nuclei, involved in limbic motor functions.

Because the thalamus is so complexly interconnected with all other parts of the brain, a thalamic model of executive function is misleading, to some extent. A combination of frontal lobe and thalamic circuits are essential, for example, for anticipatory planning, one of the more recent and complex attributes of cognition (Van der et al., 2002).

In 1989, Roger Penrose published his first book on consciousness, *The Emperor's New Mind* (1989b). Based on Godel's incompleteness theorems, Penrose argued that the brain could perform functions that no computer or system of algorithms could. From this, it could follow that consciousness itself might be fundamentally nonalgorithmic and incapable of being modeled as a classical Turing machine type of computer. By contrast, the idea that it could be explained mechanistically was prevalent in the field of artificial intelligence at that time.

Roger Penrose saw the principles of quantum theory as providing an alternative process through which consciousness could originate. He further argued that this nonalgorithmic process in the brain required a new form of the quantum wave reduction, later given the name objective reduction (OR), which could link the brain to the fundamental space-time geometry. At this stage, he had no precise ideas as to how such a quantum process might be instantiated in the brain (Penrose, 1989a).

Penrose went on to consider what it was in the human brain that might not be driven by algorithms. The physical law is described by algorithms, so it was not easy for Penrose to come up with physical properties or processes that are not described by them. He was forced to look to quantum theory for a plausible candidate. In quantum theory, the fundamental units, the quanta, are in some respects quite unlike objects that are encountered in the large-scale world described by classical physics. When sufficiently isolated from the environment, they can be viewed as waves. These are different from matter waves, such as waves in the sea however. The quantum waves are essentially waves of probability, the varying probability of finding a particle at some specific position. The peak of the wave indicates the location with maximum probability of a particle being found there. The different possible positions of the particle are referred to as superpositions or quantum superpositions. We are speaking here of the isolated form of the quanta. When the quanta are the subject of measurements or of interaction with the environment, the wave characteristic is lost, and a particle is found at a precise point. This change is commonly referred to as the collapse of the wave function.

When the collapse happens, the choice of position for the particle is random. This is a drastic departure from classical physics. There is no cause-and-effect process and no system of algorithms that can describe the choice of position for the particle. This provided Penrose with a candidate for the physical basis of the suggested noncomputable process that he proposed as possibly existing in the brain.

Penrose now proposed that existing ideas on the wave function collapse might only apply to situations in which the quanta are the subject of measurement or of interaction with the environment. He considered the case of quanta that are not the subject of measurements or interactions but remain isolated from the environment and proposed that these quanta may be subject to a different form of wave function collapse.

In this area, Penrose draws on both Einstein's general theory of relativity and on his own notions about the possible structure of space-time (Penrose, 1989a,b). General relativity states that space-time is curved by massive objects. Penrose, in seeking to reconcile relativity and quantum theory, has suggested that at the very small scale, this curved space-time is not continuous but constitutes a form of network. Penrose postulates that each quantum superposition has its own piece of space-time curvature. According to his theory, these different bits of space-time curvature are separated from one another and constitute a form of blister in space-time.

Stuart Hameroff was inspired by Penrose's book to contact Penrose regarding his own theories about the mechanism of anesthesia and how it specifically targets consciousness via action on neural microtubules. Hameroff's contribution to the theory was derived from studying brain cells (neurons). His interest centered on the cytoskeleton, which provides an internal supportive structure for neurons, and particularly on the microtubules (Hameroff, 1987), which are the important component of the cytoskeleton. As neuroscience has progressed, the role of the cytoskeleton and microtubules has assumed greater importance. In addition to providing a supportive structure for the cell, the known functions of the microtubules include transport of molecules, including neurotransmitter molecules bound for the synapses, and control of the cell's movement, growth, and shape (Hameroff, 1987). Hameroff (1987) proposed that microtubules were suitable candidates to support quantum processing.

The two met in 1992, and Hameroff suggested that the microtubules were a good candidate site for a quantum mechanism in the brain. Penrose was interested in the mathematical features of the microtubule lattice, and over the next two years the two collaborated in formulating the orchestrated objective reduction (Orch-OR) model of consciousness.

Mainstream theories assume that consciousness emerges from the brain and focus particularly on complex computation at connections known as synapses that allow communication between brain cells (neurons).

In the case of the electrons in the tubulin subunits of the microtubules, Hameroff has proposed that great numbers of these electrons can become involved in a state known as a Bose-Einsten condensate. These occur when large numbers of quantum particles become locked in phase and exist as a single quantum object. These are quantum features at a macroscopic scale, and Hameroff suggests that a feature of this kind quantum activity, which is usually at a very tiny scale, could be boosted to be a large-scale influence in the brain. Hameroff has proposed that condensates in microtubules in one neuron can link with microtubule condensates in other neurons and glial cells via gap junctions (Hameroff, 1987, 2008, 2010).

In addition to the synaptic connections between brain cells, gap junctions are a different category of connections, where the gap between the cells is sufficiently small for quantum objects to cross it by a process known as quantum tunneling. Hameroff proposes that this tunneling allows a quantum object, such as the Bose-Einstein condensates, to cross into other neurons and thus extend across a large area of the brain as a single quantum object. He further postulates that the action of this large-scale quantum feature is the source of the gamma synchronization observed in the brain, and sometimes viewed as a neural correlate of consciousness (Bennett & Zukin, 2004). In support of the much more limited theory that gap junctions are related to the gamma oscillation, Hameroff quotes a number of studies from recent years (Buhl, Harris, Hormuzdi, Monyer, & Buzsáki, 2003; Fries, Schröder, Roelfsema, Singer, & Engel, 2002).

Antonio Damasio theorized extended consciousness to arise in the structures in the human brain he described as image spaces and dispositional spaces (2004). Image spaces imply areas where sensory impressions of all types are processed, including the focused awareness of the core consciousness. Dispositional spaces include convergence zones, which are networks in the brain where memories are processed and recalled and where knowledge is merged with immediate experience. The image processing in the cerebrum is regionally specific to various senses but is highly distributed and interconnected, with images such as visual, spatial, and perhaps linguistic impressions stored in diverse areas then assembled when recalled as a thought.

Most humans are so proficient at reading printed words that they cannot easily ignore them. In fact, it takes considerable attentional effort to do so. This tendency to quickly read a word is used in the Stroop task. The Stroop ask is a psychological test of our mental (attentional) vitality and flexibility.

The task takes advantage of our ability to read words more quickly and automatically than we can name colors, if a word is printed or displayed in a color different from the color it actually names. The cognitive mechanism involved in this task is called directed attention; you have to manage your attention by inhibiting or stopping one response in order to say or do something else.

Recent data indicate that, under a specific posthypnotic suggestion to circumvent reading, greatly suggestible subjects successfully eliminated the Stroop interference effect. Stroop data were collected from six greatly hypnotizable and six not as suggestible subjects using an optical setup that guaranteed either sharply focused or blurred vision. The highly suggestible performed the Stroop task when naturally vigilant, under posthypnotic suggestion not to read, and while visually blurred. The less suggestible ran naturally vigilant, while looking for another place and visually blurred. Although visual accommodation was precluded for all subjects, posthypnotic suggestion effectively eliminated Stroop interference and was comparable to looking away in controls. "These data strengthen the view that Stroop interference is neither robust nor inevitable and support the hypothesis that posthypnotic suggestion may exert a top-down influence on neural processing" (Raz, 2012; Raz et al., 2003).

Although humans are theorized to share extended consciousness with some animals, theorized neural mechanisms for extended consciousness do not provide answers to philosophical or cosmological questions about consciousness, such as why we perceive ourselves as a limited part of a larger universe.

There are many theories of consciousness. Perhaps the largest division is between general metaphysical theories that aim to locate consciousness in the overall ontological scheme of reality and more specific theories that offer detailed accounts of its nature, features, and role. The line between the two sorts of theories blurs a bit, especially insofar as many specific theories carry at least some implicit commitments on the more general metaphysical issues. Nonetheless, it is useful to keep the division in mind when surveying the range of current theoretical offerings (Van Gulick, 2004).

Even if our neurophysiological knowledge should one day enable us to identify the exact neurochemical correlation of a psychic phenomenon, we must not forget that neurochemical knowledge is not sufficient to explain all the subjective experiences in people. A major turning point in philosophers' interest in neuroscience came with the publication of Patricia Churchland's *Neurophilosophy* (1986). The Churchlands (Pat and husband Paul) were already notorious for advocating eliminative materialism. In her (1986) book, Churchland distilled eliminativist arguments of the past, unified the pieces of the philosophy of science underlying them, and sandwiched the philosophy between a five-chapter introduction to neuroscience and a seventy-page chapter on three then-current theories of brain function. She was unapologetic about her intent. She was introducing philosophy of science to neuroscientists and neuroscience to philosophers (Bickle, 2003).

Consciousness depends on spontaneously emitted pulses from brainstem neurons that ascend in a complex mesh of activating circuits to awaken neurons in the limbic system, thalamus, and cerebral cortex. Without this ascending activation, humans lapse into a coma. Four neurotransmitters appear to be most important in creating consciousness: norepinephrine, serotonin, dopamine, and acetylcholine. Drugs such as anesthetics that interrupt consciousness interfere with cortical activation. Pulses of electrical activation are accompanied by pulses of chemicals released to topically activate regions of the brain. The thalamus, in turn, activates the cerebral cortex and links all subsystems in meaningful packages of activity that deliver monitor images of their activity to consciousness. The cortical neurons return signals to the thalamus, so the cortical activation can be regarded as a looping system that recurs and resonates (Vertes, 2002).

The physicist and mathematician John Taylor observed, "the study of consciousness is like a black hole for those that study it. Once the scientific study is done they lose sight of their normal scientific activity and give an explanation of the phenomena that does not correspond to a scientific explanation" (Taylor, 2000).

Our ordinary state of consciousness is not something natural or given, but a highly complex construction, a specialized tool for coping with our environment and the people in it (Tart, 1972). Many have tried to explain consciousness, but the explanations always seem to fall short of the target. The ambiguity of the term "consciousness" is often exploited by both philosophers and scientists writing on the subject (Chalmers, 1995).

In his neurophysiological studies, the scientist Antonio Damasio offers a thought-provoking view of consciousness centered on feelings. Through his arguments, we found that there is much to learn from neuropathology about different levels of consciousness. There is more work to do on psychological levels and the corresponding neural structures (Mosca, 2000).

Several techniques can be used to achieve a mental and physical state of relaxation and the different states of consciousness. Hypnosis is a state of heightened awareness and focused concentration. Some call it a trance; some call it an altered state of consciousness, during which your attention is turned inward, allowing you to be more open to new feelings and to the inner self.

2. CONSCIOUSNESS IN RELIEF OF PAIN AND SUFFERING

The field of pain and suffering has undergone a great revolution, and this volume reflects these exciting advances. We are so accustomed to viewing pain as a sensory phenomenon that we have long ignored the fact that injury does more than produce pain; it also disrupts the brain's homeostatic regulation system, thereby producing stress and initiating complex programs to reinstate homeostasis. Stress and suffering can be defined as an activation of the limbic system of the central nervous system (CNS) that then activates neurohumoral mechanisms of arousal. Stress produced by painful experiences initiates a cascade of neurophysiological, humoral, and phenomenological events that challenge our understanding but also provide valuable clues in dealing with chronic pain (Melzack, 1998, 1999).

Pain and suffering, especially associated with advancing and incurable illness, inevitably cause distress for patients, families, and caregivers. A psychological and spiritual approach to care aims to improve the quality of life for patients with a life-limiting illness. We can reduce suffering through early identification, assessment, and optimal management of pain, providing to the patient physical, psychological, social, and spiritual needs.

The psychological counterparts to the chronic pain state include depression, anxiety, and other affective states and are keys to understanding the disability associated with this condition (Cleeland & Syrjala, 1992).

The oldest and persistent questions of humanity are why sorrow, why suffering? How can individuals triumph over adversities? What can be done to transform despair to hope, pain to comfort, and sorrow to joy? What are the roles of religion, science, and medicine?

What are the explanations of neuroscience? How is it that the instruments used by neuroscientists (e.g. neuroimaging, cell recordings, genetic manipulations, simulations) yield knowledge? What is a neuroscientific explanation of consciousness? What is the meaning of pain, sickness, and death? Why is the world full of troubles and pain?

Valerie Hardcastle (1997) focused her study on the anatomy and physiology of the pain transmission system. Hardcastle proposes a dissociable dual system of pain transmission consisting of a pain sensory system closely analogous in its neurobiological implementation to other sensory systems and a descending pain inhibitory system. She argues that this dual system is consistent with recent neuroscientific discoveries and accounts for all the pain phenomena that have tempted philosophers toward particular theories of pain experience.

The neurobiological uniqueness of the pain inhibitory system, contrasted with the mechanisms of other sensory modalities, renders pain processing atypical. In particular, the pain inhibitory system dissociates pain sensation from stimulation of nociceptors (pain receptors). Hardcastle concludes from the neurobiological uniqueness of pain transmission that pain experiences are atypical conscious events and hence not a good place to start theorizing or generalizing (Bickle, 2003).

Ronald Melzack is a legend in the field of pain science. Together with Patrick Wall, he introduced the gate control theory from which thousands of research studies have sprung (Melzack & Wall, 1965). Melzack's later neuromatrix theory of pain proposes that pain is a multidimensional experience, produced by characteristic "neurosignature" patterns of nerve impulses, generated by a widely distributed neural network–the "body-self neuromatrix"– in the brain. These neurosignature patterns may be triggered by sensory inputs, but they may also be generated independently of them. The neuromatrix, which is genetically determined and modified by sensory experience, is the primary generating mechanism of the neural pattern, responsible for the production of pain. The neuromatrix theory is evolving and the brain functions and mechanisms in this schema still need to be elucidated.

The pain theories have traveled from the peripheral pain fibers to pain as a "feeling" state. This is paralleled by the evolution of the treatment of pain in pharmacology and psychology. The science of pain continues to explore the genetic, endocrine, and immune systems, all of which may contribute to the neuromatrix (Melzack, 2001, 2002; Melzack & Wall, 1965).

Perhaps one of the hardest things in life is coping with illness, pain, and suffering. Chronic pain and suffering can have devastating effects on patients' quality of life. The specialty of pain management has developed in medicine and other disciplines to address the need for comfort, functional restoration, and treatment of associated problems. The treatment of pain and suffering includes a broad range of interventions that together help the patient and family maintain a good quality of life while living with the disease, and allow the patient with advanced illness to face the end of life with comfort ensured, values and decisions respected, and family supported.

Should the anxiety symptoms associated with the stress in chronic pain require only treatment with an anxiolytic drug? Tranquillizer and analgesic medications are intensively marketed and continue to be heavily prescribed worldwide. Inevitably, this practice can result in an increased psychological and physical dependence on these types of medications. For well over 2000 years, noninvasive therapy in pain was practiced in every culture as a folk tradition. It was all there: heat, cold, massage, manipulation, acupuncture, reflexology, mindfulness, prayer, meditation, and so on. Therapists need to consider when they should incorporate different psychological approaches in their management of people with pain and suffering.

In this book, I will consider the treatment of pain and suffering with modified states of consciousness, mindfulness, meditative states, and clinical hypnosis therapy that could be used to help pharmacological and anesthesic therapies, or in some cases substitute them completely.

Hypnosis, relaxation, and meditative techniques are used to achieve a state of mental and physical relaxation. Mental relaxation means alleviation of anxiety; physical relaxation means a reduction in skeletal muscle tension and relief of suffering. Simple relaxation techniques should be used for episodes of brief pain, or in cases of chronic pain, during procedures, as well as when the patient's ability to concentrate is compromised by severe pain, a high level of anxiety, or fatigue. Relaxation is a state of physical and emotional calmness, the opposite of stress or "fight or flight" response. When you are relaxed, your muscles are free of tension, and you feel little or no anxiety or irritability. The hypnotic trance is a consciousness state of heightened awareness and focused concentration that can be used to manipulate the perception of pain and has been effective in the treatment of cancer-related pain (Reeves, Redd, Storm, & Minagawa, 1983; Spiegel & Bloom, 1983; Syrjala, Cummings, & Donaldson, 1992). Hypnosis is a condition of altered consciousness state and attention in an individual, achieved by an induction process. Hypnosis may help by altering the pain sensations, by directing the person's attention away from the pain, or by suggesting pain relief.

Our ordinary state of consciousness is not something natural or given but a highly complex construction, a specialized tool for coping with our environment and the people in it, a tool that is useful for doing some things but not very useful, and even dangerous, for doing other things. Hypnosis is a different state of consciousness (Tart, 1972). As an adjunct to psychotherapy, hypnosis can help clients enter a relaxed, comfortable, trance state for obtaining specific therapeutic outcomes. With clinical hypnosis, the therapist can make suggestions designed to help the client formulate specific internal processes (feelings, memories, images and internal self-talk) that will lead to mutually agreed upon outcomes. Hypnotic suggestions can influence behavior when the listener is:

1. Relaxed, receptive, and open to the suggestions
2. Experiences visual, auditory, and/or kinesthetic representations of the suggestions
3. Anticipates and envisions that these suggestions will result in future outcomes.

What are the conscious and unconscious sensations that accompany neural activities of the brain? What is the bridge between pain perception

and the experience of anxiety and suffering? Moreover, how can we cure suffering and pain in all their aspects, not only physical but also mental? How
does a neurochemical phenomenon like pain, which starts from a biological
state, transform into a psychological and suffering sensation? Even if our neurophysiological knowledge should one day enable us to identify the exact
neurochemical correlation of a psychic phenomenon, we must not forget that
neurochemical knowledge, is not sufficient to explain all the subjective experiences in people. In the past, philosopher John Searle wrote that "to study
the brain without studying consciousness is like studying the stomach without studying digestion" (Searle, 1992).

Some very interesting and excellent protocols regarding pain and suffering therapy have been written. For the management of pain, the Agency for
Health Care Policy and Research (AHCPR) was established in December
1989 under the Omnibus Budget Reconciliation Act of 1989 (Public Law
101-239) to enhance the quality, appropriateness, and effectiveness of health
care services. AHCPR carried out its mission by conducting and supporting
general health services' research, including medical effectiveness research.
The guidelines assisted practitioners in the prevention, diagnosis, treatment,
and management of clinical conditions.

AHCPR also classified the nonpharmacological and noninvasive management in pain. They said that psychological interventions should be introduced early during illness as part of a multimodal approach to pain management. Psychological therapies can be used concurrently with drugs and
other modalities to manage pain. These interventions can be carried out by
professional staff and often by the patient or family members.

One goal is to help the patient gain a sense of control over pain and suffering.

A simple rationale underlies such an intervention; how people think
affects how they feel, and changing how they think about pain can change
their sensitivity to it and their feelings and reactions toward it (Agency for
Health Care Policy and Research [AHCPR], 1989; McGrath, 1990). These
interventions should be introduced early throughout illness, so that patients
can learn and practice these strategies while they have sufficient strength and
energy. When introduced early, they are more likely to succeed, which fos-
ters the patient's motivation to continue using them.

For most people, suffering is a hard and difficult word, a word to be kept
out of one's thoughts. For this reason, when it touches us, we are not pre-
pared to deal with it. For professional people who live constantly in close
contact with all types of suffering, it may become more difficult to be able to
efficiently help those who are challenged in facing inevitably difficult life
events.

Many dictionaries define suffering only from a physical point of view, but suffering also includes the mind and the soul. One of the best-written books, on the subject of suffering, is the book of Job in the Bible, the source of ideas for many philosophers, even though its meaning may be difficult to understand. Therefore, suffering must be analyzed from all aspects that make up the human being. The aspects of suffering are derived from

- a physical pain (illness)
- difficult situations of life
- stress
- physical trauma
- psychological trauma
- a state of depression
- social problems
- spiritual suffering

As a doctor I talk about suffering when physical pain includes mental and spiritual suffering. Sources of pain are often multiple, with the combination of chronic neuropathic, inflammatory, chemical, mechanical, ischemic, or acute pain. These may be from the primary pathology, from treatment modalities, from bedsores and skin ulcers, from preexisting concurrent disease, in critical care by the discomfort of an endotracheal tube or an intravenous line, or in palliative care for dying patients. Pain may be considered as contributing significantly to an overall sense of suffering.

Psychosocial and spiritual processes strongly influence the impact and expression of pain and these need to be taken into account in assessing and treating pain. This needs a holistic approach to the patient (Kolcaba & Fisher, 1996), as well as some novel approaches to the treatment of suffering.

3. INTRODUCTION TO CONSCIOUSNESS, HIGHER CONSCIOUSNESS, AND AWARENESS

In everyday life, as each of us lives in our "normal" state of consciousness, our awareness is usually focused on the particular thoughts, emotions, or perceptions we experience on the surface level of reality. They are the experiences and perceptions we move through in our life, in the outer world, or the thoughts and feelings that we have in our inner world. As we move through life, we perceive, think, act, and feel with the assistance of our "thinking mind," the active portion of our mind that deals with this surface level of reality, through the use of thoughts, feelings, interpretations of perceptions, and actions.

Higher consciousness is our awareness state: it is the state or ability to perceive, to feel, or to be conscious of events, objects, or sensory patterns. In this level of consciousness, sense data can be confirmed by an observer without necessarily implying knowledge. More broadly, it is the state or quality of being aware of something. Although all these particular components of our life are important, when we remain identified with–and therefore limited to–these surface activities, we are far less able to perceive and act from a more fundamental level of greater awareness. The tendency of our "thinking mind" to remain preoccupied with the particulars of life inhibits our ability to move to the level of pure consciousness that is actually the source of all these particular states of mind.

Neural systems that regulate attention serve to attenuate awareness among complex animals whose central and peripheral nervous systems provide more information than cognitive areas of the brain can assimilate. Within an attenuated system of awareness, a mind might be aware of much more than is being contemplated in a focused extended consciousness. Extended consciousness is said to arise in the brain of humans with substantial capacity for memory and reason. The perception of a historic and future self arises from a stream of information from the immediate environment and from neural structures related to memory.

The scientist Antonio Damasio (1994) theorized extended consciousness to arise in the structures in the human brain he described as image spaces and dispositional spaces. Image spaces imply areas where sensory impressions of all types are processed, including the focused awareness of the core consciousness. Dispositional spaces include convergence zones, networks in the brain where memories are processed and recalled and where knowledge is merged with immediate experience.

During relaxation, clinical hypnosis states, and meditative states, higher consciousness and awareness move you back to your calm center. Awareness helps you lose habits that have held you pinned to the world's way of doing things so long. Relaxation techniques, clinical hypnosis, and imagery are used to achieve a state of mental and physical relaxation in consciousness stages. Relaxation techniques include simple focused-breathing exercises, progressive muscle relaxation (PMR), meditation, and music-assisted relaxation (AHCPR, 1992; McCaffery & Beebe, 1989). Hypnosis works with the subconscious mind to create results. Your subconscious is the part of your mind that stores all of your experiences, dreams, and beliefs.

The hypnotic trance is a essentially a state of heightened and focused concentration, and thus it can be used to manipulate the perception of pain and suffering. The use of hypnosis involves control over the focus of attention and can be used to make the patient less aware of the noxious stimuli (Broome, Lillis, McGahe, & Bates, 1992). Pleasant mental images can be used to aid relaxation and awareness, for example, visualizing a peaceful scene, such as waves softly hitting the beach, or taking slow, deep breaths as one visualizes pain leaving the body. Both pleasant imagery and PMR have been shown to decrease self-reported pain intensity and pain distress (Graffam & Johnson, 1987).

In the practice of clinical hypnosis, relaxation, mindfulness, and meditative stages, we seek to free ourselves from this mental "chatter" in which our "thinking mind" engages and instead seek connection to a higher level of our being. We free ourselves from the surface level of the mind, and by doing so, we make it easier for ourselves to come into connection with a higher consciousness, a reality. These states are processes by which we seek to recondition our conscious awareness so that we release our attachment to the surface level of reality and instead allow the awareness to gravitate toward a state of pure awareness, pure consciousness.

As we pass through these stages in the proper manner, the experience of pure awareness itself moves more to the forefront, instead of a primary identification with the highly active surface level of the mind. In learning and practice of modified stages of consciousness, we can develop some higher sense of self-consciousness and awareness, a pure awareness beyond habitual identifications with the thoughts, feelings, and perceptions of the surface level of the mind. They are, in the beginning, the journey inward and provide an inward awareness of self.

At the beginning of an inner self-practice, our higher consciousness often begins to draw inward, and progresses inward. During our practices, there are moments when our higher consciousness is focused outward, moments when we are aware of our existence in the outer universe, perhaps with a sense of the sky or heavens above, of being in the universe. It is an instantaneous reversal in the focus of awareness, and there is often a sense of elation or euphoria at this point when the inward higher consciousness expands.

This point is not a point in time or space, but it is a state of being. It is subtle, yet discernible with practice. This precise point of change in awareness is called the point of pure being. The purpose of this book is to awaken in us the skylike nature of mind and to introduce us to that which we really are, our unchanging pure higher consciousness and awareness that underlies the whole of life. These states of mind are intensely personal and spiritual experiences.

The desired purpose of each technique is to channel our awareness into a more positive direction by totally transforming one's state of mind; to turn inward, to concentrate on the inner self.

In this world, we are constantly under physical and/or mental stress. The reason for this stress is that we have become slaves of endless desires and uncontrolled emotions such as hatred, jealousy, anger, and so on. We feel powerless and limited in what we can do.

> When you abandon every desire, that rises up within you, and when you become content with things as they are, then you experience inner peace. When your mind is untroubled by misfortune, when you desire no pleasures, when your emotions are tranquil, and when you are free from fear and anger, then you experience inner calm. When you are free from all attachments, when you are indifferent to success and failure, then you experience inner serenity. When you can withdraw your senses from pleasures of the senses, just as a tortoise withdraws its limbs, then you experience inner wisdom. When no pleasure and no desire can touch the soul, then you experience the highest state of consciousness. (Bhagavad-Gita, 2.55-61)

> The stillness and silence of consciousness stages, we glimpse and return to that deep inner nature that we have so long ago lost sight of amid the busyness and distraction of our minds.

> Consciousness stages and meditation, then, are "bringing the mind home." (Rinpoche, 2002)

REFERENCES

Agency for Health Care Policy and Research (AHCPR). (1989). Acute Pain Management: Operative and Trauma, AHCPR Pub. No. 92-0032; for Clinicians–Acute Pain Management Procedures, AHCPR Pub. No. 92-0019; and in Infants, Children, and Adolescents Procedures, AHCPR Pub. No. 92-0020.

Balduzzi, D., & Tononi, G. (2009, August). Qualia: The geometry of integrated information. *PLOS Computational Biology, 5*(8):e1000462. Epub Aug 14.

Bennett, M. V., & Zukin, R. S. (2004, February 19). Electrical coupling and neuronal synchronization in the mammalian brain [Review]. *Neuron, 41*(4), 495–511.

Bickle, J. (2003). *Philosophy and neuroscience: A ruthlessly reductive account.* Norwell, MA: Kluwer Academic Press.

Broome, M., Lillis, P., McGahe T., & Bates, T. (1992). The use of distraction and imagery with children during painful procedures. *Oncology Nursing Forum, 19,* 499–502.

Buhl, D. L., Harris, K. D., Hormuzdi, S. G., Monyer, H., & Buzsáki, G. (2003, February). Selective impairment of hippocampal gamma oscillations in connexin-36 knock-out mouse in vivo. *Journal of Neuroscience, 23*(3), 1013–1018.

Chalmers, D. J. (1995). Facing up to the problem of consciousness. *Journal of Consciousness Studies, 2*(3), 200–219.

Churchland, P. (1986). *Neurophilosophy.* Cambridge, MA: MIT Press.

Cleeland, C. S., & Syrjala, K. L. (1992). How to asses cancer pain. In D.C. Turk & R. Melzack (Eds.), *Handbook of pain assessment* (pp. 360–387). New York: Guilford Press.

Damasio, A. (1994). *Descartes' error: Emotions, reason, and the human brain.* New York: Avon Books.

Dennett, D. (1991). *Consciousness explained.* London: Penguin Books.

Fries, P., Schroder, J.-H., Roelfsema, P. R., Singer, W., & Engel, A. K. (2002). Oscillatory neuronal synchronization in primary visual cortex as a correlate of stimulus selection. *Journal of Neuroscience, 22,* 3739–3754.

Graffam, S., & Johnson, A. (1987). A comparison of two relaxation strategies for the relief of pain and its distress. *Journal of Pain and Symptom Management, 2*(4), 229–231.

Hameroff, S. R. (1987). *Ultimate computing: Biomolecular consciousness and nano technology.* Philadelphia: Elsevier Science Publishers. Available at http://www.quantum consciousness.org/ultimatecomputing.html

Hameroff, S. R. (2008). That's life!–The geometry of πelectron clouds. In D. Abbott, P. C. W. Davies, & A. K. Pati (Eds.), *Quantum aspects of life* (pp. 403–426). London: Imperial College Press. Available at http://www.quantumconscious ness.org/documents/Hameroff_received-1-05-07.pdf

Hameroff, S. (2010, January). The "conscious pilot"–dendritic synchrony moves through the brain to mediate consciousness. *Journal of Biological Physics, 36*(1), 71–93.

Hardcastle, V. G. (1997, June). Consciousness and the neurobiology of perceptual binding [Review]. *Seminars in Neurology, 17*(2), 163–170.

Kolcaba, K. Y., & Fisher, E. M. (1996, February). A holistic perspective on comfort care as an advance directive. *Critical Care Nursing Quarterly, 18*(4), 66–76.

McCaffery, M., & Beebe, A. (1989). *Pain: Clinical manual for nursing practice.* St. Louis: Mosby.

McGrath, P. A. (Ed.). (1990). *Pain in children: Nature, assessment, and treatment.* New York: The Guilford Press.

Melzack, R. (1998). Pain and stress: Clues toward understanding chronic pain. In M. Sabourin, F. Craik & M. Robert (Eds.), *Advances in psychological science* (Vol. 2, Biological and Cognitive Aspects, pp. 63–85). London: Psychology Press, Hove.

Melzack, R. (1999). Pain and stress a new perspective. In R. J. Gatchel & D. C. Turk (Eds.), *Psychosocial factors in pain* (pp. 89–106). New York: Guilford Press.

Melzack, R. (2001). Pain and the neuromatrix in the brain. *Journal of Dental Education, 65,* 1378–1382.

Melzack, R. (2002). *Evolution of Pain Theories.* Program and Abstracts of the 21st Annual Scientific Meeting of the American Pain Society, March 14–17, Baltimore, Maryland. Abstract 102.

Melzack, R., & Wall, P. D. (1965). Pain mechanisms: A new theory. *Science, 150,* 971–979.

Mosca, A. (2000). A review essay on Antonio Damasio's *The Feeling of What Happens: Body and Emotion in the Making of Consciousness. PSYCHE, 6*(10). [AU: Please supply page numbers.]

Penrose, R. (1989a). *Shadows of the mind: A search for the missing science of consciousness.* Oxford, UK: Oxford University Press.

Penrose, R. (1989b). *The emperor's new mind: Concerning computers, minds and the laws of physics.* Oxford, UK: Oxford University Press.

Raz, A. (2012, September). Translational attention: From experiments in the lab to helping the symptoms of individuals with Tourette's syndrome. *Consciousness and Cognition, 21*(3), 1591–1594.

Raz, A., Landzberg, K. S., Schweizer, H. R., Zephrani, Z. R., Shapiro, T., Fan, J., & Posner, M. I. (2003, September). Posthypnotic suggestion and the modulation of Stroop interference under cycloplegia. *Consciousness and Cognition, 12*(3), 332–346.

Reeves, J. L., Redd, W. H., Storm, F. K., & Minagawa, R. Y. (1983). Hypnosis in the control of pain during hyperthermia treatment of cancer. In J. J. Bonica, U. Lindblom & A. Iggo (Eds.), *Proceedings of the Third World Congress on Pain,* Edinburgh (Vol. 5, Advances in Pain Research and Therapy, pp. 857–861). New York: Raven Press.

Rinpoche, S. (2002). *The Tibetan book of living and dying* (2nd ed.). San Francisco: HarperCollins.

Searle, J. (1992). *The rediscovery of the mind.* Cambridge, MA: MIT Press.

Tart, C. T. (1972). States of consciousness and state-specific sciences. *Science, 176,* 1203–1210.

Taylor, J. (2000, February). The enchanting subject of consciousness (or is it a black hole?). *PSYCHE, 6*(2).

Van der Werf, Y. D., Witter, M. P., & Groenewegen, H. J. (2002, September). The intralaminar and midline nuclei of the thalamus. Anatomical and functional evidence for participation in processes of arousal and awareness [Review]. Brain Research. *Brain Research Reviews, 39*(2–3), 107–140.

Van Gulick, R. (2004). Higher-order global states (HOGS): An alternative higher-order model of consciousness. In R. J. Gennaro (Ed.), *Higher-order theories of consciousness: An anthology* (pp. 67–92). Amsterdam: John Benjamins B.V.

Vertes, R. P. (2002, January 7). Analysis of projections from the medial prefrontal cortex to the thalamus in the rat, with emphasis on nucleus reuniens. *Journal of Comparative Neurology, 442*(2), 163–187.

SUGGESTED READINGS

Armstrong, D. M. (1978). Naturalism, materialism and first philosophy. *Philosophia, 8,* 261–276.

Benson, H. (1975). *The relaxation response.* New York: William Morrow.

Blackmore, S. (2003). *Consciousness: An introduction.* London: Hodder & Stoughton.

Boccio, F. J. (2004). *Mindfulness yoga: The awakened union of breath, body and mind.* Somerville, MA: Wisdom Publishers.

Bonica, J. J. (Ed.). (1990). *The management of pain* (2nd ed.). Philadelphia: Lea & Febiger.

Bower, B. (2007, September 15). Consciousness in the raw: The brain stem may orchestrate the basics of awareness [Online]. *Science News.*

Brahm, A. (2005). *Mindfulness, bliss, and beyond: A meditator's handbook.* Somerville, MA: Wisdom Publications.

Brugnoli, A. (2004). *Stato di coscienza totalizzante, alla ricerca del profondo Se.* Verona, Italy: La Grafica Editrice.

Brugnoli, A. (2005). *Stati di coscienza modificati neurofisiologici.* Verona, Italy: La Grafica Editrice.

Brugnoli, M. P. (2009). *Clinical hypnosis, spirituality and palliation: The way of inner peace.* Verona, Italy: Del Miglio Editore.

Brugnoli, M. P., Brugnoli, A., & Norsa, A. (2006). *Nonpharmacological and noninvasive management in pain: Physical and psychological modalities.* Verona, Italy: La Grafica Editrice.

Capra, F. (1996). *The web of life: A new scientific understanding of living systems.* New York: Anchor Books. Available at http://www.worldcat.org/oclc/37800841 &referer=brief_results

Capra, F. (2000). *The Tao of physics.* Boston: Shambhala Publications.

Carruthers, P. (2000). *Phenomenal consciousness.* Cambridge: Cambridge University Press.

Chalmers, D. (1996). *The conscious mind.* Oxford: Oxford University Press.

Chochinov, H. M., Krisjanson, L. J., Hack, T. F., Hassard, T., McClement, S., & Harlos, M. (2006, June). Dignity in the terminally ill: Revisited. *Journal of Palliative Medicine, 9*(3), 666–672.

Cleeland, C. S. (1987). Nonpharmacologic management of cancer pain. *Journal of Pain and Symptom Control, 2,* 523–528.

Cowan, N. (1995). *Attention and memory: An integrated framework.* New York: Oxford University Press.

Crick, F., & Koch, C. (1995a). Are we aware of neural activity in primary visual cortex? *Nature, 375,* 121–123.

Crick, F., & Koch, C. (1995b). Cortical areas in visual awareness [Reply]. *Nature, 377,* 294–295.

Dalai Lama. (1999). *The Dalai Lama's book of wisdom.* London: Thorsons.

De Zazzo, J., & Tully, T. (1995). Dissection of memory formation. From behavioural pharmacology to molecular genetics. *Trends in Neuroscience, 18,* 212–218.

Dermietzel, R. (1998). Gap junction wiring: A "new" principle in cell-to-cell communication in the nervous system? *Brain Research Reviews, 26,* 176–183.

Desimone, R., & Duncan, J. (1995). Neural mechanisms of selective visual attention. *Annual Review of Neuroscience, 18,* 193–222.

Easwaran, E. (2007). *The Bhagavad Gita.* Berkeley, CA: Nilgiri Press.

Erickson, M. H. (1959). Hypnosis in painful terminal illness. *American Journal of Clinical Hypnosis, 1,* 1117–1121.

Erickson, M. H., Rossi, E. L., & Rossi, S. I. (1976). *Hypnotic realities: The induction of clinical hypnosis and forms of indirect suggestion.* New York: Irvington Publishers.

Farthing, G. W. (1992). *The psychology of consciousness.* Englewood Cliffs, NJ: Prentice-Hall.

Frost, S. E. (1989). *Basic teachings of the great philosophers.* New York: Anchor Books.

Fuster, J. M. (1997). *The prefrontal cortex: Anatomy, physiology, and neuropsychology of the frontal lobe* (2nd ed.). Philadelphia: Lippincott, Williams & Wilkins.

Galarreta, M., & Hestrin, S. (1999). A network of fast-spiking cells in the neocortex connected by electrical synapses. *Nature, 402,* 72–75.

Gibran, K. (1992). *Sabbia e Spuma e Il Vagabondo* [*Sand and foam and the wanderer*]. Rome, Italy: Newton Compton Editori.

Gibran, K. (1993). *Il Profeta* [*The prophet*]. Verona, Italy: Editrice Demetra.

Goldstein, J. (1983). *The experience of insight.* Boston: Shambhala.

Guenther, H. V., & Kawamura, L. S. (1975). *Mind in Buddhist psychology: The necklace of clear understanding by Ye-shes rGyal-mtshan* [Tibetan Translation Series] [Kindle Edition]. Berkeley, CA: Dharma Publishing.

Gunaratana, B. H. (2002). *Mindfulness in plain English.* Somerville, MA: Wisdom Publications.

Hameroff, S. R., & Watt, R. C. (1982). Information processing in microtubules. *Journal of Theoretical Biology, 98,* 549–561. Available at http://www.quantum consciousness.org/documents/informationprocessing_hameroff_000.pdf

Handel, D. L. (2001, February). Complementary therapies for cancer patients: What works, what doesn't, and how to know the difference. *Texas Medicine, 97*(2), 68–73.

Hendler, C. S., & Redd, W. H. (1986). Fear of hypnosis: The role of labeling in patients' acceptance of behavioral interventions. *Behavior Therapy, 17*(1), 2–13.

His Divine Grace A.C. Bhaktivedanta Swami Prabhupada. (1972). *Bhagavad-Gita.* Krishna Store.

Hoopes, A. (2007). *Zen yoga: A path to enlightenment through breathing, movement and meditation.* Tokyo: Kodansha International.

Hormuzdi, S. G., Filippov, M. A., Mitropoulou, G., Monyer, H., & Bruzzone, R. (2004). Electrical synapses: A dynamic signaling system that shapes the activity of neuronal networks. *Biochimica et Biophysica Acta, 1662,* 113–137.

Huai-chin, N. (1993). *Working toward enlightenment: The cultivation of practice.* York Beach, ME: Samuel Weiser.

Jackson, F. (1982). Epiphenomenal qualia. *Philosophical Quarterly, 32,* 127–136.

Jensen, M. P., & Patterson, D. R. (2005, April). Control conditions in hypnotic-analgesia clinical trials: Challenges and recommendations. *International Journal of Clinical and Experimental Hypnosis, 53*(2), 170–197.

Kaiser, J., & Lutzenberger, W. (2003). Induced gamma-band activity and human brain function. *Neuroscientist, 9,* 475–484.

Kallio, S., & Revonsuo, A. (2003). Hypnotic phenomena and altered states of consciousness: A multilevel framework of description and explanation. *Contemporary Hypnosis, 20*(3), 111–164.

Kihlstrom, J. F. (1997). Convergence in understanding hypnosis? Perhaps, but perhaps not quite so fast. *International Journal of Clinical and Experimental Hypnosis, 45,* 324–332.

Knudsen, E. I. (2007). Fundamental components of attention. *Annual Review of Neuroscience, 30*(1), 57–78.

Lazar, S. W., Bush, G., Gollub, R. L., Fricchione, G. L., Khalsa, G., & Benson, H. (2000, May 15). Functional brain mapping of the relaxation response and meditation. *NeuroReport, 11*(7), 1581–1585.

LeBeau, F. E. N., Traub, R. D., Monyer, H., Whittington, M. A., & Buhl, E. H. (2003). The role of electrical signaling via gap junctions in the generation of fast network oscillations. *Brain Research Bulletin, 62,* 3–13.

Lehmann, D., Grass, P., & Meier, B. (1995). Spontaneous conscious covert cognition states and brain electric spectral states in canonical correlations. *International Journal of Psychophysiology, 19,* 41–52.

Leroy, E. B. (1933). *Les visions du demi-sommeil.* Paris: Alcan.

Levine, J. (1983). Materialism and qualia: The explanatory gap. *Pacific Philosophical Quarterly, 64,* 354–361.

Levitan, A. (1992). The use of hypnosis with cancer patients. *Psychiatry and Medicine, 10,* 119–131.

Loscalzo, M., & Jacobsen, P. B. (1990). Practical behavioural approaches to the effective management of pain and distress. *Journal of Psychosocial Oncology, 8,* 139–169.

Manzotti, R., & Gozzano, S. (2004). Verso una scienza della coscienza. *Networks 3–4:* i–iii. Available at http://www.swif.uniba.it/lei/ai/networks/

Marshall, W., Simon, C., Penrose, R., & Bouwmeester, D. (2003). Towards quantum superpositions of a mirror. *Physical Review Letters, 91*(13), 130401-1–130401-4.

Mathieu, V. (1969). *Storia della filosofia e del pensiero scientifico.* Brescia, Italy: Editrice La Scuola.

McCaul, K. D., & Malott, J. M. (1984). Distraction and coping with pain. *Psychology Bulletin, 95*(3), 516–533.

McFarlane, T. J. (1995). Quantum mechanics and reality [Online]. Available at www.integralscience.org

Merker, B. (2007, September). Consciousness in the raw. *Science News* Online. Available at http://www.sciencenews.org/articles/20070915/bob9.asp

Nagel, E. (1961). *The structure of science.* London: Routledge.

Nagel, T. (1974). What is it like to be a bat? *Philosophical Review, 4,* 435–450.

Nhat Hanh, T. (1999) *The heart of the Buddha's teaching.* New York: Broadway Books.

Rovelli, C. (2006, October 13). Graviton propagator from background-independent quantum gravity. *Physical Review Letters, 97*(15), 151301.

Russel, R. (1961). *Brain, memory, learning.* Oxford, UK: Oxford University Press.

Searle, J. R. (1990). Consciousness, explanatory inversion and cognitive science. *Behavioral and Brain Sciences, 13,* 585–642.

Sellars, R. W. (1919). The epistemology of evolutionary naturalism. *Mind, 28*(112), 407–426.

Shapiro, D. (1977). A biofeedback strategy in the study of consciousness. In N. E. Zinberg (Ed.), *Alternate states of consciousness* (pp. 145–137). New York: The Free Press.

Siegel, R. D. (2010). *The mindfulness solution: Everyday practices for everyday problems.* New York: The Guilford Press.

Spiegel, D. (1985). The use of hypnosis in controlled cancer pain. *CA: A Cancer Journal for Clinician, 4,* 221–231.

Syrjala, K. L. (1990). Relaxation techniques. In J. J. Bonica (Ed.), *The management of pain* (2nd ed., pp. 1742–1750). Philadelphia: Lea & Febiger.

Travis, C. (2004). The silence of the senses. *Mind, 113,* 57–94.

Vogels, T. P., Rajan, K., & Abbott, L. F. (2005). Neural network dynamics. *Annual Review of Neuroscience, 28,* 357–376.

Weiss, A. (2004). *Beginning mindfulness: Learning the way of awareness.* Novato, CA: New World Library.

Chapter II

PAIN AND SUFFERING: NEUROPHYSIOLOGICAL AND BEHAVIORAL ASSESSMENT

1. PAIN DEFINITION

The International Association for the Study of Pain (IASP) is an international professional organization promoting research, education and policies for the knowledge and management of pain. The often-quoted IASP definition of pain as "an unpleasant sensory and emotional experience associated with actual or potential tissue damage, or described in terms of such damage" (International Association for the Study of Pain [IASP], 2009).

The inability to communicate verbally does not negate the possibility that an individual is experiencing pain and is in need of appropriate pain-relieving treatment. Pain and suffering are universal human experiences. We all know what it is like. Few of us, however, know enervating and debilitating chronic pain. What is it that distinguishes the disease chronic pain from the inevitable and sometimes incessant pain that we all endure? It is difficult to make a certain distinction. Unfortunately, there is as yet no adequate definition of the disease. The reasons for this are several, and they are worth exploring.

Serious chronic illnesses are a major health issue in modern society. Any illness is called "chronic" if it is long lasting or even lifelong. The opposite of chronic is "acute," referring to diseases that come on quickly and often do not last long (if they last, they are said to become "chronic"). In the United States, more than 90 million people have a chronic illness, and the top five

---

*This often-quoted definition was first formulatd by an IASP Subcommittee on Taxonomy (bonica, 1979).

chronic illnesses (heart disease, cancer, stroke, COPD and diabetes) together cause more than two thirds of all deaths. In chronic disease anxiety/depression, self-focused attention, pain, and suffering, are significant predictors of panic-fear symptoms, lower self-efficacy, and more perceived interference in well-being of the patient.

Pain and suffering are always subjective. Everyone learns the application of the word through experiences related to injury in early life. Biologists recognize that those stimuli that cause pain are liable to damage tissue. Accordingly, pain is that experience we associate with actual or potential tissue damage. It is unquestionably a sensation in a part or parts of the body, but it is also always unpleasant and therefore, also an emotional experience. Experiences that resemble pain but are not unpleasant, for examples, pricking, should not be called pain. Unpleasant abnormal experiences (dysesthesias) may also be pain but are not necessarily so because, subjectively, they may not have the usual sensory qualities of pain (IASP, 2009).

2. NEUROPHYSIOLOGY AND NEUROPSYCHOLOGY OF PAIN

Pain is a complex phenomenon involving both neurophysiological and psychological components. The transmission of pain-related information from the periphery to the cortex depends on signal integration at three levels of the nervous system: the spinal medulla, brainstem, and telencephalon. In fulfilling its task of safeguarding human health, pain may develop as a result of damaged or altered primary afferent neurons (stimulus dependent) or arise spontaneously without any apparent causal stimulus (stimulus independent).

Hyperalgesia (i.e., an exaggerated perception of pain after a painful stimulus) is due to an anomaly in the processing of nociceptive and behavioral inputs in the central and peripheral nervous systems leading to the activation of the primary afferents by stimuli other than the usual stimuli.

The neuromatrix theory of pain proposes that pain is a multidimensional experience produced by characteristic "neurosignature" patterns of nerve impulses generated by a widely distributed neural network–the "body-self neuromatrix"–in the brain (Melzack, 2005). These neurosignature patterns may be triggered by sensory inputs, but they may also be generated independently of them.

Acute pains evoked by brief noxious inputs have been meticulously investigated by neuroscientists, and their sensory transmission mechanisms are generally well-understood. In contrast, chronic pain syndromes, which are frequently characterized by severe pain associated with little or no discernable injury or pathology, remain a mystery. Furthermore, persistent psychological or physical stress is often associated with chronic pain, but the relationship is poorly understood.

The neuromatrix theory of pain provides a new conceptual framework to examine these problems. It proposes that the output patterns of the body-self neuromatrix activate perceptual, homeostatic, and behavioral programs after injury, pathology, or chronic stress. Pain, then, is produced by the output of a widely distributed neural network in the brain rather than directly by sensory input evoked by injury, inflammation, or other pathology. The neuromatrix, which is genetically determined and modified by sensory experience, is the primary mechanism that generates the neural pattern that produces pain. Its output pattern is determined by multiple influences, of which the somatic sensory input is only a part, that converge on the neuromatrix (Melzack, 2005).

Pathophysiological mechanisms involve neural pathways, and a variety of pain-producing substances and modulating mechanisms. These include acetylcholine, serotonin, histamine, bradykinin, prostaglandins, substance P, somatostatin, cholecystokinin, vasoactive intestinal polypeptide, noradrenaline, and endogenous opioid peptides. The opioid system controls pain, reward, and addictive behaviors. Opioids exert their pharmacological actions through three opioid receptors–mu, delta, and kappa–whose genes have been cloned (Oprm, Oprd1, and Oprk1, respectively). Opioid receptors in the brain are activated by a family of endogenous peptides like enkephalins, dynorphins and endorphin, which are released by neurons (Contet, Kieffer, & Befort, 2004). Opioid receptors can also be activated exogenously by alkaloid opiates, the prototype of which is morphine, which remains the most valuable painkiller in contemporary medicine. In assessing patients with pain, it is essential to evaluate the cause of the pain, and its severity, type, location, duration, quality, and response to therapies, among other factors (Lasagna, 1986).

It is the perception of pain and the individual's physical and emotional reaction to the pain perception that give us the opportunity to create treatment approaches that can provide relief. An endogenous CNS pain-modulating network with links in the midbrain, medulla, and spinal cord has been discovered. This system produces analgesia by interfering with afferent transmission of neural messages produced by intense stimuli. Although other neurotransmitters are involved, the analgesia produced by this system depends on the release of endogenous opioid substances, generically referred to as endorphins. The system is set in motion by clinically significant pain, such as that resulting from bony fractures or postoperative pain. The analgesia network monitors the pain and controls it at the level of the spinal cord.

In 2010, a group of Japanese scientists discovered the association between personality, pain threshold, and a single nucleotide polymorphism (rs3813034) in the 3′-untranslated region of the serotonin transporter gene (SLC6A4). In 181 healthy Japanese volunteers they examined the relationship among personality, sensitivity to pain, and a single nucleotide polymorphism (rs3813034) in the 3′-untranslated region (3′ UTR) of the serotonin transporter (5-HTT) gene (SLC6A4). Pain sensitivity was assessed by using cold and pressure thresholds. Personality was assessed by the Temperament and Character Inventory (TCI). Males without the T allele (G/G) showed a significantly higher spiritual acceptance (ST3) score than those who had the T allele (T/T and T/G) did. Females with the T allele (T/T and T/G) showed considerably stronger transpersonal identification (ST2) and self-transcendence (ST) scores than did those without the T allele (G/G) (Aoki, Ikeda, Murayama, Yoshihara, Ogai, & Iwahashi, 2010).

Complex psychological factors play an important role in the variability of perceived pain, partly because of their ability to trigger this pain-suppressing system. The patient with pain in chronic diseases and in palliative care, should be reassured. It is understood that the patient is suffering, and an appropriate cause for this suffering and the most effective treatment will be sought. The physicians can offer a useful service in the diagnosis and treatment of pain in many complex cases.

3. CLASSIFICATION OF PAIN TYPES

In 1994, responding to the need for a more useful system for describing chronic pain, the IASP classified pain according to specific characteristics: (1) region of the body involved (e.g., abdomen, lower limbs), (2) system whose dysfunction may be causing the pain (e.g., nervous, gastrointestinal), (3) duration and pattern of occurrence, (4) intensity and time since onset, and (5) etiology.

The work of the Task Force on Taxonomy in the era of 1979 to 1994 has been continued by the Committee on Taxonomy, which has worked to update both pain terms and the classification of pain syndromes. All of the terms have been carefully reviewed and their utility assessed in reference to new knowledge about both clinical and basic science aspects of pain. The Scheme for Coding Chronic Pain Diagnoses (updated in 2011 by the IASP Taxonomy Working Group) and List of Topics and Codes is as follows:

A. Relatively Generalized Syndromes
B. Relatively Localized Syndromes of the Head and Neck

C. Spinal Pain, Section 1: Spinal and Radicular Pain Syndromes
D. Spinal Pain, Section 2: Spinal and Radicular Pain Syndromes of the Cervical and Thoracic Regions
E. Local Syndromes of the Upper Limbs and Relatively Generalized Syndromes of the Upper and Lower Limbs
F. Visceral and Other Syndromes of the Trunk Apart From Spinal and Radicular Pain
G. Spinal Pain, Section 3: Spinal and Radicular Pain Syndromes of the Lumbar, Sacral, and Coccygeal Regions
H. Local Syndromes of the Lower Limbs

There are two basic types of pain: acute and chronic. Acute pain occurs for brief periods of time and is associated with temporary disorders. It is always an alarm signal that something may be wrong, however. Chronic pain is continuous and recurrent. It is associated with chronic diseases and is one of their symptoms. Pain intensity depends not only on the type of stimulus that caused it but also on the subjective perception of the pain.

Chronic pain may be divided into "cancer" and "benign." In chronic pain, guidelines often are not universally accepted by those involved in pain management, and pain treatment seems to be driven mainly by tradition and personal experience. Other factors include poor communication among patients, nurses, and physicians; the side effects of analgesic drugs; and limited individualization of therapy. Difficulty in maintaining the balance between adequate pain relief and acceptable tolerability, particularly with strong opioids, can lead to the establishment of a "vicious circle" that alternates between lack of efficacy and unpleasant side effects, prompting discontinuation of treatment. The medical community's understanding of the physiological differences between nociceptive pain and neuropathic pain, which is often more severe and difficult to treat, could be improved.

Neuropathic pain is a complex, chronic pain state that usually is accompanied by tissue injury. With neuropathic pain, the nerve fibers themselves may be damaged, dysfunctional, or injured. These damaged nerve fibers send incorrect signals to other pain centers. The impact of nerve fiber injury includes a change in nerve function at both the site of injury and areas around the injury.

What causes neuropathic pain in chronic diseases? Neuropathic pain often seems to have no obvious cause; however, some common causes of neuropathic pain include

- cancer (primary tumor or metastatic disease)
- amputation

- back, leg, and hip problems
- chemotherapy
- diabetes
- facial nerve problems
- HIV infection or AIDS
- multiple sclerosis
- shingles
- spine surgery

What are the symptoms of neuropathic pain? Symptoms may include shooting and burning pain and tingling and numbness.

The Neuropathic Pain Special Interest Group of the IASP recently sponsored the development of evidence-based guidelines for the pharmacological treatment of neuropathic pain. Tricyclic antidepressants, dual reuptake inhibitors of serotonin and norepinephrine, calcium-channel alpha(2)-delta ligands (i.e., gabapentin and pregabalin), and topical lidocaine were recommended as first-line treatment options based on the results of randomized clinical trials. Opioid analgesics and tramadol were recommended as second-line treatments that can be considered for primary use in certain clinical circumstances (Dworkin et al., 2010). The increasing number of negative clinical trials of pharmacological treatments for neuropathic pain and ambiguities in the interpretation of these negative trials must also be considered in developing treatment guidelines.

Chronic neuropathic pain is a prevalent problem that eludes cure and adequate treatment. The persistence of intense and aversive symptoms in chronic diseases, inadequacy of available treatments, and the impact of such pain on all aspects of functioning underscore the important role of several psychosocial factors in causing, maintaining, and amplifying the perception of pain severity, coping adequacy, adaptation, impaired physical function, and emotional distress responses (Turk, Audette, Levy, Mackey, Stanos, 2010).

Older people are at high risk of neuropathic pain because the incidence of many diseases that cause neuropathic and chronic pain increases with age. Depending on their underlying health, older adults with chronic pain may have to cope with multiple coexisting diseases, polypharmacy, and impaired functional ability.

4. PAIN MANAGEMENT

Pain management in patients must reflect aged heterogeneity, multimorbidity, and polypharmacy; selection of treatment in an effort to maximize patients' functional abilities in addition to relieving their pain; more careful dosing (usually lower) and monitoring of pharmacotherapy relative to younger patients due to age-related changes in pharmacokinetics and pharmacodynamics; and underrepresentation of older adults in clinical trials of neuropathic pain treatments, which further compromises the physicians ability to make informed treatment decisions (Schmader et al., 2010).

Anesthesiologists have always played a leading role in research into pain and its treatment. Their efforts, however, have been focused on acute or postoperative pain problems. It was the American anesthesiologist John J. Bonica who fought for an increased interest in chronic pain. The establishment of the first Multidisciplinary Pain Center at the University of Washington in Seattle, the foundation of the IASP, and Melzack and Wall's now old gate-control theory were the driving forces behind rapid developments in research and treatment in the area of chronic pain.

The classic anesthesiological topics, such as operative anesthesia, emergency medicine, and intensive care, have been extended to include acute pain services and chronic pain treatment facilities. This reflects the understanding that anesthesiological knowledge and techniques can be valuable to patients in severe acute pain and those in lingering long-term chronic pain phases in chronic diseases and in palliative care. Special ways of administering narcotic analgesics, such as epidural infusion or patient-controlled analgesia, have already alleviated the pain problems of many patients.

Anesthesiological techniques are also crucial in diagnosis. Sequential differential blockade and simple nerve blocks can be helpful in the diagnosis and classification of the pain problems. Interventional procedures (typically used for chronic pain) include epidural steroid injections, facet joint injections, neurolytic blocks, spinal cord stimulators, and intrathecal drug delivery system implants.

The art and science of anesthetic practice has existed as a unique medical discipline for less than 150 years. During that time, the focus has changed from helping the patient tolerate surgical stress by rendering him insensible to pain to controlling stress and the patient's physiological responses to the perioperative period by careful titration of powerful pharmacological means and the appreciation of sound medical judgment.

Anesthesiologists can not only use their nerve blocking and analgesic-prescribing skills, but also can coordinate some of the other treatment strategies, such as relaxation techniques and hypnosis. By joining with colleagues skilled in behavioral, psychiatric, and surgical management of pain states, the anesthesiologist can give a useful approach to these problems (Murphy, 1986). The anesthesiologist's goals are to render the patient pain free and amnesic to preserve vital functions during the operations and procedures, and to offer to the patient during regional anesthesia a quiet, relaxed state of consciousness.

5. PAIN EVALUATION

The pain evaluation consists of pain assessment and pain treatment.

A. Pain Assessment

- Ask about pain
- Surgical or procedural pain
- Pain score
- Physical exam
- Diagnostic studies
- Pain mechanisms

  Nociceptive
  Somatic
  Visceral

  Neuropathic

The patient's pain should be acknowledged to be a very real problem for the patient. Attempts to differentiate between "real" and "unreal" pain and "organic" and "psychosomatic" are usually fruitless and only succeed in challenging such patients to attempt to prove further the "reality" of their suffering.

The patient can appreciate that there may not always be a technological or invasive solution to the problem, such as the use of a nerve block or a pill, so the patient must be willing to undergo psychological and behavioral evaluation. Many factors may contribute to the symptoms. Concomitant depression, impaired cortical function, and chronic anxiety may all be conditions in which the patients use the language and behavior of pain to communicate their distress and suffering.

Physiological indications of acute pain in adults are

- dilated pupils
- increased perspiration
- increased rate/force of heart rate
- increased rate/depth of respirations

- increased blood pressure
- decreased urine output
- decreased peristalsis of GI tract
- increased basal metabolic rate

Sometimes during acute pain, growth hormone levels significantly increased within minutes, and beta endorphin and prolactin were elevated proportionately with severity of injury. Cortisol was inversely correlated with injury severity, possibly reflecting impaired release from the adrenal cortex after very severe injury (Hetz, 1996).

In the final analysis, pain is communicated as a behavior, for it is only by word, grimacing, posturing, and other behavioral signals that we know another individual is in pain. The pain behaviors in the cognitively Impaired are

- facial expression
- slight frown, frightened face
- rapid blinking
- verbalizations, vocalizations
- verbally abusive
- calling out, chanting, grunting
- body movements
- rigid, tense
- fidgeting
- increased pacing, rocking
- changes in interpersonal interactions
- aggressive, combative, resisting care
- decreased social interaction
- socially inappropriate, disruptive
- changes in activity patterns or routines
- refusing food
- increased rest periods
- sleep pattern changes
- mental status changes
- crying, tears
- increased confusion
- irritable

Patients may acquire behavioral aspects of their pain problems in chronic diseases and in palliative care and along with psychological and tissue-damaging problems. Thus, such patients are unlikely to respond to therapy directed primarily at the tissue-damaging aspects but may well need the combined efforts of conventional therapy aimed at the degenerative disease, psychological support, pharmacological treatment, and some behavior modification in an attempt to restore normal function.

The possible physiological and psychological signs of acute pain in the neonates and in children are (Stallard et al., 2002):

Physiological Variables

- Heart rate, respiratory rate, pressure breathing
- Shallow respirations
- Vagal nerve tone (shrill cry)
- Pallor or flushing
- Diaphoresis, palmar sweating
- O_2 saturation
- EEG changes

Behavioral Variables

Vocalizations

- Crying (often with apneic spells)
- Whimpering, groaning, moaning

State Changes

- Changes in sleep/wake cycles
- Changes in activity level
- Agitation or listlessness

Bodily Movements

- Limb withdrawal, swiping, or thrashing
- Rigidity
- Flaccidity
- Clenching of fists

Facial Expression (Most Reliable Sign)

- Eyes tightly closed or opened
- Mouth opened

- Furrowing or bulging of brow
- Quivering of chin
- Deepened nasolabial fold

Acute pain signals pass through the thalamus, and then on to the sensory cortex. Chronic pain travels through the hypothalamus, which is connected to the limbic system, where emotional states (emotion-related symptoms such as anxiety or depression) seems to originate.

No aspect of our mental life is more important to the quality and meaning of our existence than emotions are. In view of the proliferation of increasingly fruitful exchanges between researches of different stripes, it is no longer useful to speak of the philosophy of emotion in isolation from the approaches of other disciplines, particularly psychology and neurology (De Sousa, 1987). If the view that emotions are a kind of perception that can be sustained, then the connection between emotion and cognition will have been secured.

There is yet another way of establishing this connection, compatible with the perceptual model. This is to draw attention to the role of emotions as providing the framework for cognitions of the more conventional kind. De Sousa (1987) and Amélie Rorty (1980) proposed this sort of account according to which emotions are not so much perceptions as they are ways of seeing, species of determinate patterns of salience among objects of attention, lines of inquiry, and inferential strategies. Emotions make certain features of situations or arguments more prominent, giving them a weight in our experience that they would have lacked in the absence of emotion (De Sousa, 1987; Roberts, 1988).

Pain is considered to be chronic if it has remained essentially unrelieved for six months or longer. Chronic pain can be of many types and locations and may or may not have specific tissue damage associated with it. This is to contrast it with temporary acute pain that is related to specific tissue damage and reduces in intensity as the damaged area heals.

Chronic pain differs from acute pain in several important ways. It is now believed that different neural circuits are traveled by chronic and acute pain. In chronic pain there exits a relationship between emotions, psychological state, and the intensity of the pain experience. Stress, depression, or anxiety can all increase the intensity of the pain experience. Consequently, procedures that reduce stress, depression, and anxiety can have the opposite effect and can reduce the intensity of the pain experience.

While pain is going on, the body tries to immobilize the inflamed tissue (muscle or joint area) by putting extra fluid there (edema), much as a garden hose becomes stiff if the flow is stopped. Eventually, the chronic stiffness and disuse cause muscle atrophy. The body begins to deposit calcium in the tissues and around the joints, in effect making an internal cast and mechanically immobilizing the area. Therefore, the longer a pain patient does not use an area, the harder it will be to ever use it, and the more painful it will become. Taking medicine for pain can also be a factor that prolongs and maintains the chronic pain condition. Most painkillers have powerful effects on other parts of the CNS. A percentage of chronic pain patients may become addicted to pain medications. Patients may also have to increase their dose periodically in order to get the same level of relief (this is called developing a tolerance to the drug). Their pain level escalates, and severe autonomic arousal develops with blockade or sudden discontinuance of the analgesic drug (an example of physical dependence causing withdrawal or abstinence syndrome). Chronic pain patients may be controlling and focused on their medication, understandably, because the drug is the only thing that has brought them any feeling of relief, and it is the only thing that gives them a feeling of control over their pain management.

Chronic pain is different from acute pain in several ways. It is now believed that different neural pathways are traveled by chronic and acute pain. Acute pain passes through the thalamus and then on to the sensory cortex; chronic pain travels through the hypothalamus, which is connected to the limbic system where emotional functioning (emotions or problems, such as anxiety or depression) seems to originate.

In chronic pain, there is a relationship between emotions, psychological state and the intensity of the pain experience. A variety of methods are available to help the acute and chronic pain patient manage depression, anxiety, and stress level, including relaxation techniques and hypnosis. Usually, some combinations of these with therapies are applied for the best results.

Typically, a pain evaluation consists of several approaches to discovering which factors play the largest role in maintaining the pain. We perform psychological testing to determine any underlying causes of depression or anxiety, which should be treated in addition to the pain and which could be helping to maintain it.

AHCPR Recommendations for the Examination of Pain

- Health professionals should ask about pain, and the patient's self-report should be the primary source of assessment.
- Clinicians should assess pain with easily administered rating scales and should document the efficacy of pain relief at regular intervals after starting or changing treatment. Documentation forms should be readily accessible to all clinicians involved in the patient's care. (Panel Consensus)

- Clinicians should teach patients and their families to use assessment tools in their homes in order to promote continuity of effective pain management across all settings. (Panel Consensus)
- The initial evaluation of pain should include
  - detailed history, including an assessment of pain intensity and characteristics
  - physical examination
  - psychosocial assessment
  - diagnostic evaluation of signs and symptoms associated with the common cancer pain syndromes (Panel Consensus)
- Clinicians should be aware of common pain syndromes. Prompt recognition may hasten therapy and minimize the morbidity of unrelieved pain.
- Changes in pain patterns or the development of new pain should trigger a diagnostic evaluation and modification of the treatment plan. (Panel Consensus)
- Health professionals should ask about pain, and the patient's self-report should be the primary source of assessment. The self-report should include a description of the pain; its location, intensity/severity, and aggravating and relieving factors; and the patient's cognitive response to pain.

Neither behavior nor vital signs should be used in lieu of a self-report (Beyer, McGrath, & Berde, 1990). It is best to use brief, easy-to-use assessment tools that reliably document pain intensity and pain relief and to relate these to other dimensions of pain, such as mood. One routine clinical approach to pain assessment and management is summarized by the mnemonic "ABCDE":

A. Ask about pain regularly. Assess pain systematically.
B. Believe the patient and family in their reports of pain and what relieves it.
C. Choose pain control options appropriate for the patient, family, and setting.
D. Deliver interventions in a timely, logical, and coordinated fashion.
E. Empower patients and their families.

Three commonly used self-report assessment tools are

- Simple Descriptive Pain Intensity Scale
- 0–10 Numeric Pain Intensity Scale

- Visual Analog Scale (VAS)

If the patient understands the scale and is capable of answering and if end points and adjective descriptors are carefully selected, each of these instruments can be valid and reliable (Gracely & Wolskee, 1983; Houde, 1982; Sriwatanakul, Kelvie, & Lasagna, 1982).

Knowing factors that aggravate or relieve pain helps clinicians to design a pain treatment plan. The initial pain assessment should elicit information about changes in activities of daily living, including work and recreational activities, sleep patterns, mobility, appetite, sexual functioning, and mood.

A psychosocial assessment should emphasize the effect of pain on patients and their families, as well as patients' preferences among pain management methods. Patients who are able to answer should be asked about the effectiveness of past and present pain treatments, such as antineoplastic therapy or specific pharmacological and nonpharmacological therapies.

B. Pain Treatment

The recommendations about the assessment and management of pain (IASP and WHO), include the use of the following.

Analgesics and Adjuvant Medicines: WHO's Pain Ladder

WHO has developed a three-step "ladder" for pain relief. If pain occurs, there should be prompt oral administration of medicines in the following order:

1. Nonopioids (aspirin and paracetamol)
2. Then, as necessary, mild opioids (codeine)
3. Then, strong opioids, such as morphine, until the patient is free of pain

To calm fears and anxiety, additional medicines—"adjuvants"—should be used. To maintain freedom from pain, drugs should be given "by the clock"; that is every 3–6 hours, rather than "on demand." This three-step approach of administering the right drug in the right dose at the right time is inexpensive and 80 to 90 percent effective. Surgical intervention on appropriate nerves may provide further pain relief if drugs are not wholly effective.

Palliative and Ablative Surgery and Anesthesiology

- Nerve blocks
- Local anesthetics

- Epidural
- Intrathecal
- Cordotomy: anteriolateral spinothalamic tract is ablated

Physical Modalities

- Physiatry. Physical medicine and rehabilitation (physiatry/physiotherapy) employs diverse physical techniques such as thermal agents and electrotherapy, as well as therapeutic exercise and behavioral therapy, alone or in tandem with interventional techniques and conventional pharmacotherapy to treat pain, usually as part of an interdisciplinary or multidisciplinary program.
- Transcutaneous electrical nerve stimulation (TENS)
- Palliative radiation
- Acupuncture. Acupuncture involves the insertion and manipulation of needles into specific points on the body to relieve pain or for therapeutic purposes.
- Laser Therapy

Nonconventional Remedies and Herbals

The Psychological and Cognitive/Behavior Strategies

Because the mechanisms of pain in chronic diseases and in palliative care may be complex, involving several causes, such patients often have difficulty obtaining an adequate diagnostic evaluation. Sometimes we ignore the psychological and behavioral components of pain. To evaluate patients with complaints pain encountered in palliative medicine, therefore, the specific psychological, social, and environmental characteristics as well as a conventional medical examination should be reviewed. There are several ways in which anesthesiologists, depending on their inclinations, can become involved in the management of pain patients in this setting. The patient can appreciate that there may not be only one solution to this problem, such as the use of nerve block, an operation, or a pill. In chronic diseases and in palliative care, acute and chronic pain and depression are often associated in the same patient. Furthermore, the successful treatment of the depression is often associated with pain relief.

6. THE PSYCHOLOGICAL AND COGNITIVE/BEHAVIOR STRATEGIES IN PAIN THERAPY AND PALLIATIVE CARE

A. The Dignity Therapy in Palliative Care

Dignity therapy is a novel psychotherapeutic intervention for patients near the end of life (Harvey Chochinov, CancerCare, University of Manitoba, Canada). It is designed to address psychosocial and existential distress among terminally ill patients and invites patients to discuss issues that matter most or that they would most want remembered. Sessions are transcribed and edited, with a returned final version that they can bequeath to a friend or family member. The objective of this study is to establish the feasibility of dignity therapy and to determine its impact on various measures of psychosocial and existential distress.

The outline of the dignity therapy interview guide is based on themes and subthemes that arise from the dignity model. Therapeutic sessions, running between thirty and sixty minutes, are offered either at the patients' bedside for those in hospital or, for outpatients, in their residential setting, at home, or at a long-term care facility (Chochinov et al., 2005).

B. Psychotherapy

Psychotherapy is a general term referring to therapeutic interaction or treatment contracted between a trained professional and a client, patient, family, couple, or group. The problems addressed are psychological in nature and of no specific kind or degree but rather depend on the specialty of the practitioner. Psychotherapy aims to increase the individual's sense of his or her own well-being. Psychotherapists employ a range of techniques based on experiential relationship building, dialogue, communication, and behavior change that are designed to improve the mental health of a client or patient, or to improve group relationships (such as in a family).

Psychotherapy is a word of Greek origin, deriving from Ancient Greek *psyche* meaning breath, spirit, soul) and *therapeia* (healing, medical treatment). According to the Oxford English Dictionary, psychotherapy first meant "hypnotherapy." The original meaning, "the treatment of disease by 'psychic' [i.e., hypnotic] methods," was first recorded in 1853 as "psychotherapeia, or the remedial influence of mind." The modern meaning, "the treatment of disorders of the mind or personality by psychological or psychophysiological methods," was first used in 1892 by Frederik van Eeden, translating "Suggestive Psycho-therapy" for his French "Psychothérapie Suggestive."

Most forms of psychotherapy use spoken conversation. Some also use various other forms of communication, such as the written word, artwork, drama, narrative story, or music. Psychotherapy with children and their parents often involves play, dramatization (i.e. role-play), and drawing, with a coconstructed narrative from these nonverbal and displaced modes of interacting.

Psychotherapy occurs within a structured encounter between a trained therapist and client(s). Purposeful, theoretically based psychotherapy began in the nineteenth century with psychoanalysis. Since then, scores of other approaches have been developed and continue to be created. There are several main broad systems of psychotherapy:

- *Psychoanalysis.* This was the first practice to be called a psychotherapy. It encourages the verbalization of all the patient's thoughts, including free associations, fantasies, and dreams, from which the analyst formulates the nature of the unconscious conflicts that are causing the patient's symptoms and character problems.
- *Behavior Therapy and Applied Behavior Analysis.* This system focuses on changing maladaptive patterns of behavior to improve emotional responses, cognitions, and interactions with others.
- *Cognitive Behavior Therapy.* This therapy generally seeks to identify maladaptive cognition, appraisal, beliefs, and reactions with the aim of influencing destructive negative emotions and problematic dysfunctional behaviors. Cognitive and behavior therapy is the use of stress reduction and relaxation, to reduce chronic pain in some patients (Kabat-Zinn, Lipworth, & Burney, 1985; Kabat-Zinn, 1982; Kwekkeboom, Cherwin, Lee, & Wanta, 2010). Applied behavior analysis views chronic pain as a consequence of both respondent and operant conditioning, in which a patient learns to display pain behavior in the presence of specific environmental antecedents and consequences. Biofeedback based on behavioral principles has shown some success for chronic pain, demonstrating greater improvement in one study than peers undergoing cognitive behavior therapy and conservative medical treatment have (Flor & Birbaumer, 1993).
- *Psychodynamic Therapy.* This is a form of depth psychology whose primary focus is to reveal the unconscious content of a client's psyche in an effort to alleviate psychic tension. Although its roots are in psychoanalysis, psychodynamic therapy tends to be briefer and less intensive than traditional psychoanalysis is.
- *Existential Therapy.* This is based on the existential belief that human beings are alone in the world. This isolation leads to feelings of mean-

inglessness that can be overcome only by creating one's own values and meanings. Existential therapy is philosophically associated with phenomenology.

- *Humanistic Therapy.* Emerged in reaction to both behaviorism and psychoanalysis, this therapy is known as the Third Force in the development of psychology. It is explicitly concerned with the human context of the development of the individual with an emphasis on subjective meaning, a rejection of determinism, and a concern for positive growth rather than pathology. It posits an inherent human capacity to maximize potential–"the self-actualizing tendency." The task of humanistic therapy is to create a relational environment where this tendency might flourish. Humanistic psychology is philosophically rooted in existentialism.
- *Brief Therapy.* Brief therapy is an umbrella term for a variety of approaches to psychotherapy. It differs from other schools of therapy in that it emphasizes (1) a focus on a specific problem and (2) direct intervention. It is solution based rather than problem oriented. It is less concerned with how a problem arose than with the current factors sustaining it and preventing change.
- *Systemic Therapy.* This system seeks to address people not at an individual level, as is often the focus of other forms of therapy, but as people in relationship, dealing with the interactions of groups, and their patterns and dynamics (includes family therapy and marriage counseling). Community psychology is a type of systemic psychology.
- *Transpersonal Therapy.* This addresses the client in the context of a spiritual understanding of consciousness.
- *Body Psychotherapy.* This addresses problems of the mind as being closely correlated with bodily phenomena, including a person's sexuality, musculature, breathing habits, physiology, and so on. This therapy may involve massage and other body exercises as well as talking.

There are hundreds of psychotherapeutic approaches or schools of thought. By 1980, there were more than 250; by 1996, there were more than 450. The development of new and hybrid approaches continues around the wide variety of theoretical backgrounds. Many practitioners use several approaches in their work and alter their approach based on client need.

C. Clinical Hypnosis

Clinical hypnosis is practiced for both chronic and acute pain conditions: (1) hypnotic analgesia consistently results in greater decreases in a variety of pain outcomes compared to no treatment or standard care, (2) hypnosis frequently out-performs nonhypnotic interventions (e.g., education, supportive therapy) in terms of reductions in pain-related outcomes, and (3) hypnosis performs similarly to treatments that contain hypnotic elements (such as PMR) but is not surpassed in efficacy by these alternative treatments (Stoelb, Molton, Jensen, & Patterson, 2009; Jensen, 2009).

Many chronic pain patients often have reversed diurnal rhythms whereby they catnap during the day, reclining on couches, and spend the night awake and restless. Hypnosis can often be quite successful in reestablishing a normal sleep pattern in such patients, often resulting in an improved sense of well-being and pain relief.

A 2007 review of thirteen studies found evidence for the efficacy of hypnosis in the reduction of pain in some conditions. The authors concluded that "although the findings provide support for the general applicability of hypnosis in the treatment of chronic pain, considerably more research will be needed to fully determine the effects of hypnosis for different chronic-pain conditions" (Elkins, 2007).

The neural mechanisms underlying the antinociceptive effects of hypnosis still remain unclear. A group of scientists in 2009, using a parametric single-trial thulium-YAG laser fMRI paradigm, assessed changes in brain activation and connectivity related to the hypnotic state as compared to normal wakefulness in thirteen healthy volunteers. Behaviorally, a difference in subjective ratings was found between normal wakefulness and hypnotic state for both nonpainful and painful intensity-matched stimuli applied to the left hand. In normal wakefulness, nonpainful range stimuli activated the brainstem, and contralateral primary somatosensory and bilateral insular cortices. Painful stimuli activated additional areas encompassing the thalamus; bilateral striatum; and anterior cingulate, premotor, and dorsolateral prefrontal cortices. In hypnosis, intensity-matched stimuli in both the nonpainful and painful range failed to elicit any cerebral activation. The interaction analysis identified that the contralateral thalamus, bilateral striatum, and anterior cingulate cortex activated more in normal wakefulness compared to hypnosis during painful versus non-painful stimulation (Vanhaudenhuyse et al., 2009).

Clinical hypnosis in pain therapy and palliative care may be useful to

- have a good relaxation of body and mind
- facilitate mechanical ventilation and physiological tidal volume in critical care
- reduce anxiety (in palliative care increases breathing in patients)
- reduce panic
- have a good acute and chronic pain relief

- altered perception of pain
- facilitate new patterns of thoughts, feelings, and consciousness
- reduce depression
- reduce sleep disturbances
- reduce preoperative anxiety
- reframe or redefine a problem or situation
- bypass normal ego defenses
- suggest solutions and new options
- provide a gateway between the conscious and the unconscious mind
- increase communication
- facilitate retrieval of resource experiences
- improve mind-body relationship
- improve psychology of self and self-realization
- understand the higher self
- understand the evolution of consciousness
- lighten up the "spiritual" dimension in dying patients
- accept death and dying

Pain and anxiety can cause hypoventilation (decreased tidal volume) and hypoxemia (decreased PaO_2) and increase airway resistance. Posture, pain, and anxiety may restrict or interfere with movements of the diaphragm: tidal volume is reduced and breathing will be rapid and shallow. Rapid shallow breathing may cause a decrease in functional residual capacity and promote atelectasis. If tidal volume is decreased and respiratory rate does not increase proportionately, minute ventilation will decrease, PaO_2 may decrease, and $PaCO_2$ may increase (Miller, 1986). With hypnosis, most symptoms may be reduced significantly.

Pain is a necessary physical sensation to warn a person of damage. Research indicates that after the organism notes the disease or injury site, pain interferes with healing and retards the eventual course leading to vitality. Reduction of pain and suffering is one of the primary targets of all treatment because reduction of pain is the beginning of recovering quality of life. Many researchers and clinicians have demonstrated that management of pain is a natural capacity housed in each person. Yet pain is a deeply subjective experience. Successful treatment utilizes hypnotic trance to help patients relearn subcortical activity in the brain and then to alter (self-talk) it.

Symptoms are defined as preverbal conditioned reflexes that at some sensate level make sense to patients and are subconsciously designed and then used to prevent awareness of experienced or subconscious distress.

Relaxation and hypnotic trances attempt to accelerate a patient's ability to reorganize thinking, to have a unique experience, and simultaneously to learn the responsibility of personal pain relief through self-involvement.

Anton Mesmer and other physicians reported on the use of "animal magnetism" for pain relief in the 1700s; the era of hypnoanesthesia began as early as 1821. Cloquet performed a breast amputation using mesmerism in a demonstration to the French Academy of Medicine in 1829, but it was a Scottish surgeon, James Esdaile, who became most famous for the use of hypnosis as a surgical anesthetic (Esdaile, 1847; Kroger, 1963).

Esdaile reported on hundreds of painless operations performed with mesmerism between 1840 and 1850. In the preface to his book *Mesmerism in India* (1847), Esdaile wrote that "painless surgical operations and other medical advantages" were the "natural birthright" that mesmerism provided his patients in Bengal. Esdaile's work overlapped the development of chemical anesthesia with the first use of nitrous oxide in 1844, ether in 1846, and chloroform in 1847. By the 1860s, chemical anesthesia had essentially eliminated the use of hypnoanesthesia, although dramatic examples of its use are still seen today.

In April 2000, the *International Journal of Clinical and Experimental Hypnosis* published a special issue entitled "The Status of Hypnosis as an Empirically Validated Clinical Intervention." Within this issue, Guy Montgomery and colleagues presented a meta-analysis of eighteen studies of hypnotically induced analgesia (Montgomery, DuHamel & Redd, 2000). As had been found in several earlier studies, this report supported hypnotic analgesia as a valid and reliable phenomena, with 75 percent of the clinical and experimental subjects reporting pain relief. The authors conclude that, based on the criteria set forth by Chambless and Hollon (1998), "hypnotically suggested analgesia should be considered a well established treatment." Patterson and Jenson (2003) supported this position for both acute and chronic pain conditions (Willmarth & Willmarth, 2005). Hypnosis is used for this purpose as an addition to or substitute for chemical anesthesia in many surgical procedures because it is completely nontoxic and shows excellent results for the hypnotizable subject (Patterson, 2010).

The greatest limit to its use in today's palliation is the lack of education by hospital personnel in its use and their resulting failure to recommend its use for patients. There are also too few hypnotherapists with specific training and experience in this field. Clinical hypnosis is very useful in chronic diseases and in palliative care.

The special problems in palliative care are

- fear of increasing functional deficits
- concerns with cognitive function
- high number of cognitively impaired

- fear of hastening death in the frail elderly
- more depression
- decreased socialization
- sleep disturbances
- communication barrier due to sensory or cognitive impairment
- reluctance to report pain
- pain may be perceived as metaphor for serious disease or death

From a clinical perspective, the use of clinical hypnosis to alter perception can be applied to the perception of pain in a number of effective ways. This is true not only for the sensation of pain but also for the cognitive and emotional factors including attention, attitude, affect, attribution, and arousal.

Although hundreds of creative suggestions and metaphors for pain control have been presented in the literature, Hilgard and Hilgard (1994) propose three general classes of pain management approaches. These include

1. direct suggestion of pain reduction
2. alteration of the experience of pain
3. redirection of attention (Willmarth & Willmarth, 2005)

We could use specific suggestions to help the patients achieve this state in palliative care. The author explains that hypnosis is not mind control; the patient is not going to be asked to do anything embarrassing. It is not like taking a powerful drug that leaves the patient zonked out. It is more like focused attention, focused concentration, in which the patient is able to let himself or herself relax and be the person in charge.

Chronic pain often requires more effort, but hypnosis provides many individuals with a way to experience focused, narrow attention, which redirects attention to thoughts or memories more pleasant than the pain. This "hallucination" may itself create physiological change (Willmarth & Willmarth, 2005). Dabney Ewin, a surgeon and gifted hypnotist, notes that if patients with severe burns can be placed in a trance soon after their injury and can imagine cool or cold conditions on the skin, the course of the injury changes (Ewin, 1986).

Once hypnotized, suggestions can be made specifically related to recovery from procedures in chronic diseases and palliative care. First, suggest them this state "Now, every time you are lying in bed at night, go deep into this state. . . ." Second, they will be trained to enter this state while starting a procedure and to remain in this state throughout the procedure: "Now, when you lie on the gurney, and you feel its vibrations under your body, you automatically go deep. . . ." Third, the patient is taught to to access this state while lying in the recovery room and/or his or her own bedroom to activate the recovery suggestions (Ewin, 1986).

The way to work with patients is to train them to use all of these processes every day in the quietness of their own beds. A hypnosis tape or CD custom made for the patient can be very helpful. In chronic diseases, heightened anxiety increases the chances of pain, analgesic consumption, and also hospital stay and recovery. Hypnosis can help the patient have less anxiety before and less pain later.

There are good neurophysiological studies to prove that hypnosis is potentially a powerful tool to alter perception of pain and associated anxiety. It is entirely possible to substantially alter pain perception during surgical procedures by inducing hypnotic relaxation, transforming perception in parts of the body, or directing attention elsewhere. The key concept is that this psychological procedure actually changes pain experience as much as many analgesic medications and far more than placebos (McGlashan, Evans & Orne, 1969; Raz, Fan & Posner, 2005; Spiegel, Kraemer & Carlson, 2001).

There is recent evidence from studies of the placebo effect that activity in the anterior cingulate gyrus is linked to that in the periaqueduct gray, a brainstem region that is crucial to pain perception (Wager, Scott & Zubieta, 2007). Hypnotic analgesia is real, no less palpable an analgesic than medication is, although the pathways are different and do not seem to involve endogenous opiates (Spiegel & Albert, 1983). Rather, hypnosis seems to involve brain activation via dopamine pathways (Lichtenberg, Bachner-Melman, Gritsenko & Ebstein, 2000; Raz, 2005; Spiegel & King, 1992). Thus, it is not surprising that hypnosis, which mobilizes attention pathways in the brain, can be used effectively to reduce pain perception and attendant anxiety.

D. Meditative States and Mindfulness

Mindfulness therapy is simply being "aware," aware of what you are choosing to think moment by moment, and then learning simple techniques to evaluate your own thoughts for what they really are: just glitches in your mind. Mindfulness is the detachment from our mind, from our self. Once you become aware of your inner thoughts, you will learn how to stop your own reactions to the "stressors" (triggers) in your own life.

Mindfulness is a common translation of a term from Buddhist psychology that means awareness or bare attention. It is frequently used to refer to a way of paying attention that is sensitive, accepting, and independent of any thoughts that may be present. Differences can be discerned in how different practitioners, many different religions, and ancient philosophies use mindfulness. Some of these reflect the hazards of translation, and others reflect long-standing ambiguities within Buddhist psychology.

In this book, the author explains numerous distinct types of mindfulness in many different philosophies and religions that we can use in pain therapy and in palliative care as spiritual care, not only at the end of life, but also in our everyday life.

REFERENCES

Aoki, J., Ikeda, K., Murayama, O., Yoshihara, E., Ogai, Y., & Iwahashi, K. (2010, May). The association between personality, pain threshold and a single nucleotide polymorphism (rs3813034) in the 3'-untranslated region of the serotonin transporter gene (SLC6A4). *Journal of Clinical Neuroscience, 17*(5), 574–578.

Beyer, J. E., McGrath, P. J., & Berde, C. B. (1990). Discordance between self-report and behavioral pain measures in children aged 3–7 years after surgery. *Journal of Pain and Symptom Management, 5*(6), 350–356.

Bonica, J. J. (1979). The need of a taxonomy. *Pain, 6*(3), 247–252.

Chambless, D. L., & Hollon, S. D. (1998). Defining empirically supported therapies. *Journal of Consulting and Clinical Psychology, 66,* 7–18.

Contet, C. S., Kieffer, B. L., & Befort, K. (2004). Mu opioid receptor: A gateway to drug addiction. *Current Opinion in Neurobiology, 14,* 1–9.

De Sousa, R. (1987). *The rationality of emotion.* Cambridge, MA: MIT Press.

Dworkin, R. H., O'Connor, A. B., Audette, J., Baron, R., Gourlay, G. K., Haanpää, M. L., ..., Wells, C. D. (2010, March). Recommendations for the pharmacological management of neuropathic pain: An overview and literature update. *Mayo Clinic Proceedings, 85*(3 Suppl), S3–S14.

Elkins, G. (2007). Hypnotherapy for the management of chronic pain. *International Journal of Clinical and Experimental Hypnosis, 55*(3), 275–287.

Esdaile, J. (1847). *Mesmerism in India, and its practical application in surgery and medicine.* Hartford, CT: Silas Andrus and Son.

Ewin, D. (1986). The effect of hypnosis and mind set on burns. *Psychiatric Annals, 16,* 115–118.

Flor, H., & Birbaumer, N. (1993). Comparison of the efficacy of cicctromyographic biofeedback, cognitive behavior therapy, and conservative medical treatment for chronic skeletal pain. *Journal of Consulting and Clinical Psychology, 61*(4), 653–658.

Gracely, R. H., & Wolskee, P. J. (1983). Semantic functional measurement of pain: Integrating perception and language. *Pain, 15*(4), 389–398.

Hetz, W., Kamp, H. D., Zimmermann, U., Von Bohlen, A., Wildt, L., & Schuettler, J. (1996). Stress hormones in accident patients studied before admission to hospital. *Journal of Accident and Emergency Medicine, 13*(4), 243–247.

Hilgard, E. R., & Hilgard, J. R. (1994). *Hypnosis in the relief of pain.* New York: Brunner/Mazel.

Houde, R. W. (1982). Methods for measuring clinical pain in humans. *Acta Anaesthesiologica Scandinavica, 74*(Suppl), 25–29.

IASP definition. (2009). Pain. Available at http://www.iasp-pain.org/AM/Template.cfm?Section=General_Resource_Links&Template=/CM/HTMLDisplay.cfm&ContentID=3058#

Jensen, M. P. (2009, December). Hypnosis for chronic pain management: A new hope. *Pain, 146*(3), 235–237. Epub 2009 July 10.

Kabat-Zinn, J. (1982). An outpatient program in behavioral medicine for chronic pain patients based on the practice of mindfulness meditation: Theoretical considerations and preliminary results. *General Hospital Psychiatry, 4*(1), 33–47.

Kabat-Zinn, J., Lipworth, L., & Burney, R. (1985). The clinical use of mindfulness meditation for the self-regulation of chronic pain. *Journal of Behavioral Medicine, 8*(2), 163–190.

Kroger, W. S. (1963). *Clinical and experimental hypnosis.* Philadelphia: Lippincott.

Kwekkeboom, K. L., Cherwin, C. H., Lee, J. W., & Wanta, B. (2010, January). Mind-body treatments for the pain-fatigue-sleep disturbance symptom cluster in persons with cancer. *Journal of Pain and Symptom Management, 39*(1), 126–138.

Lasagna, L. (1986). The management of pain. *Drugs, 32*(Suppl 4), 1–7.

Lichtenberg, P., Bachner-Melman, R., Gritsenko, I., & Ebstein, R. P. (2000). Exploratory association study between catechol-O-methyltransferase (COMT) high/low enzyme activity polymorphism and hypnotizability. *American Journal of Medical Genetics, 96,* 771–774.

Melzack, R. (2005, June). Evolution of the neuromatrix theory of pain. The Prithvi Raj Lecture. Presented at the Third World Congress of World Institute of Pain, 2004, Barcelona. *Pain Practice, 5*(2), 85–94.

McGlashan, T. H., Evans, F. J., & Orne, M. T. (1969). The nature of hypnotic analgesia and placebo response to experimental pain. *Psychosomatic Medicine, 31,* 227–246.

Miller, R. D. (1986). *Anesthesia* (2nd ed.). New York: Churchill Livingstone.

Montgomery, G. H., DuHamel, K. N., & Redd, W. H. (2000). A meta-analysis of hypnotically induced analgesia: How effective is hypnosis? *International Journal of Clinical and Experimental Hypnosis, 48,* 138–153.

Murphy, T. M. (1986). Treatment of chronic pain. In R. D. Miller (Ed.), *Anesthesia.* New York: Churchill Livingstone.

Patterson, D. R. (2010). *Clinical hypnosis for pain control.* Washington, DC: APA Books.

Patterson, D. R., & Jensen, M. P. (2003). Hypnosis and clinical pain. *Psychological Bulletin, 129,* 495–521.

Raz, A. (2005). Attention and hypnosis: neural substrates and genetic associations of two converging processes. *International Journal of Clinical and Experimental Hypnosis, 53,* 237–258.

Raz, A., Fan, J., & Posner, M. I. (2005, July 12). Hypnotic suggestion reduces conflict in the human brain. *Proceedings of the National Academy of Sciences of the United States of America, 102*(28), 9978–9983.

Rorty, A. (1980). *Explaining emotions.* Los Angeles, CA: University of California Press.

Schmader, K. E., Baron, R., Haanpää, M. L., Mayer, J., O'Connor, A. B., Rice, A. S., & Stacey, B. (2010, March).Treatment considerations for elderly and frail patients with neuropathic pain. *Mayo Clinic Proceedings, 85*(Suppl 3), S26–S32.

Spiegel, D., & Albert, L. (1983). Naloxone fails to reverse hypnotic alleviation of chronic pain. *Psychopharmacology, 81,* 140.

Spiegel, D., & King, R. (1992). Hypnotizability and CSF HVA levels among psychiatric patients. *Biological Psychiatry, 31,* 95–98.

Spiegel, D., Kraemer, H., & Carlson, R. (2001). Is the placebo powerless? *New England Journal of Medicine, 345,* 1276.

Sriwatanakul, K., Kelvie, W., & Lasagna, L. (1982). The quantification of pain: An analysis of words used to describe pain and analgesia in clinical trials. *Clinical Pharmacology and Therapeutics, 32*(2), 143–148.

Stallard, P., Williams, L., Velleman, R., Lenton, S., McGrath, P. J., & Taylor, G. (2002, July). The development and evaluation of the pain indicator for communicatively impaired children (PICIC). *Pain, 98*(1–2), 145–149.

Stoelb, B. L., Molton, I. R., Jensen, M. P., & Patterson, D. R. (2009, March 1). The efficacy of hypnotic analgesia in adults: A review of the literature. *Contemporary Hypnosis, 26*(1), 24–39.

Turk, D. C., Audette, J., Levy, R. M., Mackey, S. C., & Stanos, S. (2010, March). Assessment and treatment of psychosocial comorbidities in patients with neuropathic pain. *Mayo Clinic Proceedings, 85*(Suppl 3), S42–S50.

Wager, T. D., Scott, D. J., & Zubieta, J. K. (2007). Placebo effects on human (micro)-opioid activity during pain. *Proceedings of the National Academy of Sciences of the United States of America, 104,* 11056–11061.

Willmarth, E. K., Kevin, J., & Willmarth, K. J. (2005, Spring). Biofeedback and hypnosis in pain management. *Biofeedback, 33,* 1.

SUGGESTED READINGS

American College of Emergency Physicians. (1995). Pediatric equipment guidelines. *Annals of Emergency Medicine, 25,* 307–309.

American College of Emergency Physicians. (1997). Emergency care guidelines. *Annals of Emergency Medicine, 29,* 564–571.

Agency for Health Care Policy and Research (AHCPR). (1989). Acute Pain Management: Operative and Trauma, AHCPR Pub. No. 92-0032; for Clinicians–Acute Pain Management Procedures, AHCPR Pub. No. 92-0019; and in Infants, Children, and Adolescents Procedures, AHCPR Pub. No. 92-0020.

Bandura, A. (1963). *Social learning and personality development.* New York: Holt, Rinehart & Winston.

Benedetti, G. (1969, April). The unconscious from the neuropsychological viewpoint [Review]. *Der Nervenarzt, 40*(4), 149–155.

Biondi, M. (1984). I 4 canali del rapporto mente-corpo: dalla psicofisiologia dell'e-mozione alla psicosomatica scientifica. *Med Psic, 29,* 421–456.

Brugnoli, A. (2005). *Stati di coscienza modificati neurofisiologici.* Verona, Italy: La Grafica Editrice.

Burish, T. G., Carey, M. P., Redd, W. H., & Krozely, M. G. (1983, Summer). Behavioral relaxation techniques in reducing the distress of cancer chemothera-py patients. *Oncology Nursing Forum, 10*(3), 32–35.

Cunningham, R. S. (2006, August). Clinical practice guideline use by oncology advanced practice nurses. *Applied Nursing Research, 19*(3), 126–133.

Craig, K. D. (1992). The facial expression of pain: Better than a thousand words? *APS Journal, 1*(3), 153–162.

Dahlquist, L. M., Gil, K. M., Armstrong, F. D., Ginsberg, A., & Jones, B. (1985, December). Behavioral management of children's distress during chemotherapy. *Journal of Behavior Therapy and Experimental Psychiatry, 16*(4), 325–329.

Eccles, J. C. (1966, July14). The ionic mechanisms of excitatory and inhibitory synaptic action. *Annals of the New York Academy of Sciences, 137*(2), 473–494.

Erickson, M. H. (1978a). *La mia voce ti accompagnerà.* Rome, Italy: Casa Editrice Astrolabio.

Erickson, M. H. (1978b). *Le nuove vie dell'ipnosi.* Rome, Italy: Casa Editrice Astrolabio.

Erickson, M. H., Rossi, E. L., & Rossi, S. I. (1976). *Hypnotic realities: The induction of clinical hypnosis and forms of indirect suggestion.* New York: Irvington Publishers.

Erickson, M. H., & Rossi, E. L. (1976, January). Two level communication and the microdynamics of trance and suggestion. *American Journal of Clinical Hypnosis, 18*(3), 153–171.

Erickson, M. H., & Rossi, E. L. (1980). *The nature of hypnosis and suggestion* (Vol. 1). New York: Irvington Publishers.

Fourie, D. P. (1997, June). "Indirect" suggestion in hypnosis: Theoretical and exper-imental issues. *Psychological Reports, 80*(3, Pt 2), 1255–1266.

Guantieri, G. (1985). *II linguaggio del corpo in ipnosi.* Il Segno.

Held, J. P. (1961). Neurology. *Vie Med, 42*(13), 45–48.

Hernandez-Peon, R. & Hagbarth, K. E. (1955, January). Interaction between afferent and cortically induced reticular responses. *Journal of Neurophysiology, 18*(1), 44–55.

Jensen, M., & Patterson, D. R. (2006, February). Hypnotic treatment of chronic pain. *Journal of Behavioral Medicine, 29*(1), 95–124.

Kröner-Herwig, B. (2009, March). Chronic pain syndromes and their treatment by psychological interventions. *Current Opinion in Psychiatry, 22*(2), 200–204.

Liossi, C., & Hatira, P. (2003). Clinical hypnosis in the alleviation of procedure-relat-ed pain in pediatric oncology patients. *The International Journal of Clinical and Experimental Hypnosis, 51,* 4–28.

Matthes, H. W., Maldonado, R., Simonin, F., Valverde, O., Slowe, S., Kitchen, I., ..., Kiefer, B. L. (1996). Loss of morphine-induced analgesia, reward effect and with-drawal symptoms in mice lacking the mu-opioid-receptor gene. *Nature, 383*(6603), 819–823.

Matthews, W. J., & Langdell, S. (1989, April). What do clients think about the metaphors they receive? An initial inquiry. *American Journal of Clinical Hypnosis, 31*(4), 242–251.

McDonald, D. D., Laporta, M., & Meadows-Oliver, M. (2007, January). Nurses' response to pain communication from patients: A post-test experimental study. *International Journal of Nursing Studies, 44*(1), 29–35.

Merskey, H., & Bogduk, N. (1994). *Classification of chronic pain. Descriptions of chronic pain syndromes and definitions of pain terms* (2nd ed.). Seattle, WA: International Association for the Study of Pain Press.

Petter, G. (1989). *Dall'infanzia alla preadolescenza.* Barbera, Italy: Giunti.

Solomon, R. (1980). Emotions and choice. In A. Rorty (Ed.), *Explaining emotions* (pp. 251–281). Los Angeles, CA: University of California Press.

Stevens, A. L. (1950, June). Work evaluation in rehabilitation. *Occupational Therapy and Rehabilitation, 29*(3), 157–161.

Tan, G., Fukui, T., Jensen, M. P., Thornby, J., & Waldman, K. L. (2010, January). Hypnosis treatment for chronic low back pain. *International Journal of Clinical and Experimental Hypnosis, 58*(1), 53–68.

Taylor, S. E., Lichtman, R. R., & Wood, J. V. (1984, March). Attributions, beliefs about control, and adjustment to breast cancer. *Journal of Personality and Social Psychology, 46*(3), 489–502.

The Comprehensive Omnibus Budget Reconciliation Act of 1986, Emergency Medical Treatment and Active Labor Act. 42 USC §1395dd (1988 Suppl II 1990).

Traynor, J. R., & Elliott, J. (1993). Delta-opioid receptor subtypes and cross-talk with mu-receptors. *Trends in Pharmacological Sciences, 14*(3), 84–86.

Valente, S. M. (2006, February). Hypnosis for pain management. *Journal of Psychosocial Nursing and Mental Health Services, 44*(2), 22–30.

Vanhaudenhuyse, A., Boly, M., Balteau, E., Schnakers, C., Moonen, G., Luxen, A., ..., Faymonville, M. E. (2009, September). Pain and non-pain processing during hypnosis: A thulium-YAG event-related fMRI study. *NeuroImage, 47*(3), 1047–1054.

Chapter III

THE RELATIONSHIP BETWEEN CLINICAL HYPNOSIS AND MINDFULNESS: A NEW CLASSIFICATION OF MODIFIED STATES OF CONSCIOUSNESS

In neurophysiology, an altered state of consciousness, also called altered state of mind, is any condition that is significantly different from a normal waking beta wave state. The expression was used as early as 1966 by Arnold M. Ludwig and brought into common usage in 1969 by Charles Tart. It describes induced changes in one's mental state, almost always temporary.

The material in this chapter was originated from an intuition based on self-knowledge by my father, Dr. Angelico Brugnoli, M.D., born in Verona, Italy, in 1929. He was a pioneer in clinical hypnosis in Italy: in 1965, he founded, with some colleagues and friends, the Italian Institute for the Study of Psychotherapy and Clinical Hypnosis "H. Bernheim." I was very lucky to be one of their students and to have Angelico Brugnoli as father and master.

He has been studying the different modalities of modified states of consciousness for many years and I am very grateful to him for explaining his intuitions for a new approach and classification to me.

There are some states in which consciousness seems to be abolished, including sleep and coma. There are also a variety of circumstances that can change the relationship between the mind and the world, producing what are known as altered or modified states of consciousness, clinical hypnosis, mindfulness, and other meditative states. Some modified states occur naturally; others can be produced by drugs or brain damage. Altered states can be accompanied by changes in thinking, disturbances in the sense of time, feelings of loss of control, changes in emotional expression, alterations in body image, and changes in meaning or significance. The two most widely accepted modified states are sleep and dreaming. Although dream sleep and nondream sleep appear very similar to an outside observer, each is associated with a distinct pattern of brain activity, metabolic activity, and eye movement and also with a distinct pattern of experience and cognition. During ordinary nondream sleep, people who are awakened report only vague and sketchy thoughts, and their experiences do not cohere into a continuous narrative.

As explained in the first chapter, the author prefers to talk about modified states of consciousness and in this classification will describe only the physiological states of consciousness, obtained with hypnosis, meditative states, and mindfulness, and not the pathological states or those induced by drugs.

We can now begin to look at a conceptual framework that the author has been developing for several years about the nature of consciousness, and particularly about the nature of states and stages of consciousness.

Popular ideas about consciousness suggest the phenomenon describes a condition of being aware of one's awareness, or self-awareness. Efforts to describe consciousness in neurophysiological terms have focused on describing networks throughout the brain that develop awareness of the qualia, developed by other networks. This book also discusses a new methodological classification in research, from the neurophysiological point of view, of the different stages of consciousness.

Many people make distinctions among only a few states of consciousness because they experience just a few. Everyone, for example, probably distinguishes among ordinary waking state, dreaming, and dreamless sleep. Still others, who have personally experimented with modified states, may want to distinguish between meditative and hypnosis-induced states. Consciousness is not just a bunch of different levels; it is a group of different states, of which the best worked out are those involving wakefulness, the different stages of sleep, and the different stages of concentration.

INTRODUCTION: THE MODIFIED
STATES OF CONSCIOUSNESS

The physiological mechanisms that underlie consciousness and unconsciousness, are the sleep/wake mechanisms. Sleep is a state of physiological reversible unconsciousness. The change from that state to awake state is mediated by the reticular activating mechanism.

In 1929, the German psychiatrist Hans Berger discovered that the electrical activity within the brain could be recorded as brain waves and that these waves changed as awake gave way to sleep. This discovery of the electroencephalogram (EEG), as it is now known, made the objective study of sleep possible. Loomis provided the earliest detailed description of various stages of sleep in the mid-1930s, and in the early 1950s, Aserinsky and Kleitman identified rapid eye movement: the REM sleep.

Sleep is generally divided into two broad types: nonrapid eye movement (NREM) sleep and REM sleep two. Based on EEG changes, NREM is divided further into four stages (stage I, stage II, stage III, stage IV). NREM and REM occur in alternating cycles, each lasting approximately 90 to 100 minutes, with a total of four to six cycles.

By detecting synchronous activity of cortical neurons and recording voltage fluctuations in terms of the amplitude of the resulting waves and their frequency, the EEG is thus used to differentiate the neurophysiological changes in alertness and sleep stages. For the analysis of the stages of sleep and awake state, EEG frequencies are conveniently grouped into bands:

- *Delta: 0.5 to 4 Hz.* Delta is the frequency range up to 4 Hz. It tends to be the highest in amplitude and the slowest waves. It is seen normally in adults in slow wave sleep.
- *Theta: 4 to 8 Hz.* Theta is the frequency range from 4 Hz to 8 Hz regardless of their sources. Cortical theta is seen normally in young children. It may be seen in drowsy, meditative, or sleeping states or in arousal in older children and adults but not during the deepest stages of sleep. Cortical theta rhythms, observed in human scalp EEG, are a different phenomenon, with no clear relationship to the hippocampus.

Theta frequency EEG activity is also manifested during some short term memory tasks (Vertes, 2004). Studies suggest that they reflect the "online" state of the hippocampus, one of readiness to process incoming signals (Buzsáki, 2002). Conversely, theta oscillations have been correlated to various voluntary behaviors (exploration, spatial navigation, etc.) and alert states (piloerection, etc.) in rats (Vanderwolf, 1969), suggesting that it may reflect the integration of sensory information with motor output (Bland & Oddie, 2001). A large body of evidence indicates that theta rhythm is likely involved in spatial learning and navigation (Buzsáki, 2005).

- *Alpha: 8 to 12 Hz.* Alpha is the frequency range from 8 Hz to 12 Hz. Hans Berger named the first rhythmic EEG activity he saw the "alpha wave." It is brought out by closing the eyes and by relaxation. It was noted to attenuate with eye opening or mental exertion.
- *Sigma: 12 to 14 Hz.* Sleep spindles (sometimes referred to as "sigma bands" or "sigma waves") may represent periods when the brain is inhibiting processing to keep the sleeper in a tranquil state.

- *Beta: 14 to 30 Hz.* Beta is the frequency range from 14 Hz to about 30 Hz. It is seen usually on both sides in symmetrical distribution and is most evident frontally. Low amplitude beta with multiple and varying frequencies is often associated with active, busy, or anxious thinking and active concentration.
- *Gamma: 30 to 50 Hz.* Gamma is the frequency range approximately 26 to 100 Hz. Gamma rhythms are thought to represent binding of different populations of neurons together into a network for the purpose of carrying out a certain cognitive or motor function.

EEG data are combined with those from concurrent recording of eye movements, from the electro-oculogram (EOG), and muscle tone from the electromyogram (EMG) to define the states of sleep and wakefulness. In contrast to wakefulness (beta and gamma waves), sleep is characterized by higher voltages and slower waves, a pattern called synchronized EEG. NREM sleep is the usual term for this state. In humans, NREM sleep is further subdivided into four Stages I through IV, which depend on the extent of EEG slowing, especially in the delta frequency range. Stage II is notable for the presence of spindles, which are waxing and waning bursts of frequencies, in the sigma band. Stages III and IV, with delta waves providing more than 50 percent of the signal, are further grouped under the term slow wave sleep (SWS).

During this state, the EOG can show gradual rolling eye movements, and there is low or minimal muscle activity. Slow sleep is interrupted by periods of REM (i.e., active or paradoxical) sleep, when, despite all the overt signs of continuing sleep, the activity of the brain is remarkably different. In fact, the EEG in humans during REM sleep is essentially identical to that recorded during wakefulness, but the EOG reveals rapid bursts of eye movements, hence the name of the state. Importantly, and in all species, the EMG shows the complete loss of muscle tone (i.e., atonia) that is a characteristic of REM sleep. The reverse change, from wakefulness to sleep, is also an active process effected by an arousal inhibitory mechanism based on a partial blockade of the thalamus and upper brainstem associated with thalamic sleep spindles and also with cortical subdelta activity (<1 Hz). The deactivation of the thalamus, has been demonstrated both electrically and by positron emission tomography (PET) during deep sleep (Evans, 2003). The structure of sleep across the night, as expressed by the hypnogram, is characterized by repeated transitions between the different states of vigilance: awake, light, and deep NREM sleep and REM sleep.

Normally, awake state or wakefulness is associated with instant awareness (defined as the ability to integrate all sensory information, from the external environment and the internal environment of the body). Awareness may be a function of the thalamocortical network in the cerebral hemispheres that forms the final path, of the sleep/wake mechanism. Anatomical and physiological studies suggest that there may be a double thalamocortical network being one relating to cortical and thalamic areas, with specific functions, and the other being global, involving all cortical areas and so-called nonspecific thalamic nuclei. The global system might function as a cortical integrating mechanism, permitting the spread of information between the specific cortical areas and thus underlying awareness. The global system may also be responsible for much of the spontaneous and evoked electrical activity of the brain. The cognitive change between sleep and wakefulness is accompanied by changes in the autonomic system, the cerebral blood flow, and the cerebral metabolism.

Awareness is an essential component of total consciousness (defined as continuous awareness of the external and internal environment, both past and present, together with the emotions arising from it). In addition to awareness, full consciousness requires short-term and explicit memory and intact emotional responses (Evans, 2003). At the cellular level, it has been proposed that, under the influence of circadian and homeostatic factors, transitions between wake and sleep may be determined by mutually inhibitory interaction between sleep-active neurons, in the hypothalamic preoptic area and wake-active neurons in multiple arousal centres. These two fundamentally different behavioral states are separated by the sleep onset and the sleep inertia periods, each characterized by gradual changes in which neither true wake nor true sleep patterns are present (Merica & Fortune, 2004).

The process of automatic sleep stage scoring consists of two major parts: feature extraction and classification. Features are normally extracted from the polysomnographic recordings, mainly EEG signals. The EEG is considered a nonstationary signal, which increases the complexity of the detection of different waves in it. Your brain waves move fast when you are awake. These are known as "beta" waves. When you lie down, close your eyes, and become drowsy, your brain wave tend to start slowing down; this is known as the "alpha" state. Five minutes into the alpha state, your body slips into the Stage I sleep.

The Stages of Sleep

Stage I

Stage I sleep is also referred to as drowsiness or presleep and is the first or earliest stage of sleep. The earliest indication of transition from wakefulness to stage I sleep (drowsiness) usually consists of a combination of (1) drop out of alpha activity and (2) slow rolling eye movements. Stage I is light sleep. You experience a drifting in and out of sleep. You can be easily awakened. Your eye movement and body movements slow down. You may experience sudden jerky movement of your legs or other muscles. These are known as hypnic myoclonia or myoclonic jerks. These "sleep starts" can give a sensation of falling. They are caused by the motor areas of the brain being spontaneously stimulated.

Stage II

Stage II is the predominant sleep stage, during a normal night's sleep. The distinct and principal EEG criterion to establish stage II sleep is the appearance of sleep spindles. The presence of sleep spindles is necessary and sufficient to define stage II sleep. Another characteristic finding of stage II sleep is the appearance of K complexes, but because K complexes are typically associated with a spindle, spindles are the defining features of stage II sleep. Except for slow rolling eye movements, all patterns described under stage I persist in stage II sleep.

Around 50 percent of your time sleeping is spent in stage II sleep. During this stage, eye movement stops, and your brain waves (a measure of the activity level of the brain) become slower. There will also be brief bursts of rapid brain activity, called sleep spindles. The criteria of stage II sleep–spindles and K complexes–are usually easy to identify and are less subject to over interpretation or misinterpretation than are the patterns of stage I sleep. Sleep spindles have a frequency of 12 to 16 Hz (typically 14 Hz).

Stage III

Stages III and IV of sleep are usually grouped together as "slow wave sleep" or "delta sleep." Stage III is the first stage of deep sleep. The brain waves are a combination of slow waves and faster waves. During stage III sleep, it can be very difficult to wake someone up. If you are woken up during this stage, you may feel groggy and disoriented for several minutes.

Stage IV

Stage IV sleep is the second stage of deep sleep. In this stage, the brain is making the slow delta waves almost exclusively. The distinction between stage III and stage IV sleep is only quantitative and has to do with the amount of delta activity. Stage III is defined by delta activity that occupies 20 to 50 percent of the time, whereas in stage IV, delta activity represents greater than 50 percent of the time. In this stage, it is also very difficult to wake someone up. Both stages of deep sleep are important for feeling refreshed in the morning. If these stages are too short, sleep will not feel satisfying.

The REM Stage of Sleep

REM sleep is defined by (1) rapid eye movements, (2) muscle atonia, and (3) EEG desynchronization (compared to slow wave sleep).

REM sleep normally is not seen on routine EEGs because the normal latency to REM sleep (100 minutes), is well beyond the duration of routine EEG recordings (approximately 20–30 minutes).

Sleep typically and predictably proceeds from one stage to the next (Carskadon & Dement, 2005). As sleep progresses, a stepwise descent from wakefulness to stage I, through to stage IV, sleep occurs, followed by an abrupt ascent back through a stage II, like an EEG with spindles towards stage I with irregular theta activity. At stage I, however, the first REM sleep episode usually occurs, about 70 to 90 minutes after sleep onset in the human. Following the first REM sleep episode, the sleep cycle repeats, with the appearance of NREM sleep. Then, about 90 minutes after the start of the first REM sleep period, another episode occurs. This rhythmic cycling persists throughout the night. Hence the sleep cycle duration is about 90 minutes in humans, and, on average, REM sleep episodes last for about 20 minutes, gradually increasing in duration throughout the night. Over the course of the night, delta wave activity declines, and as sleep progresses, the EEG of NREM sleep is comprised increasingly of waves of higher frequencies and lower amplitude.

These descriptions of the physiological basis for consciousness and sleep stages constitute an important first step toward the integration of behavioral and neurophysiological evidence and theory of modified states of consciousness and the relationship among sleep, hypnosis, and meditative states.

All the electrical changes in our brain are in practice electrochemical. That is, complex chemical changes underlie the electrical correlates of attention. To take just one instance, the passage of electrical signals from nerve cell to nerve cell depends on a range of neurotransmitter substances. Each of the neural systems already discussed depends on the action of one, or sometimes combinations, of these neurochemicals. One transmitter substance, noradrenaline, is particularly prominent in alerting processes, along with its close relative transmitter substance dopamine. The total amount of another transmitter substance, acetylcholine, in the brain, is found to be inversely related to the level of CNS activity.

Neurophysiology of Concentration and Attention

Neural systems regulate attention to activate consciousness, concentration, and awareness. The author calls this framework for studying consciousness a new systems approach because she takes the position that consciousness, as we know it, is not a group of isolated psychological functions but a system—an interacting, dynamic configuration of neurophysiological and neuropsychological components—that performs various functions in greatly changing environments. Knowledge about the nature of the components is useful, but to understand any system fully, we must also consider the environments with which it deals and the goals of its functioning. So in trying to understand human consciousness, we must get the feel of the whole system as it operates in its world, not just study isolated parts of it.

In this book, we will not examine pathological modified states of consciousness, such as coma states or states of modified consciousness through drugs or medicines. A wide variety of unusual experiences in different states of consciousness, of changes in time, emotion, memory, sense of identity, cognitive processes and feelings will be studied.

Our ordinary state of consciousness is not something natural or given but a highly complex construction. As we look at consciousness closely, we see that it can be analyzed into many parts. These parts function together in a pattern, however. They form a system (Tart, 1972). The term states of consciousness has come to be used too loosely to mean whatever is on one's mind at the moment.

To understand the constructed system we call a state of consciousness, we begin with some theoretical postulates based on human and neurophysiological experience.

One postulate is the existence of a basic awareness. Because some volitional control over the focus of awareness is possible, we generally refer to it as attention/awareness. We must also recognize the existence of self-awareness, the awareness of being aware.

In recent years, there has been significant neurophysiological uptake of meditation and related relaxation techniques as a means of alleviating stress and maintaining good health. Despite its popularity, little is known about the neural mechanisms by which meditation works, and there is a need for more rigorous investigations of the underlying neurobiology. Several EEG studies have reported changes in spectral band frequencies during hypnosis and meditation inspired by techniques that focus on concentration.

In 2009, Lagopoulos and colleagues examined EEG changes during nondirective (concentrative) meditation. The investigational paradigm involved 20 minutes of acme meditation, during which the subjects were asked to close their eyes and adopt their normal meditation technique, as well as a separate 20-minute quiet rest condition during which the subjects were asked to close their eyes and sit quietly in a state of rest. Both conditions were completed in the same experimental session with a 15-minute break in between. Significantly increased theta wave power was found for the meditation condition, when averaged across all brain regions. On closer examination, it was found that theta was considerably greater in the frontal and temporal central regions, as compared with the posterior region. There was also a significant increase in alpha power under the meditation condition compared with the rest condition, when averaged across all brain regions, and it was found that alpha was considerably greater in the posterior region, as compared to the frontal region (Lagopoulos et al., 2009). These findings from this study suggest that nondirective meditation techniques alter theta and alpha EEG patterns significantly more than regular relaxation in a manner that is perhaps similar to methods based on mindfulness or concentration.

Gentle and medium self-hypnosis is a natural state of mind we go into everyday. Getting caught up in a good book or movie or studying for an exam and losing track of time are simple examples of being in the hypnosis state. A person doing positive statements or, for that matter, visualizing a scene or desired outcome is using a form of self-hypnosis.

To go into hypnosis and enter the subconscious mind, you must bypass the critical factor of the conscious mind, the thought stream. This can be done quickly, easily, and effectively. One does not need to be relaxed to go into a trance; relaxation is a by-product of having been in hypnosis. Why? Because you have relaxed the body and mind together, which allows the nervous system to flush out all the pent-up stress and tension. When the mind relaxes, it can let go. Why is hypnosis the same as meditation?

Meditation describes a state of concentrated attention to some object of thought or awareness. It usually involves turning the attention inward to the mind itself. The neurophysiological shifts, the same EEG patterns, the bodily tranquility, the pleasures of mental freedom are all part of all the modified stages of consciousness.

There are many different states of hypnosis and meditation and there are many neurophysiological correlations. The definition of true meditation is the absence of all thought and to just be. If a person is mulling over a problem during meditation, he or she is, in reality, now contemplating the situation and is no longer considered to be doing meditation. These techniques can be used, as clinical hypnosis is, for stress and pain management. With the activation of spiritual consciousness in people who are dying, they are excellent ways to reduce suffering.

The contraindications for the use of relaxation, hypnosis, and meditative stages are the same general cautions that apply to the use of other fantasy or imagery tools. The use of this way may be ill-advised with patients who have difficulty distinguishing between fact and fantasy. Patients with a dissociative history, such as in dissociative identity disorder, may find the experiences too threatening or disorienting because of the tendency for altered states to weaken or lower the protective barriers of dissociative amnesia.

The similarities and differences between hypnosis and meditation, are used to shed light on perennial questions:

1. Does hypnosis involve an altered state of consciousness?
2. Does a hypnotic induction increase awareness?

A model for hypnosis should include altered states as well as capacity for imaginative involvement and expectations. Hypnosis is a great way to enhance meditation and awareness. You can use the scientific approach of hypnosis to enter your subconscious mind. Once in a trance, you can release the old thinking patterns. Once you have done that and your mind is clear, you can move into a quiet state of meditation and awareness. You have re-connected with yourself as a spirit.

That is the meditative state. Relaxation, hypnosis, self-hypnosis, and mindfulness are the doors to get there. Clinical hypnosis, consciousness, and mindfulness through meditative states are already part of psychological and spiritual care in chronic diseases.

In everyday life, as each of us lives in our "normal" state of consciousness, our awareness is usually focused on the particular thoughts, emotions, or perceptions we experience at the surface level of reality. They are the experiences and perceptions we move through in our life in the outer world or the thoughts and feelings that we have in our inner world. As we move through life, we perceive, think, act, and feel with the assistance of our "thinking mind," the active portion of our mind, that deals with this surface level of reality through the use of thoughts, feelings, interpretations of perceptions, and actions. Our awareness is usually identified with, preoccupied with, and attached to whichever of these specific activities we engage in through the use of this thinking mind. Although all these particular components of our life are important, when we remain identified with, and therefore, limited to, these surface activities and these surface appearances of our deeper being, we are far less able to perceive and act from a more fundamental level of greater awareness. The tendency of our thinking mind to remain preoccupied with the particulars of life inhibits our ability to move beyond the level of pure consciousness that is actually the source of all these particular states of mind.

In the practice of deep hypnosis and meditation, we seek to free ourselves from this mental chatter in which our thinking mind engages and instead seek connection to the higher level of our being. Meditation is a process by which we seek to recondition our conscious awareness so that we release our attachment to the surface level of reality and instead allow the awareness to gravitate toward a state of pure awareness, pure consciousness. Mindfulness is the meditative state that we can reach in many different religions and prayers.

In the learning and practice of meditation, mindfulness, and self-hypnosis, we can develop some inner sense of self-awareness, a pure awareness beyond habitual identifications with the thoughts, feelings, and perceptions at the surface level of the mind. It is an instantaneous reversal in the focus of awareness, and there is often a sense of elation or euphoria at this point where the inward awareness expands. This point is not a point in time or space, but it is the pure state of being. It is subtle, yet discernible with practice. This precise point of change in awareness, is called the point of pure being.

The purpose of hypnosis and self-hypnosis, meditation and mindfulness in pain therapy and palliative care is to awaken in us the skylike nature of mind and to introduce us to that which we really are, our unchanging pure awareness, which underlies the whole of life and death. Clinical hypnosis, meditation, and prayers are intensely personal and spiritual experiences. The desired purpose of each meditation technique is to channel our awareness into a more positive direction by totally transforming one's state of mind. In the stillness and silence of meditation, we glimpse and return to that deep inner nature that we have so long ago lost sight of amid the busyness and distraction of our minds.

We do not know who we really are or what aspects of ourselves we should identify with, or believe in. So many contradictory voices, dictates, and feelings fight for control over our inner lives that we find ourselves scattered everywhere, in all directions, leaving nobody at home (Rinpoche, 2002).

> When you abandon every desire that rises up within you, and when you become content with things as they are, then you experience inner peace. When your mind is untroubled by misfortune, when you desire no pleasures, when your emotions are tranquil, and when you are free from fear and anger, then you experience inner calm.

When you are free from all attachments, when you are indifferent towards success and failure, then you experience inner serenity.

When you can withdraw your senses from pleasures of the senses, just as a tortoise withdraws its limbs, then you experience inner wisdom.

When no pleasure and no desire can touch the soul, then you experience the highest state of consciousness. (Bhagavad-Gita, 2.55–61)

Different stages of consciousness can be experimented with through hypnosis and meditative stages, which must be done through psychophysical states of concentration.

Let us now look at the basic elements of this new systems approach, the basic postulates, about what lies behind the phenomenal manifestations of experience. The slow path toward the states of consciousness, will not only cure our pain and suffering but will also benefit us in knowing ourselves, our higher consciousness and our internal personal world and of all the hidden qualities that every person has within their rational and intuitive mind.

There are many types of mental concentration and consciousness, states linked to hypnosis and meditative states, and there are many different relationships among meditative states, mindfulness, relaxation, self-hypnosis, and hypnosis. When our mind is focused, our energies are not dissipated on irrelevant activities or thoughts. This is why developing concentration is essential to anyone who aspires to take charge of his or her life. Concentration has been defined as "the ability to direct one's thinking in whatever direction one would intend." We all have the ability to concentrate some of the time. At other times, however, our thoughts are scattered, and our minds race from one thing to another. To deal with such times, we need to learn and practice concentration skills and strategies. To concentrate, we have to learn a skill, and as with any skill this means practice, repeated day after day, until we achieve enough improvement to feel that we can concentrate when we need to. Our ability to concentrate depends on

- commitment
- enthusiasm for the task
- skill at doing the task
- our emotional and physical state
- our psychological state
- our environment

This power can be described as focused attention. It is the ability to direct the attention to one single thought or subject, to the exclusion of everything else.

Attention is one of the most intensely studied topics within psychology and cognitive neuroscience. In his textbook *Principles of Psychology,* William James remarked, "Everyone knows what attention is. It is the taking possession by the mind, in clear and vivid form, of one out of what seem several simultaneously possible objects or trains of thought. Focalization, concentration, of consciousness are of its essence" (1890).

While breathing, we do not need to pay attention to each inhalation and exhalation. We become conscious about the process of breathing only when we have some difficulty with breathing, such as when our nose is clogged because of a cold, or when we are in an unventilated room. It is the same with thinking. We become conscious of the constant onslaught of our thoughts and of our inability to calm them down only when we need to concentrate, solve a problem, or study. We are also acutely aware of them when we have worries or fears. Concentration is exclusively to focus on, to give one's attention to, the task at hand by habitually bringing one's digressed attention back to quicker focus than that of attention and to focus that attention more accurately. Concentration or concentrating is also being able to refocus attention if and when one is much distracted or immediately after any rest. The strength of the ability to concentrate or focus of attention for concentration is by mental conditioning. Concentration, attention, focus, involve the thought. The thought outwardly directs itself creatively when uncontrolled.

Focus and refocus and attention and concentration, however, are aided by a network of nerve fibers within the brainstem. Because this reticular activating system dispatches signals to other parts of the brain, the brain is capable of being stimulated for attention, also by conscious attitude. Attention is a very basic function that often is a precursor to all other neurological and cognitive functions. As is frequently the case, clinical models of attention differ from investigation models. One of the most used models for the evaluation of attention in patients with very different neurological pathologies is the model of Sohlberg and Mateer (1989). This hierarchic model is based on the recovering of attention processes of brain-damaged patients after coma. Five different kinds of activities of growing difficulty are described as the model, connecting with the activities that patients could do as their recovering process advanced.

Attention is part of focus, concentration, a component of intelligence. Attention, the focus of attention, only lasts a few seconds and is the act or process of focusing on one or more particulars in the content of one's consciousness to give special clearance to the essentials by restricting one's sensory input, from the environment's unwanted aspects. Attention is never entire; it digresses but can be refocused at will.

Concentration and attention are subject to will. When one is trying to concentrate—paying attention—waves of electricity called alpha rhythms are given by one's brain at a frequency of 8 to 12 Hz on an EEG. Practice helps improve attention.

Attention is best described as the sustained focus of cognitive resources on information while filtering or ignoring extraneous information.

FOCUSED ATTENTION. This is the ability to respond discretely to specific visual, auditory, or tactile stimuli.

Sustained Attention. This refers to the ability to maintain a consistent behavioral response during continuous and repetitive activity.

SELECTIVE ATTENTION. This level of attention refers to the capacity to maintain a behavioral or cognitive set in the face of distracting or competing stimuli. Therefore, it incorporates the notion of freedom from distractibility"

ALTERNATING ATTENTION. It refers to the capacity for mental flexibility that allows individuals to shift their focus of attention and move between tasks having different cognitive requirements.

DIVIDED ATTENTION. This is the highest level of attention, and it refers to the ability to respond simultaneously to multiple tasks or multiple task demands.

This model has been shown to be very useful in evaluating attention in very different pathologies, correlates strongly with daily difficulties and is especially helpful in designing stimulation programs such as attention process training, a rehabilitation program for neurological patients, of the same authors (Solberg & Mateer, 1989).

The external manifestations of attention are accompanied by physiological changes, particularly within the brain and nervous system. These physiological changes can be studied by examining responses to novel stimuli. Growing out of Pavlov's research, the orienting response to novel stimuli has come to be characterized by a broad complex of physiological changes. These include changes in heart rate, in the electrical conductivity of the skin, in the size of the pupils in the eyes, in the pattern of respiration, and in the level of tension in the muscles. If the novel signal is an interesting one, the heart transiently slows down; if it is startling, the heart transiently speeds up. Most of the other types of change reflect similar reactions. Thus, the startling signal increases the level of skin conductance and the size of the pupils, causes respiration to pause or briefly become irregular, and increases tension in certain muscles.

Sensory inputs travel through the brain via primary sensory pathways that converge on a central relay structure, the thalamus, from which they are sent to relatively specific and localized receiving areas in the higher (cortical) levels within the brain. On their way from the sensory receptors to the thalamus, the signals pass an area of the brainstem and midbrain to which the sensory pathways have lateral connections. This area, called the reticular formation, is important in changing the overall level of arousal. When it is damaged, the individual may be unarousable. It has interconnections with the higher brain centers, and it projects pathways to the cerebral cortex. Unlike the primary sensory projections, which are limited to specific sensory modalities, many of the reticular formation cells respond to signals from any of the sensory modalities. When this ascending reticular activating system is operating, the individual is alert, aroused, and attentive.

The reticular system seems to account physiologically for the sustained, tonic shifts in an individual's level of involvement with the environment, including the control of sleep wakefulness. One nonspecific route to the cerebral cortex via the thalamus–the diffuse thalamic projection system–appears to be concerned with moment to moment fluctuations in the focus of attention. Collectively, the primary sensory pathways associated areas of the cerebral cortex, and the more diffuse projection systems, cooperate in the process of registering the incoming sensory signal, evaluating its contents, and mobilizing brain resources in response to the demands made.

Inevitably, this account is an oversimplification. In the human brain, other structures, particularly the hypothalamus, are involved in regulating states of sleep and wakefulness; limbic structures, such as the hippocampus, take part in arousal when rewards, punishments, or other emotional factors are involved.

In many cases, attention produces changes in the EEG. Many animals, including humans, produce gamma waves (40–60 Hz) when focusing attention on a particular object or activity (Kaiser & Lutzenberger, 2003). Most experiments show that one neural correlate of attention is enhanced firing. If a neuron has a certain response to a stimulus, when the animal is not attending to the stimulus, then when the animal does attend to the stimulus, the neuron's response will be enhanced, even if the physical characteristics of the stimulus remain the same.

In a recent review, Knudsen (2007) describes a more general model tat identifies some core processes of attention, with working memory at the center:

- *Working memory* temporarily stores information for detailed analysis.
- *Competitive selection* is the process that determines which information gains access to working memory.

- *Through top-down sensitivity control,* the higher cognitive processes can regulate signal intensity in information channels that compete for access to working memory, and thus give them an advantage in the process of competitive selection. Through top-down sensitivity control, the momentary content of working memory can influence the selection of new information and thus mediate voluntary control of attention in a recurrent loop: the endogenous attention (Pattyn, Neyt, Henderickx & Soetens, E., 2008).
- *Bottom-up saliency filters* automatically enhance the response to infrequent stimuli or stimuli of instinctive or learned biological relevance: the exogenous attention (Pattyn et al., 2008).

Working memory is a theoretical construct, within cognitive psychology as to the structures and processes used for temporarily storing and manipulating information in short-term memory. Many theories exist both as to the theoretical structure of working memory and as to the role of specific parts of the brain involved in working memory. Most research identifies that the frontal cortex, parietal cortex, anterior cingulate, and parts of the basal ganglia are crucial for its functioning. The neural basis of working memory mostly comes from lesion experiments in animals and functional imaging in humans.

The term "working memory" was coined by Miller, Galanter, and Pribram and was used in the 1960s in the context of theories that likened the mind to a computer. Atkinson and Shiffrin (1968) also used this term, working memory to describe their short-term store. What we now call working memory has been referred to as a "short-term store," primary memory, immediate memory, operant memory, or provisional memory (Fuster, 1997). The short-term memory is the ability to remember information over a brief period of time (in the order of seconds). Most theorists today use the concept of working memory to replace or include the older concept of short-term memory, thereby marking a stronger emphasis on the notion of manipulation of information instead of passive maintenance.

Baddeley and Hitch (1974) introduced and made popular the multicomponent model of working memory. Baddeley (2003) extended the model by adding a fourth component—the episodic buffer—that holds representations that integrate phonological, visual, and spatial information and possibly information not covered by the slave systems (e.g., semantic information, musical information).

Localization of brain functions in humans has become much easier with the advent of brain imaging methods (PET and fMRI). This research has confirmed that areas in the prefrontal cortex are involved in working memory functions. During the 1990s, much debate centered on the different functions of the ventrolateral (i.e., lower) and the dorsolateral (higher) areas of the prefrontal cortex. One view was that the dorsolateral areas are responsible for spatial working memory and the ventrolateral areas for nonspatial working memory. Another view proposed a functional distinction, arguing that ventrolateral areas are mostly involved in pure maintenance of information, whereas dorsolateral areas are more involved in tasks, requiring some processing of the memorized material. The debate is not entirely resolved, but most of the evidence supports the functional distinction (Owen, 1997).

Research suggests a close link, between the working memory capacities of a person and his or her ability to control the information from the environment, which he or she can selectively enhance or ignore (Fukuda & Vogel, 2009). Such attention allows, for example, for the voluntary shifting in regard to the goals of a person's information, processing to spatial locations or objects, rather than to those that capture their attention due to their sensory saliency (such as an ambulance siren). The goal directing of attention is driven by top-down signals from the prefrontal cortex that bias processing in posterior cortical areas (Desimone & Duncan, 1995) and saliency capture by bottom-up control from subcortical structures and the primary sensory cortices (Yantis & Jonides, 1990).

The ability to override sensory capture of attention differs greatly among individuals, and this difference closely links to their working memory capacity. The greater a person's working memory capacity, the greater his or her ability to resist sensory capture (Fukuda & Vogel, 2009). Concentration means holding the mind to one form or object steadily for a long time. When our mind is focused, our energies are not dissipated on irrelevant activities or thoughts. This is why developing concentration is essential to anyone who aspires to take charge of his or her life. This skill is essential for every kind of wellbeing. Without it, our efforts get scattered, but with it, we can accomplish great things.

Concentration has many uses and benefits. It assists in studying and understanding faster; improves the memory; and helps in focusing on any task, job, activity, or goal and achieving it more easily and efficiently. It is also required for developing psychic abilities, and it is a powerful tool for the efficient use of creative visualization. When this ability is developed, the mind obeys us more readily and does not engage in futile, negative thoughts or worries. We gain mental mastery, and we experience true peace of mind.

Concentration, attention, and working memory play a very great part in the different states of consciousness. They are the basis of will. When they are properly guided and directed toward the internal world for purposes of introspection, they will analyze the mind and illumine very many astounding facts for your awareness.

The force with which anything strikes the mind is generally in proportion to the degree of attention bestowed upon it. Moreover, the great art of awareness is concentration. Concentration is focusing of external consciousness and inner consciousness. It is one of the signs of trained will. It is found in people of strong mentality. It is a rare faculty. Attention and concentration can be cultivated and developed by persistent practice. All the great people of the world who have achieved greatness have risen up through this faculty.

It is through the power of attention and concentration that our mind carries out all its activities. Concentration may be either subjective and internal or objective and external on any object. Throw your entire concentration into whatever you happen to be doing at the moment. It is easy to fasten the mind on an object that the mind likes best.

Concentration also plays an important role in meditation. Without it, the mind just jumps restlessly from one thought to another, not allowing us to meditate properly.

Concentration can be fun if approached in the right way. It should be practiced with joy, fun, optimism, and understanding of its great possibilities. It has to be approached in a positive manner and then success dawns.

Thought is a dynamic force. Thought moves. Thought creates. The mind is intimately connected with the body. The mind acts upon the body, and the body reacts upon the mind. Mind has influence over the body. A pure, healthy mind means a healthy body. Grief in the mind weakens the body. The body influences the mind also in its turn. If the body is strong and healthy, the mind also becomes strong and healthy. If the body is sick, the mind also becomes sick.

Sometimes you can find strong powers of concentration in yourself. To do so, you need to practice special exercises on a daily basis. Here is what you can gain by developing the concentration's power:

- The ability to focus your mind
- Peace of mind
- Freedom from futile thoughts
- Better memory
- Better attention
- Better consciousness
- Better awareness
- Self-confidence
- Better knowledge of Inner self
- The ability to study and comprehend more quickly
- Inner happiness

- Enhanced capability to develop psychic abilities
- Enhanced capability to develop spiritual abilities
- More powerful and efficient use of creative work
- Enhanced ability to meditate
- Pain and suffering relief
- Awareness.

When the mental rays are concentrated on the mind's illumination, the consciousness and higher self begin. Be introspective and watch the mind carefully.

We can divide the many different states of consciousness, in the distinct modalities of mind's concentration so it is easier to understand the neuro-physiological and psychological correlation between them. Concentration seems in some way, to be at the very core of mental activity. Training the mind in the variety of ways concentration is the beginning.

INTRODUCTION: THE MODIFIED STATES OF CONSCIOUSNESS

1. ACTIVE CONCENTRATION: TYPES AND TECHNIQUES
   A. Awake state, wakefulness
   B. Relaxed awakening
   C. Progressive relaxation
   D. Light sleep (consciousness and the stages of sleep)
   E. Repetitive vocal and mental prayer
   F. The exercises and physical postures of Yoga
2. PASSIVE CONCENTRATION: TYPES AND TECHNIQUES
   A. Autogenic Training of Schultz
   B. Light hypnosis, medium hypnosis, and self-hypnosis
   C. Lucid dreams, hypnagogic and hypnopompic states
   D. The REM phase of sleep
   E. Free mental prayer and mental meditation
   F. The breathing exercises
3. DEEP CONCENTRATION: TYPES AND TECHNIQUES
   A. Deep sleep
   B. Extreme thoughts: the 'flow state'
   C. Medium self hypnosis
   D. Deep hypnosis
   E. Meditative stages of contemplation and Mindfulness

4. SUPERIOR CONCENTRATION (HIGHER CONSCIOUSNESS):
TYPES AND TECHNIQUES
   A. Medium to deep self-hypnosis: Annulment of the normal consciousness;
   A. The Higher Consciousness
   B. Absorption
   C. Meditative stages: awareness, contemplation and ecstasy, living with God
5. TRUE CONCENTRATION OR AWARENESS ACTIVATION:
TYPES AND TECHNIQUES
   A. Deep self hypnosis
   B. Contemplation and mystical states leading to Spiritual Enlightenment: Samadhi, living in God

THE STAGES OF CONSCIOUSNESS

Concentration Stages	Stages of Relaxation and Hypnosis	Meditative Stages in Christianity	Meditative Stages in Buddhism (The Noble Eightfold Path)	Meditative Stages in Hindu Religion (The Yoga Saltras of Patanjali)
1. Active Concentration	• wakefulness • relaxed awakening • progressive relaxation • light sleep	repetitive vocal and mental prayer	Sila. It includes • vāc (vāca): speaking in a truthful and nonhurtful way • karman (kammanta): acting in a non-harmful way • ājīvana (ajīva): a nonharmful livelihood	Yama and niyama. Ethical and disciplined lifestyle: control, indifference, detachment, renunciation, charity, celibacy, vegetarianism, cleanliness, and nonviolence. Asanas involves the development and care of the body through the use exercises and postures yoga. Pranayama breathing exercises. Pratyahara involves meditation by means of which one withdraws consciousness from the senses.

THE STAGES OF CONSCIOUSNESS–*Continued*

Concentration Stages	Stages of Relaxation and Hypnosis	Meditative Stages in Christianity	Meditative Stages in Buddhism (The Noble Eightfold Path)	Meditative Stages in Hindu Religion (The Yoga Saltras of Patanjali)
2. Passive Concentration	• light sleep • deep relaxation • light and medium hypnosis and self-hypnosis	free mental prayer and mental meditation	Prajñā is the wisdom that purifies the mind. • ditthi: viewing reality as it is, not just as it appears to be • sankappa: intention of renunciation, freedom, and harmlessness	Pranayama breathing exercises. Pratyahara involves meditation, by means of which one withdraws consciousness from the senses.
3. Deep Concentration	• deep sleep • deep relaxation • extreme thoughts, flow • medium self-hypnosis • deep hypnosis	stage of contemplation	vyāyāma (vāyāma): making an effort to improve	Dharana, which means concentration. An object of contemplation is held fixedly in the mind.
4. Superior Concentration	• medium to deep hypnosis and self-hypnosis • annulment of the normal • higher consciousness	contemplation and ecstasy living with God	sati: awareness to see things for what they are with clear consciousness, being aware of the present reality within oneself, without any craving or aversion	Dhyana occurs when the sense of separateness of the self from the object of concentration disappears = absorption
5. True Concentration	• deep hypnosis • annulment of the normal consciousness • higher consciousness	enlightenment living in God	samādhi • understood as means of access to absorption enlightenment • cosmic consciousness	samadhi absolute, ecstatic cosmic consciousness enlightenment: cosmic consciousness

Source: Maria Paola Brugnoli, M.D. and Angelico Brugnoli, M.D.

1. ACTIVE CONCENTRATION: TYPES AND TECHNIQUES

A. Awake state, wakefulness
B. Relaxed awakening
C. Progressive relaxation
D. Light sleep (consciousness and the stages of sleep)
E. Repetitive vocal and mental prayer
F. The exercises and physical postures of Yoga

A. Awake State, Wakefulness

Wakefulness is the absence of sleep and is marked by consciousness, awareness, and activity. It occurs when the human body is completely vigilant, and above all when the cerebral cortex keeps all the circuits perfectly open to all sensory stimulation coming from the outside through the five senses and also through other superficial or deep stimulations. Awake refers to the state of being conscious and can be understood in biological terms as the behavioral manifestation of the metabolic state of catabolism. It is the daily recurring period in an organism's life during which consciousness, awareness, and all behaviors necessary for survival exist. Attention and awareness can be volitionally directed to some extent. If asked to become aware of the sensations in your left knee now, you can do so, but few would claim anything like total ability to direct attention.

The physiological mechanisms of wakefulness and sleep are highly interrelated. Wakefulness is defined by a low voltage fast frequency EEG pattern called desynchronized or activated EEG that consists primarily of frequencies in the beta and gamma ranges.

Wakefulness and EEG desynchronization require excitatory innervations of the forebrain. Being awake depends on the discharge activity in several, apparently redundant, parallel ascending neurotransmitter pathways. None of these systems, which include glutamate, acetylcholine (ACh), and the monoamines (serotonin and norepinephrine), is absolutely necessary for the expression of wakefulness, but all appear to contribute (Jones, 2005). Recent research reveals that there are distinct differences in the active brain processing and the specific neurochemical systems involved in the two states. There are specific neuronal pathways, transmitters, and receptors composing the ascending arousal system that flow from the brainstem through the thalamus, hypothalamus, and basal forebrain to the cerebral cortex (Schwartz & Roth, 2008). These scientists also discussed the mutually inhibitory interaction between the core neuronal components of this arousal system and the sleep-active neurons in the ventrolateral preoptic nucleus, which serves as a brainstem switch, regulating the stability of the sleep-wake states.

This basic attention and awareness is something we can both conceptualize and (to some extent) experience as distinct from the particular content of awareness at any time. I am aware of a plant beside me at this moment, and if I turn my head I am aware of a chair. The function of basic awareness remains in spite of various changes in its content. A second basic theoretical and experiential given is the existence, at times, of an awareness of being aware—self-awareness. The degree of self-awareness varies from moment to moment. At one extreme, I can be very aware that at this moment I am aware, that I am looking at the plant beside me. At the other extreme, I may be totally involved in looking at the plant but not be aware of being aware of it (Tart).

Active Concentration in Aware State

This is the state of consciousness often used colloquially to describe being awake and aware and responsive to the environment, in contrast to being asleep or in a coma state. In philosophical and scientific discussion, however, the term is restricted to the specific way in which humans are mentally aware, in such a way that they distinguish clearly between themselves (the thing being aware) and all other things and events. A characteristic of consciousness is that it is reflective, an "awareness of being aware." This "self-awareness" may involve thoughts, sensations, perceptions, moods, emotions, and dreams.

Active Concentration and Empathy State

There is some debate concerning how exactly the conscious experience of empathy should be characterized during active concentration. Empathy (from the Greek empatheia, "to suffer with") is commonly defined as one's ability to recognize, perceive, and directly experientially feel the emotion of another.

The human capacity to recognize the bodily feelings of another is related to one's imitative capacities and seems to be grounded in the innate capacity to associate the bodily movements and facial expressions one sees in another with the proprioceptive feelings of producing those corresponding movements or expressions oneself. The basic idea is that by looking at the facial expressions or bodily movements of another or by hearing their tone of voice, one may get an immediate sense of how they feel. When seeking to communicate with another, it may be helpful to demonstrate empathy with the other, to open up the channel of communication with the other. Empathy is not agreement or approval. It is simply understanding, the intuitive sensing of another person's underlying feelings, wants, and psychological dynamics, looking at the world from behind the other's eyes. "What would I be feeling if I were him or her?" Empathy in therapy is the expression of four basic skills:

- Pay attention: Attention is like a spotlight, illuminating its object.
- Inquire: Empathy is a process of discovery.
- Dig down: You can imagine the insecure, scared, suffering person behind the other's eyes.
- Double check: When we receive a communication, we need to tell the sender "message received."

B. Relaxed Awakening

The second type of active concentration, which is also defined as an active disinhibited concentration, occurs when the patient inhibits all the five senses and also other superficial or deep sensations. In this way, he or she always keeps those circuits open, which can well elaborate and interpret all the stimulations, that come through the activation of the limbic areas of the brain.

The relaxed awakening is referred to as relaxed wakefulness. This is the stage in which the body prepares for sleep. All people fall asleep with tense muscles, their eyes moving erratically. Then, normally, as a person becomes sleepier, the body begins to slow down. Muscles begin to relax, and eye movement slows to a roll. Humans can experience the different stages of concentration through relaxed awakening, which need to be achieved through a psychophysical concentration: physical because it is necessary to learn slowly to inhibit the rationality of the cerebral cortex and psychological in order to activate the limbic areas of the brain.

Studies of human evolution over the course of the centuries and millennia and the neurophysiological development of the brain and the mind can give us some help in providing medical therapy for the suffering of the body, a therapy that we can learn through the path toward the relaxation techniques.

How Stress Affects the Body

Your emotional and physical reactions to stress are partly determined by the sensitivity of your sympathetic nervous system. This system produces the fight or flight reaction in response to stress and excitement, speeding up and heightening the pulse rate, respiration, muscle tension, glandular function, and circulation of the blood. If you have recurrent anxiety symptoms, either major or minor lifestyle and emotional upsets may cause an overreaction of your sympathetic system. If you have an especially stressful life, your sympathetic nervous system may always be poised to react to a crisis, putting you in a state of constant tension. In this mode, you tend to react to small stresses the same way you would react to real emergencies. The energy that accumulates in the body to meet this "emergency" must be discharged in order to bring your body back into balance. Repeated episodes of the fight or flight reaction deplete your energy reserves and, if they continue, cause a downward spiral that can lead to emotional burnout and eventually complete exhaustion.

Simple Relaxation Technique

This simple relaxation technique is usually used for body and mind relaxation. This is where you will begin your journey into a new level of relaxation.

Each relaxed awakening and meditation serves a specific purpose, depending on what you want to achieve. Choose freely and feel free to perform more than one relaxation. Here are some hints to get you started:

- Make sure you are in a quiet room with no distractions.
- Allow some time for your relaxed awakening. These relaxations last from 3 to 10 minutes.
- As you listen to the words of your inner self, picture the images that are being described in your mind.
- Be open to the relaxed awakening:

  My body . . . in time passing by . . .
  is becoming more and more pleasantly calm . . .
  Even more pleasantly calm . . .
  and a feeling of great well-being . . .
  Great calm . . .
  great tranquility . . . it becomes part of me . . .
  the time goes by . . .
  I feel well . . . I feel well . . . I feel really well . . .
  and everything else does not bother me anymore . . .

- For this exercise please repeat the sentences slowly, calmly, at least ten times.

Relaxing Awakening Technique to Improve
Self Well-Being and Self-Esteem

Self-esteem is a term used in psychology to reflect a person's overall evaluation or appraisal of his or her own worth. Self-esteem encompasses beliefs (for example, "I am competent") and emotions, such as triumph, despair, pride, and shame. A person's self-esteem may be reflected in behavior, such as in assertiveness, shyness, confidence, or caution. Use these relaxation exercises to rediscover your latent self-esteem and creativity and rebuild your confidence in your skills and talents.

> I enjoy my own well-being.
> I enjoy my own self-esteem.
> I am blessed with a vivid imagination.
> I love to express myself in creative ways.
> Imagine yourself in a wonderful place . . .
> a room surrounded by windows looking out on the sky . . .
> In this room there are many small areas, and you can move freely around the room, trying each of the areas to see how you feel . . .
> these are just some of the areas into which you may choose to channel your own creativity . . . and where no one else need judge or approve.
> Only your opinion matters . . . and the joy of translating the inner world of the imagination into a form or expression that suits you.
> Imagine yourself using one of the areas in this marvelous room . . .
> Or out of the room . . .
> in order to create your response to the world around you, or your inner world . . .
> Be aware of the feeling of having time and energy to channel into this creative activity . . .
> Be aware of the focus of attention that this creates for you . . .
> nothing else seems to matter . . .
> Enjoy your creativity, well-being, and imaginative power and translate it into the world around you.

C. The Progressive Muscle Relaxation of Edmund Jacobson

Progressive muscle relaxation (PMR) is a technique of stress management developed by the physician Edmund Jacobson in the early 1920s. Jacobson argued that since muscular tension accompanies anxiety, one can reduce anxiety by learning how to relax the muscular tension. Jacobson trained his patients to voluntarily relax certain muscles in their body in order to reduce anxiety symptoms. He also found that the relaxation procedure is effective against ulcers, insomnia, and hypertension.

The PMR procedure teaches you to relax your muscles through a two-step process. First, you deliberately apply tension to certain muscle groups and then you stop the tension and turn your attention to noticing how the muscles relax as the tension flows away. Through repetitive practice, you quickly learn to recognize, and distinguish, the associated feelings of a tensed muscle and a completely relaxed muscle. With this simple knowledge, you can then induce physical muscular relaxation at the first signs of the tension that accompanies anxiety. With physical relaxation comes mental calmness in any situation.

This type of concentration is reachable almost only in a state of relaxed awakening or in the first stages of self-hypnosis, with a prevailing activity of the right-brain hemisphere and with a minimum activity of the left-brain hemisphere.

PMR entails a physical and mental component. The physical component involves the tensing and relaxing of muscle groups over the arms, legs, face, abdomen, and chest. With the eyes closed, and in a sequential pattern, tension in a given muscle group is purposefully held for approximately 10 seconds and then released for 20 seconds before continuing with the next muscle group. The mental component focuses on the difference between the feelings of tension and relaxation. Because the eyes are closed, one is forced to concentrate on the sensation of tension and relaxation.

Progressive relaxation, therefore, involves alternately tensing and relaxing the muscles. A person using PMR may start by sitting or lying down in a comfortable position. With the eyes closed, the muscles are tensed (10 seconds) and relaxed (20 seconds) sequentially through various parts of the body.

The Technique for Jacobson's Progressive Muscle Relaxation

- Assume a comfortable position. Your entire body, including your head, should be supported.
- Try to pay attention to the feelings of muscular relaxation and tension.
- When you tense a particular muscle group, do so vigorously without straining for 7 to 10 seconds.
- Concentrate on what is happening. Feel the buildup of tension in each particular muscle group. It is often helpful to visualize the particular muscle group being tensed.
- When you release the muscles, do so abruptly, and then relax, enjoying the sudden feeling of limpness.
- Allow the relaxation to develop for at least 15 to 20 seconds before going on to the next group of muscles.

Tense forcefully the following muscles:

- legs: tense energetically . . . suddenly let go . . . and breathe . . .
- thighs: tense energetically . . . suddenly let go . . . and breathe . . .
- gluteus: tense energetically . . . suddenly let go . . . and breathe . . .
- pelvis: tense energetically . . . suddenly let go . . . and breathe . . .
- abdominal: tense energetically . . . suddenly let go . . . and breathe . . .
- back: tense energetically . . . suddenly let go . . . and breathe . . .
- chest: tense energetically . . . suddenly let go . . . and breathe . . .
- neck: tense energetically . . . suddenly let go . . . and breathe . . .
- jaw: tense energetically . . . suddenly let go . . . and breathe . . .
- forehead: tense energetically . . . suddenly let go . . . and breathe . . .
- shoulders: tense energetically . . . suddenly let go . . . and breathe . . .

Let go of all the tension and relax completely . . .
Feel the immediate sensation of well-being . . .
Mentally scan your body for any residual tension . . .
If a particular area remains tense . . .
repeat one or two tense-relax cycles for that group of muscles . . .
Now imagine a wave of relaxation slowly spreading throughout your body . . .
starting at your head . . .
and gradually penetrating every muscle group . . .
all the way down to your toes . . .

The immediate effects of PMR include all the benefits of the relaxation mind-body response. Long-term effects of regular practice of PMR include

1. A decrease in generalized muscle tension
2. A decrease in generalized anxiety
3. A decrease in anticipatory anxiety related to phobias
4. Reduction in the frequency and duration of panic attacks
5. Improved ability to face phobic situations through graded exposure
6. Improved concentration
7. An increased sense of control over moods
8. Increased self-esteem
9. Increased spontaneity and creativity

There are no contraindications for PMR.

D. The Light Sleep (Consciousness and the Stages of Sleep)

Stage I is the Lightest Sleep Stage

During Stage I your body is very busy. Your muscles begin to relax, your heart rate and brain temperature rise, and your breathing begins to slow down. This stage occurs while you are still awake. EEG waves begin to take over the brain wave activities. If you were awakened during this stage of sleep, you would not feel like you were asleep. This stage lasts for only a few minutes.

Stage II is the K-Spindle Sleep Stage

Stage II is a light level of sleep in which a burst of electrical activity (spindles) intrudes into your EEG. Your brain waves seem to slow down even more. Sleep walking and sleep talking normally occur in this stage. You would feel as if you were sleep if awakened now. This stage usually lasts about 15 to 30 minutes.

As sleep begins and progresses into Stage II, spindle pacemaker GABAergic nucleus reticularis thalamic neurons, which are hyperpolarized during wakefulness, gradually depolarize. Spindle waves then arise as a discharge pattern caused by network interactions between these spindle pacemaker neurons and thalamocortical projection neurons (Steriade & McCarley, 2005). As sleep progressively deepens, spindle waves are blocked by continuing changes in input to the thalamus. These changes affect the level of depolarization of thalamic spindle pacemaker neurons as well as thalamocortical projection neurons. At this time, NREM sleep becomes increasingly characterized by high voltage, slow wave, delta activity in the cortex. The cellular basis of this activity depends on thalamocortical neurons maintained in a hyperpolarized state by the absence of depolarizing input and generating synchronous bursts of discharges (McCormick & Bal, 1997; Steriade et al., 1993). Delta waves reflect these bursts of activity, transferred through the thalamocortical network and synchronized as oscillations with cortical pyramidal cells, which are themselves discharging in a similar mode. Importantly, this burst discharge mode in thalamic cells prevents the transfer of sensory information through the thalamus to the cortex, so maintaining the block on sensory input that is characteristic of sleep.

At sleep onset in humans, the low voltage, high frequency EEG pattern of wakefulness, often with alpha waves when the eyes are closed, gradually changes to Stage I sleep as the EEG frequencies slow. Stage I, a brief transitional phase after wakefulness, is followed by Stage II sleep when EEG frequencies slow further. During Stage II, the episodic bursts of rhythmic, 12- to 14-Hz waveforms occur in the EEG. These bursts are sleep spindles, an important characteristic of sleep onset.

Sleep spindle correlations include positive correlations in the thalamus and right hippocampus. K-complex correlations include positive correlations in the frontomedian prefrontal cortex and cerebellum. Delta wave correlations include negative correlations in the thalamus, frontomedian prefrontal cortex, dorsal pons, and primary visual cortex. Each pattern of correlations may suggest a functional significance for these waveforms that relates to a waking outcome (Picchioni, Killgore, Balkin & Braun, 2009).

E. Repetitive Vocal and Mental Prayer

A review of scientific studies identified relaxation and concentration, an altered state of awareness, a suspension of logical thought, and the maintenance of a self-observing attitude as the behavioral components of meditation (Perez-De-Albeniz & Holmes, 2000). Prayer and meditation are accompanied by a host of biochemical and physical changes in the body that alter metabolism, heart rate, respiration, blood pressure and brain chemistry (Lazar et al., 2000). Three priests were tested by EEG during prayer. The results indicated three periods: generalization, bilateral desynchronization (spontaneous), and a period of suppression of main rhythms, but local pulsations were taking place.

As we know, there are three functional conditions of the brain: sleep, wakefulness and paradoxal sleep. These new conditions may therefore be marked as a new condition of the brain (V. Slezin, Laboratory of Psychophysiology, Bekhterev Institute, Russia, I. Rybina). When we pray, it is considered advantageous to spiritual growth to pray selflessly. Prayer and meditation have been used in clinical settings as a method of stress and pain reduction. Meditation has also been studied specifically for its effects on stress (Kabat-Zinn, Lipworth & Burney, 1985; Davidson et al., 2003; Ospina et al., 2007).

The Stage of Active Concentration (State of Aware Waking) Corresponds in Christianity to the First Phase of Prayer

One moment of the "repetitive vocal prayer" is the prayer of believers going to church. The Holy Rosary in honor of the Virgin Mary, one of the traditional Roman Catholic family prayers at the beginning of the last century, belongs to this kind of prayer. The recitative prayers have a pregnant and evocative meaning in great solemnities in any kind of liturgy (with music, hymns, and processions) because they happen in important and great religious events. In this phase we can include the moment of the "repetitive mental prayer," in which the believer thinks to the traditional formulas without pronouncing (or singing) them out loud.

The "Repetitive Mental Prayer"

Sit quietly in your sacred place. Relax and center yourself. Witness yourself praying to God. Witness silently, detached, without commentary, judgment, or comparisons. Say a prayer for yourself. Say a prayer for someone else. Say a prayer for everyone and everything. Do this again and again for a total of three cycles or do it for a total of twelve times or until it feels like you've done it enough. You will clearly see that you feel really good when you pray for others.

The simple prayer of St. Francis of Assisi provides a blueprint to use to pattern our living in our thoughts, speech, and actions, within our day to day relationships with our fellow beings and with all life around us. Therefore, the prayer of St. Francis is a precious document for us—an indispensable, invaluable frame of reference by which to achieve consciousness in our own daily life.

The Peace Prayer of Saint Francis

"O Lord, make me an instrument of Thy peace!
Where there is hatred, let me sow love.
Where there is injury, pardon.
Where there is discord, harmony.
Where there is doubt, faith.
Where there is despair, hope.
Where there is darkness, light.
Where there is sorrow, joy.

Oh Divine Master, grant that I may not
so much seek to be consoled as to console;
to be understood as to understand;
to be loved as to love.

For it is in giving that we receive;
it is in pardoning that we are pardoned;
and it is in dying that we are born to eternal life."

Saint Francis of Assisi
(baptized as Giovanni di Bernadone, 1182–1226 A.D., Italy

The Repetitive Vocal and Mental Prayer in Buddhism, Hinduism, and Other Religions

The same state of consciousness can be reached with the purification of the mind, exerting nonviolence, with the chastity of the body and the serenity of the mind. (*See* the meditative techniques in Chapter V, "Mindfulness and Meditative States in Spiritual Care.") It is necessary to dominate all kinds of desires, and every kind of gift must be refused. The applied study of all disciplines, the capability of enjoying small things, the abstinence from food, and the worship of God are extremely important in order to reach the active concentration in a state of aware waking.

Active concentration uses mainly the short-term memory, which is not definitively fixed in the subcortical group of neurons.

F. The Exercises and the Postures of Yoga

The practice of yoga exercises means practicing with both your body and your mind. The body is held poised and relaxed, with the practitioner experiencing no discomfort. During yoga exercises (and transcendental meditations), the medial prefrontal cortex and anterior cingulate cortex work in the generation of EEG alpha activity (Yamamoto, Kitamura, Yamada, Nakashima & Kuroda, 2006).

Asanas Yoga: Yoga Exercises and Postures

Asana (Sanskrit: sitting down) is a body position typically associated in the practice of yoga, intended primarily to restore and maintain a practitioner's well-being, improve the body's flexibility and vitality, and promote the ability to remain in seated relaxed meditation for extended periods. These are widely known as yoga postures or yoga positions, which is currently practiced for exercise and as alternative medicine.

It takes willpower and perseverance to accomplish each yoga pose and to practice it daily. The practice of yoga exercises or yoga asanas can improve your health, increase your resistance, and develop your mental awareness. Doing the yoga poses, requires you to study each pose and execute it.

In the yoga sutras, Patanjali suggests that the only requirement for practicing asanas is that it be "steady and comfortable." Asana is a body posture; it is a Sanskrit word used to describe a position of the body. Patanjali, the founder of Ashtanga yoga defines asana as "Steady and comfortable posture." Traditionally, many asanas are practiced in Hatha Yoga tradition, principally to achieve better physical and mental health. Asanas have a deep impact on the entire body and mind complex; they affect different systems within the body, such as the muscular, respiratory, circulation, digestive, excretory, reproductive, endocrine, and nervous systems.

When control of the body is mastered, practitioners free themselves from the duality of heat and cold, hunger and satiety, and joy and grief, which is the first step toward the unattachment that relieves suffering. This nondualistic perspective comes from the Sankya school of the Himalayan Masters.

How the Yoga Asanas Work

The asanas are based on five principles:

1. THE USE OF GRAVITY. The inverted postures such as the headstand, shoulder stand, and reverse posture take advantage of gravity to increase the flow of blood to the desired part of the body: in the headstand, to the brain, in the shoulder stand, to the thyroid gland; and in the reverse posture, to the gonads (sex glands).

2. ORGAN MASSAGE. The position of the asana causes a squeezing action on a specific organ or gland, resulting in the stimulation of that part of the body.

3. STRETCHING MUSCLES AND LIGAMENTS. This causes an increase in blood supply to the muscles and ligaments as well as relaxing them. It also takes pressure off nerves in the area. The stretching is involved in all the asanas, because it has such a beneficial effect on the body.

4. DEEP BREATHING. While holding the yoga posture, we breathe slowly and deeply, moving the abdomen only (abdominal or low breathing). This increases the oxygen and prana supply to the target organ or gland, thereby enhancing the effect of the asana.

5. CONCENTRATION. As well as breathing slowly and deeply, we also focus our attention on the target organ or gland. This brings the mind into play and greatly increases the circulation and prana supply to the organ or gland. This concentration has the second benefit of increasing general powers of concentration through regular practice. This benefits every aspect of life. Your mind is less distracted and swayed by external events, and you are therefore calmer and worry less. You will be able to solve day-to-day problems better and have more success in whatever activity you undertake.

Night and day, hot and cold, Inhale and exhale, work and rest–everything has an opposite. So it is with life and yoga. Below are a series of poses known as "The Salutation to the Sun." Give it a try; you are invited to experience the "joy of cycles" right now.

The Technique of Yoga Pose: Surya Namaskar or Sun Salutation

Surya Namaskara (Sūrya namaskāra) or Sun Salutations (lit. "salute to the sun") are a common sequence of Hatha Yoga asanas. Its origins lie in a worship of Surya, the Hindu solar deity. This sequence of movements and poses can be practiced on varying levels of awareness, ranging from that of physical exercise in various styles to a complete sadhana, which incorporates asana and pranayama (Sri K. Pattabhi Jois, Suryanamaskara, 2005).

Begin: Shivasana
INHALE

Laying down, heels together, arms by your side, palms facing upward. With each exhale let your entire body melt through the floor. Let go and melt until every cell in your body is completely relaxed, allowing each cell to melt over the next. Give yourself a few minutes. Now melt even more!

Next, roll to your left side and stand.

Surya Namaskar (The Sun Salutation) includes twelve different positions:

1. Inhale and maintain the standing position with hands joined together near chest, feet together, and toes touching each other. EXHALE
2. Raise the arms upward. INHALE
   Slowly bend backward, stretching arms above the head.
3. Uttanasana (Standing Forward Bend) EXHALE
   Exhale and bend forward in the waist until palms touch the ground in line with the toes. Do not bend the knees while performing. At first you may find it difficult to attain the ideal position but try to bend as much as possible without bending the knees.
4. Inhale and take the left leg back with left toes on the floor, press the waist downwards and raise the neck, stretch the chest forward, and push shoulders backwards. Keep the right leg and both the hands in the same position. Keep the right leg folded.
5. Adho Mukha Svanasana (Downward-Facing Dog)
   Hold the breath and raise the knee of left leg. Take the right leg backwards and keep it close to the left leg. Straighten both the legs and both hands. Keep the neck straight and sight fixed. Keep the toes erect. Take care that the neck, spine, thighs, and feet are in a straight line.

6. Ashtanga

   Exhaling, bend both the hands and elbows and touch forehead on the ground, touch the knees on the ground, keep both the elbows close to chest. The forehead, chest, both palms, both sets of toes, and knees should touch the ground and the rest of the body is not touching the floor. Since only eight parts rest on the ground, it is called "Ashtanga" (8-limbed yoga) position.

7. Naga-asana (Cobra)

   Inhale and straighten the elbows, stretch the shoulders upwards, press the waist downward but do not bend the arms. Keep the knees and toes on the floor. Push the neck backwards and look upward.

8. Hold the breath, bend the neck downward and press the chin in the throat, push the body backward and touch the heels on the ground, raise the waist upward, but do not move the palms on the floor.

9. Hold the breath, bring the left leg to the front and place it in between the hands while the right foot stays in place with the right knee and right toes touching the ground.

10. Exhale and bring the right leg forward as in position 3 and place it in between both the arms.

11. INHALE

    Raise the arms upward. Slowly bend backward, stretching arms above the head.

12. EXHALE

    Hands joined together near chest, feet together, and toes touching each other.

    Completing 1 Cycle:

    Shivasana–Laying down, heels together, arms by your side, palms facing upward, breathe in and out, letting your entire body melt through the floor. Let go until every cell in your body is completely relaxed, as though you are melting through the floor. Give yourself a few minutes. Now relax.

Surya Namaskar is an appreciated yoga exercise among people of all ages from children to the elderly. The Surya Namaskar postures are a very effective means to limber up. Hence, they are generally carried out before the other asanas. At the end of the twelve postures, you will feel refreshed and relaxed.

2. PASSIVE CONCENTRATION: TYPES AND TECHNIQUES

Passive concentration is the opposite of what you are probably well-acquainted with as "active" concentration. In this stage we find autogenic training, the hypnagogic and hypnopompic states, the REM phase of sleep (with dreams), and some initial stages of self-hypnosis and light and medium hypnosis, with the presence of brain activity of both the right and the left hemispheres, even if the latter is to a lesser degree.

With active concentration, you are goal (and result) oriented, with the likely notion in the background that the harder you concentrate and the harder you work, the more likely you are to achieve your goals. Passive concentration is the permissive and accepting attitude out of which you intentionally relinquish any effort and willpower during your practice of relaxation and meditation.

Indifferent toward any outcome, you become the observer of what is happening in your body. You concentrate "passively" for example on your right arm to become heavy without any effort to bring about the sensation of heaviness. You allow the sensation of heaviness to arise as you allow the pleasant sensation of deep relaxation to permeate you gradually. The more passive your concentration is, the more profound and lasting the experience of relaxation will be.

Passive concentration has similarities to "mindfulness" as a spiritual concept in some Eastern meditation traditions. Here, you learn to become the observer or "watcher" of the mind, allowing each thought, each emotion, each sensation to arise and then to dissipate into the next moment. Your awareness and your knowing that you are watching leads to detachment from and nonidentification with your mind's content.

If you want to relax, then passive concentration is essential. How do you do it? Well, in a few words, you allow sensations, images, and thoughts to just float on by: just notice them and let them go, like a leaf floating by you on a stream. You do not hold on to anything that your attention is drawn to. Just let it go. This kind of concentration is great to develop anytime you want to relax now and then.

A. Autogenic Training of Schultz

Autogenic training is the passive concentration relaxation technique developed by the German psychiatrist Johannes Schultz and first published in 1932. The technique involves daily practice of sessions that last approximately 15 minutes. Autogenic therapy (or autogenic training as it is often known), has spread to many parts of the world, and more than 3000 research papers have shown its efficacy. Autogenic training can have a positive effect on many chronic health problems, while preventing invasive treatments for many acute symptoms. Phrases for autogenic training with active concentration could be: "I want my right arm to become heavy!" or, "Right arm, become heavy!" The result, however, would be like trying to fall asleep with force.

In the 1920s, a German neuropsychiatrist named Dr Johannes Schultz became intrigued by the physiological implications of a person in a deeply relaxed state, such as when under hypnosis or when going to sleep. Taking the observations of researchers into the hypnotic state (the work of Vogt and Brodmann), Schultz constructed a set of simple autosuggestions (mental exercises) incorporating those observations. Over time, these were developed into the standard exercises of autogenic training that we know today: heaviness in the limbs, then warmth, focusing on the heartbeat or pulse, breathing, an idea of warmth in the abdomen, and coolness in the forehead. If these are the perceived sensations of mind and body in a deeply relaxed state, then Schultz simply made a conscious exercise of that perception.

Example of an Autogenic Training Session

- Sit in the meditative posture and scan the body
- "my right arm is heavy"
- "my arms and legs are heavy and warm" (repeat 3 or more times)
- "my heartbeat is calm and regular" (repeat 3 times)
- "my solar plexus is warm" (repeat 3 times)
- "my forehead is cool"
  For any exercise, please repeat the sentences slowly, with calm, for at least three to ten times.

All of the previous exercises are suitable to the passive concentration, but we will consider some examples.

My Body is Pleasantly Warm

My body . . . in the time passing by . . .
is becoming more and more pleasantly warm . . .
Even more pleasantly warm . . .
and a feeling of great well being . . .
Great calm . . . great tranquility . . .it becomes part of me . . .
the time goes by . . . I feel well . . . I feel well . . .
I feel really well . . . and everything else does not bother me anymore . . .

For this exercise, please repeat the sentences slowly with calm at least ten times.

My Forehead is Cool

This can be another exercise used for the pain relief therapy, depending on the patient's personality and character. It is also a very important exercise to control chronic headache.

This is how to carry out the technique of the cool forehead:

- Concentrating on your forehead please repeat

  My head is light . . .
  All the muscles of my face are rested . . .
  I am calm . . . calm . . .
  Perfectly calm . . . in a state of great well-being . . .
  My forehead is cool . . . pleasantly cool . . .
  Even more pleasantly cool . . .
  The coolness is all around me and gives me well-being . . .
  Wellbeing of the body and well-being of the mind . . .

- Repeat this formula between five and ten times.

  my neck and shoulders are heavy (repeat three times)
  I am at peace (repeat three times)

The mind, the body, and the spirit, are all interrelated and interdependent. All holistic practitioners know the principle of this statement, and they all know that the human being's innate capacity for self-healing is largely untapped. Autogenic training has been subject to clinical evaluation from its early days in Germany and from the early 1980s worldwide. In 2002, a meta-analysis of sixty studies was published in *Applied Psychophysiology and Biofeedback* (Stetter & Kupper, 2002) finding significant positive effects of treatment when compared to normals over a number of diagnoses, finding these effects to be similar to best recommended rival therapies, and finding positive additional effects by patients, such as their perceived quality of life.

B. Light, Medium Hypnosis and Self-Hypnosis

Practitioners of clinical hypnosis have long observed often dramatic emotional, cognitive, behavioral, and physiological changes, occurring during and as an apparent consequence of passive concentration hypnotic trance. EEG activity at the midfrontal region was recorded during pre and post baselines, live hypnotic induction, arm levitation, progressive relaxation deepening, and therapeutic ego-enhancing suggestions among sixty college student volunteers previously screened with the Stanford Hypnotic Susceptibility Scale. Comparisons across conditions for delta, theta, alpha, and beta activity were made among low, moderate, high, and very high hypnotizable groups. The results indicated significant increases in theta EEGs, across the hypnosis process with a peak at progressive relaxation and a drop in theta thereafter to termination, with highs showing significantly more dramatic effects than moderates (Stevens et al., 2004).

Light Hypnosis and Self-Hypnosis

This is the first stage of hypnotic passive concentration that anyone can enter as soon as eyes closure is achieved. During light hypnosis we can observe

- eyes closed
- movements are reduced
- posture and facial features begin to relax
- breathing begins to deepen
- body indicators of tension begin to decrease

Medium Hypnosis and Self-Hypnosis

This is the next step of hypnosis. We can observe

- deep breathing
- slumped posture
- mouth may open
- feelings of lethargy
- retardation in responsiveness
- reduction in sensory awareness

During the induction into medium hypnosis and self-hypnosis, the hypnotherapist guides the client to narrowly focus his or her attention to the point that sensory impressions are blocked out. The client can then reach the state of complete relaxation necessary for hypnosis to occur. The hypnotherapist's office usually is quiet and dimly lit to create a relaxing atmosphere. The hypnotherapist chooses a particular method or combination of methods (*see* Chapter IV, for induction based on the assessment of the client).

An induction script may use different types of verbal and visual cues, including the following.

METAPHORS AND IMAGERY. The hypnotherapist suggests images or describes a scene for the patient (e.g., "Let your mind drift to a calm and peaceful place. See the wind blowing through the trees, the flowers in the meadow."). A mental image is an experience that, on most occasions, significantly resembles the experience of perceiving some object, event, or scene but occurs when the relevant object, event, or scene is not actually present to the senses (Finke, 1989; McKellar, 1957; Richardson, 1969; Thomas, 2003). There are not infrequently, however, episodes, particularly on falling asleep (hypnagogic imagery) and waking up (hypnapompic), when the imagery, being of a rapid, phantasmagoric and involuntary character, defies perception, presenting a kaleidoscopic field in which no distinct object can be discerned.

Philosophers such as Berkeley and Hume and early experimental psychologists such as Wundt and James understood ideas in general to be mental images, and today it is very widely believed that much imagery functions as mental representations, or mental models, playing an important role in memory and thinking (Barsalou, 1999; Egan, 1992; Paivio, 1986; Prinz, 2002). Indeed, some have gone so far as to suggest that images are best understood as by definition of a form of inner, mental, or neural representation (Block, 1983; Kosslyn, 1983).

If the patient is having trouble obtaining sufficient imagery, it may be helpful to ask questions that will provide more context. Particularly if the patient is more auditory or kinesthetic than visual, these questions can survey different sensory experiences. "You might notice what you are wearing, if anything, on your feet." "What time of day or night does it seem to be?" Other questions can address such things as whether the person is indoors or not, if others are present, if there is an awareness of any smells, or if any sounds can be heard (Schenk, 1999).

Repetition of words: The therapist repeats key words or sounds (e.g., "Breathe in deeply . . . ," "As you breathe in . . . ").

Emotional cues or probes: A hypnotherapy session may be used to gather more information about painful experiences or to help patients cope with difficult emotions. The therapist integrates the inquiries or instructions into the induction script (e.g., "You are in control and will choose to experience or ignore any suggestions during the session.").

Analogies, metaphors, and associative statements: Metaphors and poetry in hypnosis, are a trance state characterized by a very relaxed, drowsy, and lethargic appearance (*see* Chapter VII). During this trance state, the person who has been hypnotized loses initiative to carry out his or her own plans, redirects attention away from the activity in which he or she was engaged toward the instructions of the hypnotist, has heightened ability to produce fantasies, and has an increased susceptibility to suggestions. The biology of cognition attributes a practical and connotative role to language but also gives importance to emotions, which together braid with language in forming the consensual domain of conversations of living organisms. In hypnosis, we use rhythm, with consciously creating recognizable patterns. The hypnotherapist uses comparisons to familiar experiences or images to help clients achieve physical relaxation (e.g., "Your legs are sinking into the couch, heavy as logs." "Feel your body, heavy and relaxed, being supported by the tree behind you, the ground beneath you."). Hypnosis and metaphors can be the power of words in the modified states of consciousness.

Rhythm is unique and privileged in communication with patients. Rhythm (or "measure") in writing is like the beat in music. In poetry, in hypnosis, and in spiritual mantras and prayers, rhythm implies that certain words are produced with more force, more fully than others, and may be held for longer duration. The repetition of a pattern of such emphasis is what produces a rhythmic and hypnotic effect. The word rhythm comes from the Greek rhythmos, meaning "measured motion."

Descriptive words in poetry and rhythm make their sound like a feeling; mindfulness of feeling is the mind experiencing awareness of the thoughts. A language more and more spontaneously and hypnotically indirect, implicit, symbolic, it can activate new mental associations.

Metaphor can rouse old and repressed ones as well as we can imagine a road network actively and continuously developing, amidst the swarming of synaptic connections and links (Hopkins). The relation between the structure and functioning of our mind, the structure and modes of operation of our physical brain, and also the structure and conduct of the outside world has been the issue of debate for ages.

We can use metaphors and poems as "indirect" Ericksonian suggestion in hypnosis and during therapeutic modified states of consciousness. With poetry and metaphor, any creative space is opened, followed, listened to, but then encircled and defined within one's way of individuation. Repetition of a sound, syllable, word, phrase, line, stanza, or metrical pattern is a basic unifying device in hypnosis.

The Technique of the Self-Hypnosis or Autogenic Hypnosis

This is a method of mental, meditative-type exercises that bring about profound relaxation in mind and body. The word autogenic means self-generating. This can be a twofold concept. First, the treatment is carried out by the client; autogenic exercises are applied by the self to the self. There is no middle-man in the shape of a therapist except in the role of guide and support in the initial teaching of the method. Second, the result of practicing the exercises is entirely spontaneous and unpredictable. The system of rebalance knows exactly what is required and will bring it about if left alone to do so.

Metaphors and hypnosis are amazing experiences that teach you feelings from inside yourself you could never ever begin to imagine. They are a way of using the mind that is so easy, so natural, so simple and yet produces an endless resource stream of truly mind-blowing proportions. I have learned to ask certain parts of myself to give me a stream of data for a specific purpose and how to interpret these data into words, or sounds, or movements, or images; I have learned how to do this consciously and how to cooperate so this can happen.

In self-hypnosis with metaphors, some factors are absolutely important:

- You must use "all five senses" in your descriptions. If you see a snow-covered mountain, for example, do not just describe how it looks. Describe its taste, its texture, its smell, and the sound of the wind howling across the peak.
- Phrase all your descriptions in the "present tense."
- Close your eyes and describe out loud anything you can "see."
- Later on in the image-streaming process, you can use it for problem solving and a great many other things besides.

A symbol is the smallest unit of metaphor, consisting of a single object, image, or word representing the essence of the quality or an attribute it stands for. The following is Jung's definition of a symbol: "A word or an image is symbolic when it implies something more than its obvious and immediate meaning. It has a wider 'unconscious' aspect that is never precisely defined or fully explained. Nor can one hope to define or explain it. As the mind explores the symbol, it is led to ideas that lie beyond the grasp of reason." This is therefore the basis for the emergence of the world experienced by each individual. Within the context of our experienced world, it is conventionally valid to say that the physical objects we perceive in the world around us, such as planets and stars, exist within the external, subjective space of consciousness. The mental objects we perceive, such as thoughts and mental images, exist in the internal, subjective space of the consciousness of each individual. Although we may believe in the existence of space independent of consciousness, all our concepts of such real, objective space arise within the space of consciousness. As for the relation between sensory images and their related objects, believed to exist in the objective world independent of consciousness, neurologist Antonio Damasio acknowledges, "There is no picture of the object being transferred from the object to the retina and from the retina to the brain."

To generalize, to our senses, the appearances are not replicas or representations of phenomena in objective, physical space. They are fresh creations arising in the space of consciousness.

Music and Sounds

The hypnotherapist speaks in a steady, evenly paced rhythm without varying voice tone. Sometimes, the therapist plays music in the background.

What we feel as music is a mental content generated by the ears and the brain responding to external vibration stimuli. These stimuli cause the musical perception but are substantially different from it. Because each individual is unique, cerebrally and psychologically, each one has its own particular way to respond to the external stimuli, thus having a more or less different experience while listening to the same music. It is not possible to express objective and absolute judgments about a tune, without a reference version of it; in a certain sense, there are as many versions as there are listeners. We may say that what we call music, and its beauty (or feeling), exists only in the subjectivity (this means in the minds) of the listeners. Music has the ability to affect our emotions, intellect, and our psychology; lyrics can assuage our loneliness or incite our passions.

Organic life is based on different kind of rhythms: the rhythm of breathing, of pulsations, of muscles in their different physiological functions, let alone the more subtle vibratory rhythm of each single cell, of each molecule, of each atom. Therefore, it should not come as a surprise that the musical rhythms exert a powerful influence on those organic and psychological rhythms, sometimes stimulating them and sometimes calming them, creating harmony and peace.

C. Lucid Dreams, Hypnagogic and Hypnopompic States

A lucid dream is a dream in which the sleeper is aware that he or she is dreaming. A lucid dreamer can actively participate in (during a state of passive concentration) and manipulate imaginary experiences in the dream environment. Lucid dreams can seem extremely real and vivid, depending on a person's level of self-awareness during the lucid dream. Lucid dreaming is also known as dream consciousness or conscious dreaming. Lucid dreaming is a modified state of consciousness, with aspects of waking and dreaming combined in a way so as to suggest a specific alteration in brain physiology. It constitutes a hybrid state of consciousness, with definable and measurable differences from waking and from REM sleep, particularly in frontal areas.

Results show lucid dreaming to have REM-like power in frequency bands delta and theta and higher than REM activity in the gamma band, the between states difference peaking around 40 Hz. Power in the 40-Hz band, is strongest in the frontal and frontolateral region. Overall coherence levels are similar in waking and lucid dreaming and significantly higher than in REM sleep throughout the entire frequency spectrum analyzed. Regarding specific frequency bands, waking is characterized by high coherence in alpha, and lucid dreaming by increased delta and theta band coherence (Voss, Holzmann, Tuin & Hobson, 2009).

Hypnagogic hallucinations and visualizations can occur as one is falling asleep, and hypnopompic hallucinations occur when one is waking up. They are considered normal phenomena.

The role of dreams as a significant source of information about the patient's inner life has been richly studied by many theorists and therapists, including Freud, Jung, Perls, and others. The visualization involves one or more of your five senses (hearing, taste, touch, smell, sight). We can use a word or phrase to stimulate the memory of those senses. A lucid dream is an emotionally charged event that stands apart from the rest of your day. To conquer the recidivism of these old familiar patterns, we must turn inward and ask, "What is the message in this lucid dream?" What aspects of my personality are symbolized by these people, objects, animals, actions, and so on? Symbols are the language of the psyche and the soul. Curiosity with emotional detachment and mindful reflection are key factors in the decoding process. This is the first step on the path to higher consciousness.

Early references to hypnagogia are to be found in the writings of Aristotle, Iamblichus, Cardano, Simon Forman, and Swedenborg (Mavromatis 1987). Romanticism brought a renewed interest in the subjective experience of the edges of sleep (Pfotenhauer & Schneider, 2006). In more recent centuries, many authors have referred to the state; Edgar Allan Poe, for example, wrote of the "fancies" he experienced "only when I am on the brink of sleep, with the consciousness that I am so" (Mavromatis, 1987).

Serious scientific enquiry began in the nineteenth century with Johannes Peter Müller, Jules Baillarger, and Alfred Maury and continued into the twentieth with Leroy (Leroy, 1933).

The advent of electroencephalography has allowed the introspective methods of these early researchers to be supplemented with physiological data. The search for neural correlates for hypnagogic imagery began with Davis and colleagues in the 1930s (Davis, Davis, Loomis, Harvey & Hobart, 1937) and continues with increasing sophistication to this day.

Although the dominance of the behaviorist paradigm led to a decline in research, especially in the English-speaking world, the later twentieth century saw a revival, with investigations of hypnagogia and related subjects playing an important role in the emerging multidisciplinary study of consciousness (Susan, 2003; Vaitl et al., 2005).

Nevertheless, much remains to be understood about the experience and its corresponding neurology, and the topic has been somewhat neglected in comparison with sleep and dreams. Hypnagogia has been described as a "well-trodden and yet unmapped territory" (Mavromatis, 1987). Important reviews of the scientific literature have been made by Leaning (1925), Schacter (1976), and Richardson and Mavromatis (1987).

Physiological studies have tended to concentrate on hypnagogia in the strict sense of spontaneous sleep-onset experiences. Such experiences are associated especially with stage I of NREM sleep (Rechtschaffen & Kales, 1968), but may also occur with presleep alpha waves (Foulkes & Schmidt, 1983; Foulkes & Vogel, 1965). Davis and associates found short flashes of dreamlike imagery at the onset of sleep to correlate with drop-offs in alpha EEG activity (Davis et al., 1937).

Hori, Hayaskie, and Morikawa regard sleep-onset hypnagogia as a state distinct from both wakefulness and sleep, with unique electrophysiological, behavioral and subjective characteristics (Hori, Hayashi, & Morikawa, 1993; Vaitl et al., 2005). Germaine and coworkers have demonstrated a resemblance between the EEG power spectra of spontaneously occurring hypnagogic images, on the one hand, and those of both REM sleep and relaxed wakefulness, on the other (Germaine & Nielsen, 1997; Nielsen, Germain & Ouellet, 1995).

To identify more precisely the nature of the EEG state that accompanies imagery in the transition from wakefulness to sleep, Hori and colleagues (1993) proposed a scheme of nine EEG stages, defined by varying proportions of alpha (stages 1–3), suppressed waves of less than 20µV (stage 4), theta ripples (stage 5), proportions of sawtooth waves (stages 6 and 7), and presence of spindles (stages 8 and 9). Germaine and Nielsen (1977) found spontaneous hypnagogic imagery to occur mainly during Hori sleep, onset stages 4 (EEG flattening) and 5 (theta ripples).

The covert-rapid-eye-movement hypothesis proposes that hidden elements of REM sleep emerge during the wakefulness-sleep transition stage (Bodizs, Sverteczki, Lazar & Halasz, 2005).

Support for this comes from Bódicz et al., who note a greater similarity between WST (wakefulness-sleep transition) EEG and REM sleep EEG than between the former and stage 2 sleep (Bodizs et al., 2005).

D. The REM Phase of Sleep

REM Sleep, Rapid Eye Movement

REM sleep is the sleep stage in which dreaming occurs. When you enter into REM sleep, your breathing becomes fast, irregular, and shallow. Your eyes will move rapidly, and your muscles become immobile. Heart rate and blood pressure increase. Men may develop erections. About 20 percent of sleep is REM sleep. This sleep phase begins about 70 to 90 minutes after you fall asleep. The first sleep cycle has a shorter phase of REM sleep. Toward morning, the time spent in REM sleep increases and the deep sleep stages decrease.

Researchers do not fully understand REM sleep and dreaming. They know it is important in the creation of long-term memories. If a person's REM sleep is disrupted, the next sleep cycle does not follow the normal order but often goes directly to REM sleep until the previous night's lost REM time is made up.

REM sleep is distinguishable from NREM sleep by changes in physiological states, including its characteristic rapid eye movements. Polysomnograms show wave patterns in REM to be similar to stage I sleep, however. In normal sleep (in people without disorders of sleep-wake patterns or REM behavior disorder), heart rate and respiration speed up and become erratic, while the face, fingers, and legs may twitch. Intense dreaming occurs during REM sleep as a result of heightened cerebral activity, but paralysis occurs simultaneously in the major voluntary muscle groups, including the sub-mental muscles (muscles of the chin and neck).

Because REM is a mixture of encephalic (brain) states of excitement and muscular immobility, it is sometimes called paradoxical sleep. It is generally thought that REM-associated muscle paralysis is meant to keep the body from acting out the dreams that occur during this intensely cerebral stage. The first period of REM typically lasts 10 minutes, with each recurring REM stage lengthening, and the final one lasting an hour. Neuroscientists think

> The function of rapid-eye-movement (REM) sleep is still unknown. One prevailing hypothesis suggests that REM sleep is important in processing memory traces. Here, using positron emission tomography (PET) and regional cerebral blood flow measurements, we show that waking experience influences regional brain activity during subsequent sleep. Several brain areas activated during the execution of a serial reaction time task during wakefulness were significantly more active during REM sleep in subjects previously trained on the task than in non-trained subjects. These results support the hypothesis that memory traces are processed during REM sleep in humans. (Maquet et al., 2000)

E. Free Mental Prayer and Mental Meditation

The Passive Concentration in Meditative Stages

There are different ways, depending on the different schools of thought, to reach this phase. For example, according to Ignacio of Loyola 's school, the most quoted in Catholicism, the best way to practice mental meditation is to analyze every single word of repetitive prayers, concentrating the thought on their intrinsic meaning without letting the mind wandering. In Buddhism and Hinduism, the same state can be reached through meditation. Meditation is integration: therefore, its main goal is to reassemble the divided part of the human being. If you say that the body is different from the mind, and that the mind is different from the soul, this means that you are disaggregating. How can meditation take us back to the integration if it is something that separates the body from the brain, the brain from the mind, or the mind from the soul? If when we close our eyes and we keep silent, we consider this meditation then we all meditate for hours during our sleep. Why do we not call it meditation? Is not that silence? During sleep, the mental function stops, but we cannot consider this meditation. All of us can meditate, but the goal is far, far from us, because we are not able to control our senses, our mind, and our intelligence.

Three main transformation take place while we meditate. In Hindu philosophy, at the beginning of his Yoga Sutra, Patanjali says that yoga is the appeasement of the mind. He then affirms that when a person tries to appease the mind, a sort of resistance develops as new thoughts and/or new ideas arise. A sort of tug-of-war starts between our attempt at control and the arising thoughts. The asana can be reached with a particular control of the physical posture, keeping the body completely free from nervous and muscular tensions, even with unusual positions. The way of meditation is the way of silence. Silencing the ceaseless chatter of a mind buzzing with thoughts is not easy. The way to silence is the way of the mantra. A mantra is a sound, syllable, word, or group of words that is considered capable of "creating transformation." Mantras (Devanāgarī) originated in the Vedic tradition of India, becoming an essential part of the Hindu tradition and a customary practice within Buddhism, Sikhism, and Jainism. In the context of the Vedas, the term mantra refers to the entire portion that contains the texts called Rig, Yajur, or Sama, that is, the metrical part as opposed to the prose Brahmana commentary. It is advisable to choose a word of four syllables and pronounce them with equal length. The recommended word in the Christian tradition is Ma-ra-na-tha. In Aramaic, the language of Jesus' time, it means "The Lord comes."

Once we commence this daily practice, a few guidelines can enable us to go deeper. First, we are not to assess our progress. The feeling of success or failure may be the biggest distraction of all. We are not to look for experiences in our meditation. We come to meditation in poverty of spirit. So be faithful to the recitation of the word or mantra during the period of meditation and to the daily practice, twice a day, morning and evening. The minimum time prescribed is 20 minutes, the optimum 30 minutes. "The way of saying your word, your mantra, is the way to stillness."

Eastern Christians call it hesychia. It is pure prayer, worship in spirit and truth. It purifies the heart of contradictory desires and unifies us. The place of unity is the heart, where we find our deepest and most natural orientation toward God as our personal source and goal.

Meditative Free Mental Prayer and Meditation (Angelico Brugnoli)

> From your immensity Lord,
> you looked at me
> and I felt comforted,
> and I could arise my eyes up to you.
> From your immensity Lord,
> you looked at me.
> From your place without space and without time, you heard me,
> and I dared to speak to you.
> From your place without space and without time, you heard me, Lord.
> You immerged into my time, Lord,
> and I could feel that you were forever close by me.
> Since you planned to create me, Lord, I felt you,
> I invoked your name from the abyss, and you helped me
> to feel as a thinking being, to feel as a being that wants,
> that wishes, that longs to be near you.
> Since you planned to create me, Lord,
> you thought of me, and I felt your warm love for me.
> Since you planned the universe, Lord,
> since beyond time and space, I was totally swallowed up by nothingness,
> Lord, you wanted me, you loved me, you heard me,
> and in this moment, I offer you my heart, my soul, my spirit.
> Since I was totally swallowed up by nothingness,
> Lord, since the elementary particles that form my body, Lord,
> drifted inert in the space but with their potential life,
> you thought of me. You wanted me.
> You loved me, Lord.
> Therefore, I devote myself to you, Lord.
> Since you wanted me,

you loved me, and you only expect that I remember you,
that I want you, and I love you as you wanted and loved me
since the elementary particles that form my body were still inert in the space.
Since, Lord, you thought of me, I started living.
Since you wanted me, I began my way of being.
Since you loved me, you gave me the heat of life.
So I am here, in this moment to entrust you
all that little moment of love,
that in my own small way I can have for you, Lord.
Accept my heart, Lord,
accept my soul, Lord,
accept my spirit, Lord, and let this little moment
of life in this world
become the instant that lasts forever together with you, Lord.
since you wanted me,
since you loved me,
Since you thought of me.
Lord, while we praise and thank you,
we want to express you all our bliss in knowing, feeling, seeing
that you are with us, that you guide us, that you live among us.
Lord of our tears,
we praise you and thank you.
As we know that tears,
as our way of being.
In order to get nearer to you,
to feel you,
to be more and more clear minded,
to appreciate you with our heart,
to feel you with our soul,
to rejoice in you with our spirit.
Lord of our tears,
we ask you to turn them into tears of joy,
when we are able to hear your voice and see your face,
when at the end of the life path that leads to you,
we will be able to hug you and live with you forever outside time,
outside space,
in a world that we cannot even imagine,
not even with the most fervent fantasy.
Lord of our tears,
turn them into tears of joy,
turn them into tears of love,
for the consciousness of being together with you,
feeling you inside our heart
while you lead our soul to be always closer

to the reasons of the spirit.
Lord of all our moments,
we praise you and thank you for the consciousness
that each moment we lived with you is a step that leads us always higher
along the path towards you.
So we humbly ask you
to warm our heart,
to strengthen our soul,
to cultivate, as a precious flower, our spirit,
so that we can be warmed by your heart,
we can be strengthened in our soul by your word,
we can be cultivated in our spirit by your thought,
that thought that created us and thus wanted us inside time and space,
so to come up to you closer and closer,
you who love the planet earth,
who love all nations,
who love each single ethnic group,
who love each of us.
Lord of our illusions,
we humbly ask you to see that our illusions
may be canceled,
so that you can remain the only and prime reason for us,
that we can absorb your energy,
we can see your light,
we can feel your light,
we can appreciate the bliss that only you can give
to the heart, to the soul, and to the spirit,
that we can feel you, as our only starting point,
our only point of far-off arrival,
each of us, from the illusion that our society creates on this planet.
Lord of our illusions,
see that we all, and each of us, do not get lost in the illusions
that our world can give.
Lord of our illusions,
see that they do nott become
just great disappointments
because in this way the illusions of our society
make of us disappointed and depressed beings, because these illusions take
away,
day after day, the energy of the heart, the energy of the soul,
the energy of the spirit, until we become always more depressed,
always more disappointed beings.
Lord of our illusions,
here assembled in your name,

we all praise and thank you
for all the advice you give us every day.
Therefore, we pray you to see that
we do not become disappointed in our same illusions.
However, instead we try to overcome our illusions
in order to enter your world and your will
so that we become more and more full of energy
in our heart, in our soul, in our spirit
that we can obtain overcoming our illusions in your name
and trying to fulfill, day after day, only your will
so that we too
can become beings satisfied for your joy, for your energy, for your will.
Lord of our illusions,
help us.
We are conscious that you only will never disappoint anyone,
that you only can give the right energy to overcome the problems of the heart,
to overcome our illusions, so that we enter your world
that give us a new life, a life without illusions,
therefore, without disappointments.
Lord of our happiness,
we thank you because we are conscious,
through all that you give us,
that it is impossible to obtain the true happiness without you.
Lord of our personal happiness,
each of us humbly asks you to see that
each of us can follow your will always and anyway,
so that we can obtain the happiness of the heart, of the soul, and of the spirit,
even if we are conscious that
we cannot obtain it in this world,
however, only going up just one step
in the path that leads to you.
Therefore, we humbly ask you to give us the strength of will
to follow your will always and anyhow,
even if apparently
alternatively, strongly in contrast with ours,
with our own or with the collective one.
Lord of our happiness,
as we are conscious that in this world, it is never possible
to obtain it fully neither through our heart, nor trough our soul, nor trough our spirit,
while we humbly praise and thank you,
we ask you to give us at least
just a moment of happiness that you only can give,
a moment of happiness of heart,

a moment of happiness of soul,
a moment of happiness of spirit,
as, for instance, in this particular moment in which
we completely immerse ourselves deep in you, with all our senses,
the normal and the hidden ones,
we completely immerse ourselves deep in you,
with the feelings of our heart,
with the moments of gratitude of our soul,
with all can exalt our spirit.
Lord of our happiness,
we completely immerse ourselves deep in you,
we trust you and your will,
trying to penetrate, as far as possible for a human being,
your way of being, in order to be better immersed in the only bliss,
that you can give whom approach you in this way,
with heart, with soul, with spirit.
We feel quite near you, Lord, in this way, we feel you ours,
we feel between us, and we are always more willing and conscious
to follow your will always and anyhow.
Lord,
help our heart to feel you more.
Help our minds to be on the same wavelength as yours.
Help our spirit to enter you in order to be fortified
until we follow the path that leads to you
each moment of our life.
From your immensity,
Lord,
you looked at me,
and I felt comforted,
and I could arise my eyes up to you.

F. The Breathing Exercises

The Techniques of Deep Breathing

A technique that is usually taught in both passive concentration meditation and hypnosis, classes alike that can instantly reduce stress, is called deep breathing–breathing exercises.

Anytime during the day or evening, if you feel overwhelmed, anxious, or stressed in any way, it would be extremely beneficial to just stop for a moment and take five to ten deep, relaxing breaths. We all started out our life doing deep breathing, but as we got older, some, because of certain factors in their life, switch over to shallow breathing. So, if you want to look at it as relearning the type of breathing you did when first born, then do so, because as an unknowledgeable newborn baby, you came into this world knowing at the subconscious level or soul level what was best for your survival. If you have difficulty in doing deep breathing, try it while lying down. The more you do it, the more it will become automatic, and the need to consciously think about it will eventually be gone.

The Pranayama

Vialatte and colleagues (2009) discovered EEG paroxysmal gamma waves during Bhramari Pranayama: the yoga breathing technique. The Pranayama can be obtained with a great and constant training aimed at a persistent and progressive control of the respiration until one is able to keep it calm, deep, quiet and regular with two or three respirations per minute. "When the Breath wanders, the mind is unsteady, but when the Breath is still, so is the mind still" (Hatha Yoga Pradipika).

Breathing is life. It is one of our most vital functions. One of the Five Principles of Yoga is Pranayama or Breathing Exercise, which promotes proper breathing. From a yogic point of view, proper breathing is to bring more oxygen to the blood and to the brain and to control prana or the vital life energy.

Pranayama Yoga also goes hand in hand with the asanas. The union of these two yogic principles is considered as the highest form of purification and self-discipline, covering both mind and body.

Breathe:

Hold the posture, but try not to tense up. Breathe.

As you inhale, imagine the breath coming up through the floor, rising through your legs and torso and up into your head.
Reverse the process on the exhale and watch your breath as it passes down from your head, through your chest and stomach, legs and feet.
Hold for five to ten breaths, relax . . . and repeat.
On your next inhale, raise your arms over head (Urdhava Hastasana, Upward Salute)
and hold for several breaths.
Lower your arms on an exhale.
As a warm up, try synchronizing the raising and lowering of your arms with your breath . . . raise, inhale; lower, exhale.

Repeat five times.

The Corpse–Savasana

Possibly the most important posture, the Corpse, also known as the Sponge, is as deceptively simple as Tadasana, the Mountain pose. It relaxes and refreshes the body and mind, relieves stress and anxiety, quiets the mind. Usually performed at the end of a session, the goal is conscious relaxation. Many people find the "conscious" part the most difficult, because it is very easy to drift off to sleep while doing Savasana.

> Begin by lying on your back, feet slightly apart, arms at your sides with palms facing up.
> Close your eyes and take several slow, deep breaths.
> Allow your body to sink into the ground.
> Try focusing on a specific part of the body and willing it to relax.
> For example, start with your feet and imagine the muscles and skin relaxing, letting go, and slowly melting into the floor.
> From your feet, move on to your calves, thighs and so on up to your face and head.
> Then simply breathe and relax.
> Stay in the pose for at least 5 to 10 minutes.

In this specific modified state, it is possible to live differently the flow of time, getting close to the flow of the rhythms, of the Great Cosmic Time.

The passive concentration state, particularly needs long-term memory, in addition to short-term memory. This kind of memory is fixed on groups of cortical and subcortical neurons or some programs active in our brain since the first two or three years of life.

Meditative Self-Hypnosis: "The Seven-Minute Practice"

- First Minute:

  Connecting ourselves to our inner self
  through the awareness of our breathing . . .
  Putting our attention on it . . . attention . . . or passive concentration.

- Five Minutes:

  Let's stay like this . . . breathing . . .
  paying attention to it . . . without effort . . . naturally.
  When something distracts us, a thought, a sound, a voice far away,
  without effort, naturally we return our attention on our breathing,
  observing it . . .
  Inhaling and exhaling each time we distance ourselves,

we gently return to it,
so the saying goes
"Hundred times I fall and one hundred and one times I get up."

- Seven Minutes:

Let's widen our awareness of ourselves . . .
and the universe . . .
so our breathing
is the breathing of the whole world . . .
So our meditation benefits all other human beings.

3. DEEP CONCENTRATION: TYPES AND TECHNIQUES

It is in deep sleep, in circular sleep with paradoxical thought (i.e., in the NREM sleep), in the state of medium self-hypnosis, or even in deep hypnosis that deep concentration prevails.

At this level the activity of the right-brain hemisphere prevails over that of the left one.

A light or medium state of self-hypnosis, with the consequent loss of the awareness of the flow of time, and the activity of the right-brain hemisphere make the achievement of this state easier. We also find, at this point, the beginning of an active participation of the subconscious.

A. The Deep Sleep

Since the early twentieth century, human sleep has been described as a succession of five recurring stages: four NREM stages and the REM stage. Stages III and IV are deep sleep stages, with stage IV being more intense than stage III is. These stages are known as SWS, or delta sleep. During SWS, especially during stage IV, the EMG records slow waves of high amplitude, indicating a pattern of deep sleep and rhythmic continuity.

What exactly is the difference between REM and NREM sleep? REM dreams and NREM dreams are very different from each other in a few major ways. The first difference between the two is that NREM dreams consist of brief, fragmentary impressions. They are also less likely to involve visual images compared to REM sleep and are more frequently forgotten. NREM dreams are like thinking about something during the day for a brief period of time, whereas REM dreams are comparable to thinking deeply about something. REM sleep consists of about two hours a night, whereas NREM sleep lasts about four to six hours.

Delta waves are produced from the brain in the third stage of sleep. These brain waves become slower when the sleep cycle begins. During this cycle, your heart rate, blood pressure, and arousal decline (NREM sleep). Stage IV is very similar to stage III because delta waves continue in the brain. During this stage of sleep, most dreams and nightmares occur (NREM sleep).

Stages III and IV are the SWS stages (deepest sleep). Your brain waves slow down tremendously. These are called delta waves. These two stages last a total of 30 to 40 minutes on top of your first sleep cycle.

During stage III your breathing becomes very slow and your heart rate slowly drops. Your brain generates stronger electrical impulses than the impulse it produces while you are awake. Stage III is the stage you are in when it takes a great deal to wake you up. Most of your dreaming takes place in this stage. Your body can not move; it is temporarily paralyzed. This is why you sometimes feel that you cannot run or scream in a nightmare, because the sleeping brain believes what it sees. This stage is where dreaming and REM sleep occur.

Stage IV is the deepest level of sleep, and your brain during this period will show large, slow EEG waves. Certain hormones and chemicals are released into the body, growth hormones are one of them. Teenagers need more stage IV sleep than older people do. Once you get over the age 70, stage IV sleep may disappear from your sleep cycle. This stage gets shorter and shorter as your rest cycle continues, and by the end of your cycle, stage IV may not exist any more. Once stage four has been reached, we descend back through stages III, II, and I before beginning REM sleep.

B. Extreme Thoughts: A Clear Mind, The Flow State

Our right brain (unlike our left, reasoning brain) is intuitive and nonreasoning and deals with ethereal matters. Extreme thoughts are right brain or intuitive mind. How can we foster a clear intuitive mind? A mind with no thoughts? A total sensing mind? The body's internal network of sensory receptors provides us with proprioception (awareness of the precise position of our body) and kinesthesia (the awareness of direction of movement) that combined function as a sixth sense, allowing us to know where we are in space and time. On yet another energy level (the spiritual), we become aware of influences and information through intuition. When we lay the groundwork for a spiritual connection to one another and to the inner self, we sharpen these higher senses of receptivity. Intuition is our greatest link to our higher selves (our spiritual selves).

How do we know when we are receiving intuitive information? How do we discern that particular type of information from the thousands of impulses we receive every day? As with the different types of information experienced by individuals, confirmations of intuition come to us in a variety of ways.

The Flow State

Flow is the mental state of consciousness in which the person is fully immersed in what he or she is doing by a feeling of energized focus, full involvement, and success in the process of the activity. Proposed by Mihály Csíkszentmihályi, the positive psychology concept has been widely referenced across a variety of fields. Colloquial terms for this or similar mental states include to be in the "zone." The concept of "being in the zone" during a performance fits within Csíkszentmihályi's description of the flow experience. We consider flow in terms of challenge level and skill level.

Csíkszentmihályi identifies the following factors as accompanying an experience of flow. According to Csíkszentmihályi (1975, 1997; Csíkszentmihályi & Rathunde, 1993), the components of flow are

- *Clear goals.* Expectations and rules are discernible and goals are attainable and align appropriately with one's skill set and abilities. Moreover, the challenge level and skill level should both be high.
- *Concentrating and focusing.* A high degree of concentration on a limited field of attention. A person engaged in the activity will have the opportunity to focus and to delve deeply into it.
- *A loss of the feeling of self-consciousness.* The merging of action and awareness.
- *Distorted sense of time.* One's subjective experience of time is altered.
- *Direct and immediate feedback.* Successes and failures in the course of the activity are apparent, so that behavior can be adjusted as needed.
- *Balance between ability level and challenge.* The activity is neither too easy nor too difficult.
- *A sense of personal control over the situation or activity.*
- *The activity is intrinsically rewarding.* There is an effortlessness of action.
- *People become absorbed in their activity.* Focus of awareness is narrowed down to the activity itself, action awareness merging.

Not all are needed for flow to be experienced.

For millennia, practitioners of Eastern religions such as Hinduism, Buddhism, and Taoism have honed the discipline of overcoming the duality of self and object as a central feature of spiritual development. Eastern spiritual practitioners have developed a very thorough and holistic set of theories around overcoming duality of self and object, tested and refined through spiritual practice instead of the systematic rigor and controls of modern science.

The phrase "being at one with things" is an example of Csíkszentmihályi's flow concept. Practitioners of the varied schools of Zen Buddhism apply concepts similar to flow to aid their mastery of art forms, including, in the case of Japanese Zen Buddhism, Aikido, Cheng Hsin, Kendo, and Ikebana. In yogic traditions such as Raja Yoga, reference is made to a state of "flow" in the practice of Samyana, a psychological absorption in the object of meditation.

When I write, I feel out of control in a lovely way. The analogy that comes to mind is flow: a heightening of senses, a rush, no concept of time, a dimming of the external world, an altered state in which creation is the unconscious though central intent.

A flow state is, in many ways, the opposite of being stressed. Instead of feeling pressured, self-conscious, oppressed by time or out of sync, this is a great "zone" in which what you are doing feels natural with great results. The term describes the highest achievements of athletes, musicians, writers, spiritual gurus, masters in practically every field of activity. Most people, in fact, have found themselves in this state of mind at some point, and it is not as hard to bring about as it might seem.

The Technique to Find a Flow State

- Focus completely on what you are doing. That means doing whatever you have to so that distractions are not on your mind. Pay attention to the results you are getting and not your role in the process.
- Recreate the flow state by repeating the same steps. Each time you practice your activity and think about how exactly you did it so well when you are finished, should make finding that flow state easier. This builds the trust in yourself needed to let go of your self-consciousness and put that awareness in a more rewarding place—on the thing you want to do well.

C. Medium Self Hypnosis
and
D. Deep Hypnosis

The Deep Concentration in Hypnosis and Self-Hypnosis

During these stages, medium self-hypnosis is as deep as deep hypnosis is, because in self hypnosis, awareness of your immediate surroundings decreases faster, and you lose the awareness of space and time.

In this stage we can observe

- decreased awareness of immediate surroundings
- very deep breathing
- suggestions are best received
- partial or total amnesia of hypnotic events
- depersonalisation, disappearance of self
- analgesia or anesthesia
- external awareness periodically closing down

Deep Hypnosis and Anesthesia in Pain Therapy

When a state of deeper hypnosis is achieved through different techniques, the patient is trained as to how to interpret the feeling of pain coming from a specific place in the body and to transform it slowly from a feeling of pain to a feeling of different nature, for example light or medium tension, moderate pressure, beneficial warmth, or a cold sensation of anesthetizing nature.

Example of Anesthesia

While in a state of relaxation, you can imagine immersing your hand in a container of melting ice cubes . . .
and from the wrist up to the tip of your fingers the ice acts on your hand like a very powerful anaesthetic . . . making it feel more and more insensitive . . .
You will feel your hand becoming more and more insensitive . . .
and the anaesthesia will increase . . .
You will also know that the anaesthesia will last until you repeat to yourself three times:
"Everything is normal."

Other techniques of deep self-hypnosis are in Chapter IV.

The ability of bringing up the meditation object of concentration to the point of access concentration and self-hypnosis just before absorption involves the building up of the mental factors of concentration skillfully, so that it becomes powerful enough to fall into absorption.

E. Meditative Stages of Contemplation and Mindfulness

Factors in Development of Deep Concentration and Contemplation

Sabom (1982) summarized a similar set of core consciousness experiences:

- a mind's "separation" from the physical body
- a dark region or void
- a brilliant source of light
- a transcendental environment
- the nearness of some other personage
- a life review
- a return to the physical body

Some important factors in development of deep concentration and contemplation are given below.

Mindfulness

As the main controlling faculty of the mind, mindfulness is of course indispensable. It brings the mind to the point of concentration skillfully. It also guards against defilements and extraneous thoughts. Then it causes us to take the appropriate action to remedy them. It also keeps the mind flexible, workable, soft, and so on.

Therefore, there must be plenty of mindfulness at various depths of consciousness. It will, however, have to be that suited to the tranquility form of concentration and not the insight form. In tranquility meditation, the concentration faculty is comparatively much stronger than is the energy faculty, and so its unique balance has to be maintained. It has also to be continuous.

Detachment

Right concentration is often referred to as concentration detached from the five senses. We can understand this if we know that our object is solely that of the mind door. Its concentration is that above the five sense doors. If we still have rampant cravings for sense pleasures, we can never get near the absorptions. If one is really detached, however, then it lifts one off from the valleys of the five senses. Detachment has the power to remove the bondages that tie us to the lower worlds. When deep concentration comes with pleasantness and joy, the detached attitude is an important consideration.

Patience

Patience is the opposite of impatience or anger, which are associated with agitation. If we preserve patience, our mind by itself will calm down. In this case, patience is synonymous with the undisturbed aspect of tranquility. It can remain with the object for longer periods of time, for with nonanger there follows equanimity, another factor of concentration. The corresponding stage in Christianity is "contemplation."

During the contemplation phase it is always necessary to be in a "passive mental position in front of God," so that He can enter in our heart. For this reason, the heart must be free from all our ambitions. It is indeed essential "to free the heart from whatever is unnecessary." Otherwise, God cannot bring His light in after the dark night of the renunciation of the common realizations of life.

Contemplation is a state similar to hypnosis or to light or medium self-hypnosis, with a prevailing activity of the right-brain hemisphere.

During the phase of ecstasy, God inundates our heart with love with a consequent feeling "real presence." We are aware that the energy that we receive is transformed into further information that then transforms itself into knowledge, consciousness, and awareness. Therefore, every moment in our life becomes of interest about who we are and where we are, becomes a joy of living and participating to the whole universe of life, and becomes minute by minute a moment of life in a "continuum time space" that will adapt and expand to the infinite within ourselves and in the macrocosm.

4. SUPERIOR CONCENTRATION (HIGHER CONSCIOUSNESS): TYPES AND TECHNIQUES

A. Medium to Deep Self-Hypnosis: Annulment of the Normal Consciousness

The path to the consciousness, the knowledge, the awareness and, in the end, to the spiritual awareness always depends from person to person, and has unique and particular characteristics. Every human being is unique in all aspect of physical, mental, and spiritual being. The annulment of the normal consciousness it is prevailing in the state of medium to deep self-hypnosis.

Time and space disappear, and we live in a particular world in which we live experiences indescribable with everyday words.

The hypnotic state is inconsistent, and changes with each individual. Changes in the hypnotic state occur in relation to a person's own experience and his or her reactions to the ongoing experience of hypnosis and its induction in relation to time, the people involved, the purposes being served, and the ongoing situation. Past studies have found that most subjects seem to respond much better to internal fixations on personally imagined object or sounds (intrapsychic behavior).

Another important factor to consider as mentioned earlier is time. Some subjects enter hypnosis quickly: others may take a great deal of time. Milton Erickson notes that on average a total of four to eight hours of hypnotic induction training is required for most subjects. Along the same lines, certain trance-induced behavior, such as the ability to speak while in a deep trance, could take countless hours of training. Such abilities require learning because subjects might yet have no understanding or realization that it is possible to speak at an unconscious level of awareness. When functioning at a deep trance level, subjects perform with unconscious understandings, independent of ordinary conscious responses. Things are taken in a literal sense, and external realities are relevant only as utilized within the hypnotic experience. Erickson has conceptualized the deep trance as somnambulistic and stuporous, hence his description of deep hypnosis: "Deep hypnosis is the level of hypnosis that permits subjects to function adequately and directly at an unconscious level of awareness without interference by the conscious mind."

Charles T. Tart said, "I think we can expand the scientific framework to take in most of the humanistic phenomena, maybe all. For instance if I say that by a certain kind of Yoga breathing exercise, I can reach a state of ecstasy, that is basically a scientifically testable statement. I've said, here's a condition, you breathe in a certain way. Here's an observable outcome: somebody says–I've got this kind of an ecstatic experience" (Tart, 1970). Through medium self-hypnosis and deep hypnosis, we can experiment with higher consciousness.

B. The Higher Consciousness

Who or what we perceive ourselves to be in any given moment directly affects what we think and believe in the world, the goals and interests we pursue, and every aspect of our spiritual lives. During Transcendental Meditation (TM) techniques, the mind effortlessly attends to a specific object and automatically transcends the normal boundaries of conscious perception, experiencing a shift from active, waking consciousness to one without boundaries—pure consciousness. Past research suggests that the TM technique produces a state of profound rest and relaxation in subjects. Objectively, measurements of blood chemistry, skin galvanic response, and EEG recordings while subjects are practicing the technique indicate profound changes occur in the physiology. Subjectively, subjects report the experience of awareness alone without an object of perception (Arenander). This experience has been described as "restful alertness." It has also been described in some of the oldest known written records.

The Vedas, more than 5000 years old, are the classic texts describing this fundamental human experience. The Vedas call this experience of awareness, without an object of perception pure awareness. According to the Vedas, this state of restful alertness or transcendental consciousness is considered to be the fundamental mode or ground state of human conscious experience. Thought processes represent fluctuations of this underlying abstract, pure field of intelligence.

A model is proposed to explain the process of transcending that is based upon cognitive and neural mechanisms similar to the well-known orienting reflex. In this model, the state of restful alertness is produced by a coordinated response of orienting and habituating processes. The prefrontal cortex and the basal forebrain interact to produce a sequence of progressive de-excitations of neuronal activity, while conscious awareness is maintained. The brainstem core, in particular the mesencephalic reticular formation and the locus coeruleus, are suggested to be involved in maintaining awareness by producing orienting reflexes to the object of perception (stimulus) used in meditation at each stage in the sequence of de-excitation and generating global neural coherence. The regulation of attentional processes during transcending is via an integrated hierarchy of control converging on the thalamocortical system (Arenander).

The coherent integration of corticaltholamic processing loops would lead to a global state of neural integration corresponding to a transcendental state of awareness (Arenander). It is no wonder that we are continually evolving our understanding and awareness of the truth of who we are and our relationship with God as we wind our way down the path of self-realization.

When we are born, there is no sense of self, no sense of differentiation or separation from anything else in our awareness. As we grow older, we become identified with our bodies, personalities, families, and all of the thoughts and beliefs that make up our experience of life. As time progresses, we take on new identities: husbands and wives, mothers and fathers, managers, lawyers, office workers. As one begins to earnestly pursue a spiritual path, it is natural to question these roles and identities and try on new ones. As we move deeper and deeper into experiencing the truth of who we are—

beyond what we can see with our eyes, hear with our ears, or believe with our mind–the pursuit of a direct and personal experience with our True Nature begins to grow, until experiencing and knowing this true self eventually becomes the primary goal in our lives.

What Is Our Higher Consciousness?

There are many great words to describe who or what your highest identity or self truly is. Below are just a few:

- Higher consciousness
- Higher self
- I am presence
- Pure being
- Nonduality
- Love
- Spirit
- Essence of life
- Cosmic consciousness
- Universal mind
- Universal love
- The TAO
- God
- Christ
- Holy Spirit
- and the list goes on . . .

Depending on your spiritual path, background, or religious influence, you may be attracted to one or more of these terms. Ultimately, these words are only ideas that point to the unlimited and infinite nature of your true self. In the end, it does not matter which words you use. It is directly experiencing your higher self that you ultimately seek in your heart.

Cosmic Consciousness, Universal Mind, and Your Higher Self

Incorporating new beliefs about your higher self or true identity is an important aspect of spiritual growth, but no matter how powerful, inspiring, or life-changing these new ideas and beliefs may be, they eventually run out of steam because who you are is beyond thought or belief.

When one reaches this stage of desire and intention, developing a spiritual practice that can consistently restore you to a direct experience of your higher self becomes essential. One realizes that spiritual belief is essentially meaningless and hollow without a personal and direct experience of the divine.

There are countless practices in the world that serve the purpose of restoring your awareness to one of pure being. Ultimately, it does not matter which practice you choose, but choosing one and applying it consistently is what will lead you to a continual and ever-present state of enlightenment . . . the state of directly experiencing your self or God in every moment. The path that has led us to this direct experience of self on an ongoing basis, and that countless others share along with us, is the path of hearing God's voice within as a means of restoring our awareness to the truth of who we are in every moment.

It is possible to experience yourself as pure energy and consciousness. You can enter a period of deep meditation or deep hypnosis and temporarily put aside the limitations of body, mind, and emotions to transcend regular human limitations into infinite or universal consciousness. Certainly, this is one of the marvelous aspects of higher consciousness. Free of the mind's chatter or any negative emotion, your consciousness soars beyond mortality for a period of cosmic consciousness, as it is often called. You are able to experience the source of life in its essence. You are able to transcend form and float free in the formless and infinite realm of conscious energy that is profoundly wonderful. Experiences of this nature revivify your whole being.

Coming back from cosmic consciousness into bodily awareness, you find your mind is fresh with insights and intuitions. Your emotions are washed free and clean, and deep calmness and joy easily establish themselves in a renewed heart. Breathing and circulation seem to work better, and you marvel at your body's increased strength and coordination.

The higher self is the "you" inside of you, the living force that grows and changes in your body throughout your time on earth. It is the "you" behind all of the defenses and images you have created for yourself . . . the you that really knows why you are here, what it is you need, and how you can get it.

By transcending to your personal core–the higher self–you discover your true nature, a blissful self of infinite worth. The spiritual needs we all have for love, compassion, meaningfulness, total acceptance, devotion, and inner peace are not grand goals to be achieved in a distant time and place. They exist here and now and exert powerful influences on our lives. Only by transcending to the higher self can you achieve total, spontaneous fulfillment of these needs.

In The Higher Consciousness State, Through Hypnosis and Meditative States You Can

- eliminate fear and other obstacles to spiritual growth
- rejoin the stream of life through willingness and trust
- utilize more fully the true solver of problems–intuition
- untangle pain from suffering
- liberate your emotional body
- experience infinite worth
- learn to heal as a conscious activity
- establish a relationship with your personal and cosmic mind
- break the circular trap of addictions and find new pleasures that surpass them
- develop a quiet mind that can experience the truth of this new reality
- attain spontaneous right action

From Self-Hypnosis to Higher Consciousness and Awareness

Through hypnosis we can activate the concentrative mental stages that will help us to develop the mental energies toward the higher consciousness. People can experience the different stages of concentration through hypnosis, which needs to be achieved through a psychophysical concentration.

- Physical because it is necessary to learn slowly to inhibit the rationality of the cerebral cortex.
- Psychological in order to activate the limbic areas of the brain.

After you break the dominance of thoughts, awareness becomes quite easy and natural. In the alpha zone, you can balance focusing and awareness. You can be with the breath half the time and watch the stream for the rest. You still have to be vigilant, but as the body settles, you get even more freedom. It becomes possible to watch the show as a spectator. This is how focusing, which is so important at the start, gradually gives way to a tolerant and versatile awareness.

As you watch what flows downstream, you become familiar over time with its huge variety and the way it changes as you relax. This is actually "you." It is the texture and contents of your mind. You become able to watch every last thought, sensation, feeling, and image, just as it is, without being entranced by it. You also see how it connects causally; how a thought leads to a feeling, which leads to a response in the body, and often to action as well. These are some of the fruits of awareness that make it worth cultivating. It matches the Christian seventh phase, in other words, with the moment of the "annihilation of the normal consciousness." According to many authors, this means slowly learning how to "live with God." In other words, we live in a state of complete annihilation of our personality, having the feeling of living experiences taking place in a different time from the terrestrial time. A time that could be defined cosmic time or unified time.

The superior concentration is fulfilled in a state of medium or deep self-hypnosis with an appreciable increase of the subconscious activity. It is a modified state of consciousness, achievable when all the mental waves merge, without any kind of thoughts, without material experiences, out of time and space.

According to many Western and Eastern schools of philosophy, superoir concentration facilitates the long-term memory, with a consequent memory of past lives. It helps the accomplishment of karma, so one can free oneself from it definitively. It is specifically in this state of superior concentration and higher consciousness that the heart starts operating, of course along with both brain hemispheres. With the term heart we mean not the hydraulic pump of our body, but instead the complex of all our cells united in a physical and mental synchrony. When we experience the awareness, we will feel it for certain because we will experience a wave of inner joyful emotions: the physics and metaphysic level have become one.

This arrival at the state of awareness can be compared to what some call illumination, samadhi, ecstasy, or nirvana. It is not perfectly clear what ecstasy is; the word in any spiritual context indicates the sensation (along with a vivid desire) of transcending, at least for a moment, the normal condition of the consciousness in order to reach a type of experience set in a different time and in a different space.

Plutarch describee the predeath experience, which is often similar to certain states of deep hypnosis and meditative stages of contemplation. The person who is near death is, without reaching the limit of letting life go, experiences an initiatory situation, or a situation similar to ecstasy. Plutarch wrote,

> At the moment of death the soul experiences feeling similar to that experimented by people facing a mystery (the unknown). . . . At the beginning, you are feeling as if you were getting lost in circular movements following fearful tracks that won't take you anywhere. Before the last moment the fear, the shivering being frightened, the cold sweats everything is felt at the maximum. And then a wonderful light comes to the eyes; you go through wonderful places with lovely echoes of sound and sights of beautiful dance, holy words and images of divine nature inspire a religious respect. It is there where the initiated is now free from anything. He can walk around crowned with a garland, celebrating the party with the other pure souls, and he is looking from above towards the crowd of

those who are not initiated and not purified in the mud and in the darkness. (Plutarch, p. 168)

Studies of human evolution over the course of the centuries and millennia and the neurophysiological development of the brain and the mind can give us some help in providing medical therapy for the suffering of the body. They are of no help, however, for the emotional suffering, a therapy that we can learn through the path toward spiritual consciousness. It is therefore, important to study the expansion of the conscience to take us toward new horizons, especially in pain therapy and in palliative care.

At least we can agree that the only material life as we see it today has no reason to exist just on its own, because we are aware that there exists an entropic relationship between all of us, and we know that together we can follow the path of spiritual awareness.

C. Absorption

Many aspirants experience difficulty concentrating their attention and keeping it fixed on one point. Their minds tend to readily wander away from a focal point, even in bands of the conscious and subconscious mind, close to the surface of waking awareness. Going to profound states of absorption in the superconscious mind is extremely difficult for these beginning meditators. Spiritual teachers use seven primary methods for helping focus the attention of meditation students on the key inner centers of the ensouling entity, the spirit, and the attentional principle. In some cases, these methods may actively lock the attention of the meditator in an altered state of consciousness, for long periods of time.

Breathing Absorption

Called remembering the holy name, ajapa japa, or pranava laya in various traditions, the attention is kept focused on subtle aspects of breathing. The attention may be variously abstracted through these methods into the union with the attentional principle (mindfulness), with the self. We concentrate our attention into habitually remaining in a specific altered state of consciousness and identifying with it.

Contemplative Mantra

Called mantra japa, the attention is focused on the spirit by a contemplative mantra. The mantra is repeated by the attention, in contrast to speaking it aloud, whispering it, or breathing it. Different contemplative mantras may be used to focus the attention on varying octaves of the spiritual path.

Guru Mantra

Chanted aloud or silently within the mind, this transformation or bija mantra can become an unbroken focus on the attention, resulting in full identification with an altered state of awareness. Some gurus often use this method of control over the attention.

Prayer Without Ceasing

This method is used in the Christian faith to hold the mind in union with the soul. One form of this method is to repeat a ritual prayer such as The Lord's Prayer or Hail Mary continuously.

Light Immersion or Absorption

This method temporarily guides the attention to inner centers within the vehicles or into the union with the attentional principle, the spirit, or the entity by holding it in a ray or beam of light.

Some spiritual teachers do not favor the grounding of attention after the meditation experience but have the meditator remain absorbed in the focal point for extended periods of time. This leads to a state of detachment from normal personality functioning, a witnessing of the activity of the mind from a higher vantage point, and, often, identification with the focal point about the method used to control the attention.

These methods of sustained absorption facilitate the shunting or sublimating of energy from the personality and energy channels of the higher self. This may permit better control of passions and behavior from a higher stratum of the mind.

D. The Meditative Stages: Awareness, Contemplation and Ecstasy, Living With God

Dhyana

"Dhyana heyah tad vrttayah"
Dhyana means absorption in meditation
heyah means eliminate
tad means that or these
vrttayah means movements of the thought

The absorption in the meditation eliminates these movements from the thought about the pain. These thoughts or movements of pain are rejected and silenced by meditation. One eliminates these movements from the thought about the pain by absorption in the meditation. It is through the tools for learning meditation and absorption in meditation that movements of the thought of pain, which besiege the unconscious mind, are dispelled, rejected, avoided, or silenced. When elements of mental distress besiege the unconscious mind, they can be eliminated with the tools fore learning meditation and absorption in the meditation. When elements of mental distress become disgusting and operative, they can be dispelled with the tools for learning meditation and absorption in the meditation. Tools of the learning of meditation and absorption in the meditation destroy the unpleasant movements of the thought, which strangle the unconscious mind. There are some kinds of distress provoking pain, however. There are several causes underlying these pains and movements of the thought. Their main cause is lack of tools for learning meditation. So long as the causes leading to distress provoking movements of the thought do not get destroyed, the flow of distress provoking movements of the thought keep on undulating and swelling in the unconscious mind.

These movements of the thought keep on moving as ripples across the surface of the unconscious mind. The flow of pain provoking movements of the thought is of three kinds. It is in form, subtle, and subtlest. Such a flow keeps on floating on the unconscious mind, the conscious mind and the interior core of the conscious mind, respectively. So long as the disciple the unconscious mind, the conscious mind, and the interior core conscious mind does not experience the lack of tools for learning meditation, pain, and distress-provoking movements of the thought will not get destroyed. Further preparatory yogic discipline is of three kinds.

The yogic discipline consists if tools for learning meditation and absorption in the meditation in the conscious mind. This discipline entails perfection and disciplining of the yogic limbs of absorption in the meditation and spiritual union.

Patanjali says that with the perfecting and disciplining of the tools for learning meditation and absorption in the meditation, the flow of pain-provoking movements of the thought in their gross form gets destroyed. These movements of the thought however continue to remain in their subtle seed form.

These tools for learning meditation and absorption in the meditation occur when a disciple enters the final field of preparatory yogic discipline. It is only by the elimination of the seeds of pain-provoking movements of the thought of the unconscious mind that these movements of the thought get completely restrained and nullified. It is only by the restraint and nullification of movements of the thought that the mind gets deactivated from their activity. It is then that the stranglehold of subtlest nature essence on the concentration meditation and self-conscious of the soul gets broken.

It is then that the individual self-conscious of soul gets into the pure form. It is in this state that knowledge about realization of true self-conscious, soul, and God essence is realized. It is in this state that knowledge about birth and death of life of subtlest nature essence over self-conscious is realized. It is in this state that the liberation from birth and death of life of mind that is subtlest nature essence is attained.

From Maha-Satipatthana Sutta (DN 22.21)

And what is right meditation (sama-samadhi). There is the case where an aspirant, quite withdrawn from sensuality, withdrawn from unskillful (mental) qualities, enters and remains in the first jhana: joy and ecstasy born from withdrawal, accompanied by applied and sustained concentration (vitakka and vicára).

> With the stilling of applied and sustained concentration (vitakka and vicára), one enters and remains in the second jhana: joy and ecstasy born of tranquillity, unification of awareness free from directed applied and sustained concentration (vitakka and vicára), internal assurance.

> With the fading of joy one remains in equanimity, (aware) and alert, physically sensitive of ecstasy. One enters and remains in the third jhana, of which the Noble Ones declare, "Equanimous and (aware), one has a pleasurable abiding."

> With the abandoning of (grasping and aversion for) pleasure and pain – as with the earlier disappearance of pleasure and pain—one enters and remains in the fourth jhana: purity of equanimity and awareness, neither pleasure nor pain.

> This is called right meditation.

Higher consciousness and awareness are the idea of having a higher appreciation, knowledge of, and consciousness of your connection between the physical plane and the spiritual plane. When you are thoughtless awareness, when your brain is just in the state of witness, and you understand everything that is divine. Words do not exist to describe the state of awareness: the "I" disappears completely, the borderline between you and the rest of the world dissolving totally. Awareness is the pure expansion of the mind.

In his commentary of Patanjali's Yoga sutras, His Holiness Sri Sri Ravi Shankar says,

With spiritual growth, there is a keenness of observation. You become totally relaxed, yet at the same time you possess sharpness of awareness, strength of intelligence. Your senses become so clear. You can see better, think better, hear better. Like a pure crystal, your senses come to reflect all objects as one Divinity.

In the state of awareness, we think neither of the past nor of the future. We are entirely in the present moment, in the state of being and do not waste the precious moments of life, thinking about times that are finished forever or yet to come. We start enjoying our self, our spirit, our own inner beauty, and the beauty of creation. We start to enjoy being.

Contemplation and Ecstasy, Living With God

"I entered into unknowing,
and there I remained unknowing
transcending all knowledge." (St. John of the Cross)

"Lead me from the Unreal to the Real.
Lead me from darkness to Light.
Lead me from death to Immortality." (Brihadaranyaka Upanishad)

"Being and non-being create each other.
Difficult and easy support each other.
Long and short define each other.
High and low depend on each other.
Before and after follow each other." (Tao Te Ching, Verse 2)

5. TRUE CONCENTRATION OR AWARENESS ACTIVATION: TYPES AND TECHNIQUES

A. Awareness

Watch your consciousness closely, this feeling and sensation of being aware and alive, and observe what you feel. I do not mean that you look at the contents of your mind. I mean becoming fully aware and conscious of the sensation of being alive and existing. Some concentration ability is required to perform this simple exercise, because the mind and its thoughts will probably try to stand in your way. This consciousness I am referring to is not the awareness of having a body, emotions, or thoughts but of something beyond. Awareness is the state or ability to perceive; to feel; or to be conscious of events, objects, or sensory patterns. In this level of consciousness, sense data can be confirmed by an observer without necessarily implying understanding. More broadly, it is the state or quality of being aware of something.

Meditation for Inner Awareness

Begin this meditation by taking a few slow . . .
deep breaths . . .
breathing in peace and stillness with each breath . . .
and then slowing exhaling... releasing any tension . . . worry or irritation . . .
Now visualize the energy in you . . .
as a feeling of energy . . . rising upwards to you as you inhale . . .
See your center transmuting negative emotional feelings into positive . . .
loving feelings as you exhale . . .
loving feelings as you inhale . . .
loving feelings as you exhale . . .
Now inhale again . . .
this time visualizing the energy rising up from you . . .
and in the interlude before exhaling . . .
dedicate the energy to helping others in some way . . .
Then exhale . . .
visualizing the energy . . . flowing out . . .
through your throat center to release creativity and energy.
Repeat this sequence a few times . . .
seeing the energy rising all the way up to you . . .
and then lift your consciousness higher . . .
invoking your soul . . .
Invoke soul consciousness through your intention to align with it . . .
and by affirming the soul as your essential identity . . .
the presence of God within . . .
the presence of God in you . . .
the presence of you in God . . .
. . . Then hold the silence for 10 to 15 minutes . . .
. . . listening inwardly to the voice of your soul . . .
the still . . . small voice that provides inspiration and guidance for your life . . .
Close the meditation by visualizing love . . .
light and spiritual power . . .
flowing out to the world . . . to where it is most needed for peace . . .
healing and transformation . . .
Use your intention to direct your attention: practice consciously focusing your attention where you choose it to go.

Give conscious attention to something that is close to your heart, that you do not usually attend to because you think you have other more pressing or important things to deal with. Meditate daily to experience the joy in your soul and to receive inner guidance in your life. The life into the soul and awareness is a life of meaning. It imbues each gesture, thought, and deed with the full integrity of being that comes from conscious connection with the source of life. It infuses all responsiveness to life in the love that is part of this connection. "I was once spiritually ill , we all pass through that, but one day the intelligence in my soul cured me" (Meister Eckhart). This, then, is the beginning of soul awareness, an awareness founded in love and in the knowledge of the sacred oneness within which we draw breath.

Although for centuries a wakeful and tranquil state or experience variously called samadhi, pure awareness, or enlightenment has been said to be a normal experience and the goal of meditation in Vedic, Buddhist, and Taoist traditions, there was little known about this behavior until recently, when the practice of TM* became available for study in Western scientific laboratories. Derived from the Vedic tradition, TM is unique because it requires no special circumstances or effort for practice. Based on a wide spectrum of physiological data on TM, we can hypothesize that meditation is an integrated response with peripheral circulatory and metabolic changes subserving increased CNS activity. Consistent with the subjective description of meditation as a very relaxed but, at the same time, a very alert state, it is likely that such findings during meditation as increased cardiac output and probable increased cerebral blood flow and findings reminiscent of the "extraordinary" character of classical reports–apparent cessation of CO_2 generation by muscle, fivefold plasma AVP elevation, and EEG synchrony–play critical roles in this putative response (Jevning, Wallace & Beidebach, 1992). Outside of neuroscience, biologists Humberto Maturana and Francisco Varela contributed their Santiago theory of cognition, in which they wrote, "Living systems are cognitive systems, and living as a process is a process of cognition." This statement is valid for all organisms, with or without a nervous system (Capra, 1996). Lagopoulos and associates (2009) found increased theta and alpha EEG activity during nondirective meditation.

This theory contributes a perspective that cognition is a process present at organic levels that we do not usually consider to be aware. Given the possible relationship among awareness and cognition and consciousness, this theory contributes an interesting perspective in the philosophical and scientific dialogue of awareness and living systems theory.

This consciousness is your inner being, and there is nothing mysterious or mystical about it. We all experience this consciousness constantly but never investigate or try to be consciously and intently aware of it. This is

*TM = Transcendental Meditation.

because the mind and the attention flow outside, and rarely inside. You are this consciousness; it is your being, and you therefore need to know about it. You did not lose consciousness during this experience. It was a happy and joyous experience, in which you became aware of something beyond your ordinary awareness. Meditation deals with contacting the consciousness within us, which by its very nature is peaceful, calm, and rejuvenating. The whole universe is nothing but pure consciousness. Scientific researches have taken us up to the point where we can convincingly say that at the quantum level it is just the play of energy that is going on in the entire universe.

Everything has a mass and thus can be converted into energy. Remember the famous Einstein equation: $E = MC^2$. The spiritual world, however, is of the view that in the ultimate analysis, at a more deeper level (something still beyond even the reach of quantum physics), everything in the whole universe is pure consciousness, known also as supreme consciousness or God. It is just the play of this consciousness that is going on. The whole universe is a manifestation of this supreme consciousness.

B. Deep Self- Hypnosis
and
C. Contemplation and Mystical States Leading to Spiritual Enlightenment: Samadhi, Living in God

Hypnosis is often thought of as a mental state in which the conscious mind ceases analyzing the meanings of expressions and permits the hypnotist to directly chat with the subconscious mind. In this state of mind, one being is more responsive to another individual's words or feelings.

Drawing on the same "relaxation response" that drives meditation, self-hypnosis helps you to relax your body, lets stress hormones subside, and distracts your mind from unpleasant thoughts. The relaxation achieved with self-hypnosis can be intense. Unlike meditation, we often use affirmations as part of self-hypnosis to manage stress and build self-confidence. Affirmations are the positive statements (based on rational thinking) that we make to ourselves to counter stress and unpleasant thoughts.

Sometimes it is possible to reach a state of deep self-hypnosis after months or, better, years of constant training in every other state we have analyzed. Even then not everybody can completely achieve this last step. Developing the power of concentration and self-hypnosis, practicing meditation and trying to be aware of your awareness, consciousness, and being are the way to the golden key that opens the door of enlightenment. Spiritual enlightenment and spiritual awakening are the primary goal of almost all spiritual practices, traditions, and religions and for any spiritual seeker. There are many names for this awakened state of consciousness depending on what culture and tradition we belong to.

> A human being is a part of a whole, called by us universe, a part limited in time and space. He experiences himself, his thoughts and feelings as something separated from the rest . . . a kind of optical delusion of his consciousness. This delusion is a kind of prison for us, restricting us to our personal desires and to affection for a few persons nearest to us. Our task must be to free ourselves from this prison by widening our circle of compassion to embrace all living creatures and the whole of nature in its beauty. (Albert Einstein)

Looking for spiritual light is part of our purpose as soul for living in this world. The goal of spiritual enlightenment is the goal in life for every human being born on this earth, and it awaits each of us just over the horizon, in our own mind. Stay on the path until the goal is reached.

We can learn to follow the light of divine spirit, through the events of our lives. In Christianity, it corresponds to the eight steps of prayer. It is the moment of the enlightenment of the living in God, as it has been narrated from all the greatest Christian mystics of all times.

It is an experience we make out of time, without time or lived, according to the latest theories of modern physics (especially the ones related to the quantum mechanics and to the Anthropic Principle) in a unified time. It is conducted in a self-hypnosis state with the surfacing or emersion of subconscious contents. It is a state of "Immersion in the Absolute." In Buddhism and Hinduism, we are at the last step of meditation, the samadhi, the most elevated state a human being can reach.

Deep inside each of us, there is a space of pure happiness. Without stress. Without worry. Without illness. Only happiness. Each of us can connect with this divine space. It can be reached through the experience of the super-conscious through contemplation, through identification with the cosmos, through interior enlightenment with the dispersion of thought inside some kind of imagined contents. All that baggage of particular experiences very often originated from spontaneous visualizations.

The Tipitaka, the Buddhist canon, is replete with references to the factors of enlightenment. Further says the Buddha, "Just as, monks, in a peaked house all rafters whatsoever go together to the peak, slope to the peak, join in the peak, and of them all the peak is reckoned chief: even so, monks, the monk who cultivates and makes much of the seven factors of wisdom, slopes to Nibbana, inclines to Nibbana, tends to Nibbana." The seven factors are

1. Mindfulness (sati)
2. Keen investigation of the dhamma (dhammavicaya)

3. Energy (viriya)
4. Rapture or happiness (piti)
5. Calm (passaddhi)
6. Concentration (samadhi)
7. Equanimity (upekkha)

When concentrated on right thoughts, with right understanding, the effects the mind can produce are immense.

Let us now deal with the enlightenment factors, one by one. The first is sati, mindfulness. It is the instrument most efficacious in self-mastery, and whosoever practices it has found the path to deliverance. It is fourfold: mindfulness consisting in contemplation of the body (kayanupassana), feeling (vedananupassana), mind (cittanupassana), and mental objects (dhammanupassana). Right mindfulness or complete awareness, in a way, is superior to knowledge, because in the absence of mindfulness, it is just impossible for a person to make the best of his or her learning.

The second enlightenment factor is dhammavicaya, keen investigation of the dhamma. It is the sharp analytical knowledge of understanding the true nature of all constituent things, animate or inanimate, human or divine. It is seeing things as they really are. The whole universe is constantly changing, not remaining the same for two consecutive moments. All things in fact are subjected to causes, conditions, and effects. All things are impermanent. What is impermanent and not lasting we see as sorrow fraught. What is impermanent and sorrow fraught, we understand as void of a permanent and everlasting soul, self, or ego entity.

The third enlightenment factor is viriya, energy. It is a mental property (cetasika) and the sixth limb of the Noble Eightfold Path, there called sammavayama, right effort.

The fourth enlightenment factor is piti, rapture or happiness. This, too, is a mental property (cetasika) and is a quality that suffuses both the body and the mind. The person lacking in this quality cannot proceed along the path to enlightenment.

Passaddhi, calm or tranquility, is the fifth factor of enlightenment. Passaddhi is compared to the happy experience of a weary walker who sits down under a tree in a shade or the cooling of a hot place by rain. It is only when the mind is tranquillized and is kept to the right road of orderly progress that it becomes useful for the individual possessor of it and for society.

The sixth enlightenment factor is samadhi, concentration. It is only the tranquilized mind that can easily concentrate on a subject of meditation. Concentration is the intensified steadiness of the mind, comparable to an unflickering flame of a lamp in a windless place. It is concentration that fixes the mind aright and causes it to be unmoved and undisturbed.

The seventh and the last factor of enlightenment is upekkha, equanimity. In the Abhidhamma, upekkha is indicated by the term tatramajjhattata, neutrality. It is mental equipoise and not hedonic indifference. Equanimity is the result of a calm concentrative mind. It is hard, indeed, to be undisturbed when touched by the vicissitudes of life, but the person who cultivates this difficult quality of equanimity is not upset. Santideva writes in Bodhicarya-vatara,

> Some there be that loathe me; then why
> Shall I, being praised, rejoice?
> Some there be that praise me; then why
> Shall I brood over blaming voice?
> Who master is of self, will ever bear
> A smiling face; he puts away all frowns
> Is first to greet another, and to share
> His all. This friend of all the world, Truth crowns.

The goal in life is spiritual enlightenment to unite the conscious mind with the soul.

What is enlightenment? The act of enlightening is defined as "the act of enlightening or casting light where there was darkness." Spiritual enlightenment is pretty much what all spiritual studies strive for. It is the hope of anyone studying the topics within spirit and sky to come to this stage of being. Imagine understanding life, the universe, and everything? It is not likely anyone of us will achieve "total" spiritual enlightenment in our lifetimes, but many have and will at least gain partial enlightenment. Spiritual enlightenment is a universal subject and quite difficult to define. It actually refers to the concept of self-realization, which can be achieved by years of dedication, meditation, and spiritual growth. Self-realization is a Hindu concept of looking into one's inner self.

The correct spiritual path for you is the one that resonates with you, that helps you to become a better person, achieve a loving, whole feeling of being connected to everyone and everything, at peace inside and in tune with our true nature as spiritual beings.

When you seek a way to open your heart, to love all including yourself, and to feel your connection with life, you have started on your path toward spiritual enlightenment.

Consciousness is personalized energy that knows itself, and its abilities go far beyond human understandings. You soul is conscious energy in all its forms. The brain is a vital organ that facilitates the link between your mind and matter, yet without a brain the physically focused portions of your consciousness would become refocused elsewhere.

How you do that is of course up to you, there are many spiritual tools that you can use to lead you to experiencing your spiritual self. Meditation, yoga, clinical hypnosis and self-hypnosis, Reiki, spiritual churches, and more. There are many earth angels who will assist you on your spiritual journey, many books written to guide you, but ultimately listening to your intuition is at the very core of all of these processes. When you can intuitively listen and trust your internal guidance, then your life will take on a new dimension.

REFERENCES

Baddeley, A. (2003). Working memory: Looking back and looking forward. *Nature Reviews: Neuroscience, 4*(10), 829–839.

Baddeley, A. D., & Hitch, G. J. L. (1974). Working memory. In G. A. Bower (Ed.), *The psychology of learning and motivation: Advances in research and theory* (Vol. 8, pp. 47–89), New York: Academic Press.

Barsalou, L. W. (1999). Perceptual symbol systems. *Behavioral and Brain Sciences, 22,* 577–660.

Blackmore, S. (2003). *Consciousness: An introduction.* London: Hodder & Stoughton.

Bodizs, R., Sverteczki, M., Sandor Lazar, A., & Halasz, P. (2005). Human parahippocampal activity: non-REM and REM elements in wake-sleep transition. *Brain Research Bulletin, 65*(2), 169–176.

Capra, F. (1996). *The web of life: A new scientific understanding of living systems.* New York: Random House.

Csikszentmihalyi, M., & Rathunde, K. (1993). The measurement of flow in everyday life: Towards a theory of emergent motivation. In J. E. Jacobs (Ed.), *Nebraska Symposium on Motivation* (Vol. 40: Developmental perspectives on motivation, p. 60). Lincoln, NE: University of Nebraska Press.

Csikszentmihalyi, M. (1997). *Finding flow.* New York: Basic Books.

Csíkszentmihályi, M. (1975). *Beyond boredom and anxiety.* San Francisco, CA: Jossey-Bass.

Davidson, R. J., Kabat-Zinn, J., Schumacher, J., Rosenkranz, M., Muller, D., Santorelli, S. F., ..., & Sheridan, J. F. (2003). Alterations in brain and immune function produced by mindfulness meditation. *Psychosomatic Medicine, 65*(4), 564–570.

Davis, H., Davis, P. A., Loomis, A. L., Harvey, E. N., & Hobart, G. (1937). Changes in human brain potentials during the onset of sleep. *Science, 86,* 448–450.

Desimone, R., & Duncan, J. (1995). Neural mechanisms of selective visual attention. *Annual Review of Neuroscience, 18,* 193–222.

Erickson, M. H. (0000). *The collected papers of Milton H. Erickson, Vol. 1.*

Foulkes, D., & Schmidt, M. (1983). Temporal sequence and unit composition in dream reports from different stages of sleep. *Sleep, 6,* 265–280.

Foulkes, D., & Vogel, G. (1965). Mental activity at sleep onset. *Journal of Abnormal Psychology, 70,* 231–243.

Fukuda, K., & Vogel, E. K. (2009). Human variation in overriding attentional capture. *Journal of Neuroscience, 29,* 8726–8733.

Fuster, J. M. (1997). *The prefrontal cortex: Anatomy, physiology, and neuropsychology of the frontal lobe* (2nd ed.). Philadelphia: Lippincott, Williams & Wilkins.

Germaine, A., & Nielsen, T. A. (1997). Distribution of spontaneous hypnagogic images across Hori's EEG stages of sleep onset. *Sleep Research, 26,* 243.

Hori, T., Hayashi, M., & Morikawa, T. (1993). Topographical EEG changes and hypnagogic experience. In R. D. Ogilvie & J. R. Harsh (Eds.), *Sleep onset: Normal and abnormal processes* (pp. 237–253). Washington, DC: American Psychological Association.

James, W. (1890). *The principles of psychology* (Vol. 1). New York: Henry Holt.

Kabat-Zinn, J., Lipworth, L., & Burney, R. (1985). The clinical use of mindfulness meditation for the self-regulation of chronic pain. *Journal of Behavioral Medicine, 8*(2), 163–190.

Kaiser, J., & Lutzenberger, W. (2003). Induced gamma-band activity and human brain function. *Neuroscientist, 9,* 475–484.

Knudsen, E. I. (2007). Fundamental components of attention. *Annual Review of Neuroscience, 30*(1), 57–78.

Lazar, S. W., Bush, G., Gollub, R. L., Fricchione, G. L., Khalsa, G., & Benson, H. (2000). Functional brain mapping of the relaxation response and meditation. *NeuroReport, 11*(7), 1581–1585.

Leaning, F. E. (1925). An introductory study of hypnagogic phenomena. *Proceedings of the Society for Psychical Research.*

Leroy, E. B. (1933). *Les visions du demi-sommeil.* Paris: Alcan.

Maquet, P., Laureys, S., Peigneux, P., Fuchs, S., Petiau, C., Phillips, C., ..., Cleeremans, A. (2000). Experience-dependent changes in cerebral activation during human REM sleep. *Nature Reviews: Neuroscience, 3,* 831–836.

Nielsen, T., Germain, A., & Ouellet, L. (1995). Atonia-signalled hypnagogic imagery: Comparative EEG mapping of sleep onset transitions, REM sleep, and wakefulness. *Sleep Research, 24,* 133.

Ospina, M. B., Bond, K., Karkhaneh, M., Tjosvold, L., Vandermeer, B., Liang, Y., ... & Klassen, T. P. (2007). Meditation practices for health: State of the research. *Evidence Report/Technology Assessment (Full Report), June* (155), 1–263.

Owen, A. M. (1997). The functional organization of working memory processes within human lateral frontal cortex: The contribution of functional neuroimaging. *European Journal of Neuroscience, 9,* 1329–1339.

Pattyn, N., Neyt, X., Henderickx, D., & Soetens, E. (2008). Psychophysiological investigation of vigilance decrement: boredom or cognitive fatigue? *Physiology & Behavior, 93,* 369–378.

Perez-De-Albeniz, A., & Holmes, J. (2000). Meditation: Concepts, effects and uses in therapy. *International Journal of Psychotherapy, 5*(1), 49–59.

Pfotenhauer, H., & Schneider, S. (2006). *Nicht völlig wachen und nicht ganz ein Traum: Die Halbschlafbilder in der Literatur.* Verlag Königshausen & Neumann.

Rechtschaffen, A., & Kales, A. (1968). *A manual of standardized terminology, techniques and scoring system for sleep stages of human subjects.* Washington, DC: Public Health Service, U.S. Government Printing.

Schacter, D. L. (1976). The hypnagogic state: A critical review of the literature. *Psychological Bulletin, 83,* 452–481.

Sohlberg, M. M., & Mateer, C. A. (1989). *Introduction to cognitive rehabilitation: Theory and practice.* New York: Guilford Press.

Tart, C. T. (1972). States of consciousness and state-specific sciences. *Science, 176,* 1203–1210.

Vaitl, D., Birbaumer, N., Gruzelier, J., Jamieson, G. A., Kotchoubey, B., Kübler, A., ... & Weiss, T. (2005, January). Psychobiology of altered states of consciousness. *Psychological Bulletin, 131*(1), 98–127.

Vertes, R. (2004). Memory consolidation in sleep dream or reality. *Neuron, 44,* 135–148.

Yantis, S., & Jonides, J. (1990). Abrupt visual onsets and selective attention: Voluntary versus automatic allocation. *Journal of Experimental Psychology. Human Perception and Performance, 16*(1), 121–134.

SUGGESTED READINGS

Alcock, J. E. (1979). Psychology and near-death experiences. *Skeptical Inquirer, 3*(3), 25–41.

Amorim, M-A., Isableu, B., & Jarraya, M. (2006). Embodied spatial transformations: body analogy for the mental rotation. *Journal of Experimental Psychology: General, 135*(3), 327–347

Anderson, J. R. (2004). *Cognitive psychology and its implications* (6th ed.). New York: Worth Publishers.

Antonelli, F. (1970). *Elementi di Psicosomatica.* Toroni, Italy: Rizzoli.

Arieti, S. (1979). *Creatività la sintesi magica.* Italy: Il Pensiero Scientifico.

Atkinson, R. C., & Shiffrin, R. M. (1968). Human memory: A proposed system and its control processes. In K. W. Spence & J. T. Spence (Eds.), *The psychology of learning and motivation* (Vol. 2, pp. 89–195). New York: Academic Press.

Attention. (2009). In *Encyclopædia Britannica.* Retrieved August 14, 2009, from Encyclopædia Britannica Online: http://www.britannica.com/EBchecked/topic/42134/attention

Austin, J. H. (1999). *Zen and the brain: Toward an understanding of meditation and consciousness.* Cambridge, MA: First MIT Press paperback edition.

Balbi, R. (1981). *Lungo viaggio al centro del cervello.* Mondadori.

Barendregt, H. P. (1988). Buddhist phenomenology. In *Atti del Congresso Temi e prospettive della logica e della filosofia della scienza contemporanea.* (Cesena 1987. Vol. 11, pp. 37–55). CLUEB, Bologna.

Bartolomeo, P. (2002). The relationship between visual perception and visual mental imagery: A reappraisal of the neuropsychological evidence. *Cortex, 38*(3), 357–378.

Bechert, H., & Gombrich, R. (Eds.). (1984). *The world of Buddhism*. London: Thames & Hudson.

Benedetti, G. (1969). *Neuropsicologia*. Feltrinelli.

Bertoletti, P. (1986). *Mito e Simbolo*. Dedalo.

Bettelheim, B. (1977). *Il mondo incantato*. Feltrinelli.

Biondi, M. (1984). I 4 canali del rapporto mente-corpo:dalla psicofisiologia dell'emozione alla psicosomatica scientifica. *Med Psic, 29,* 421–456.

Blackmore, S. (1998). Abduction by aliens or sleep paralysis? *Skeptical Inquirer, 22,* 23–28.

Bódizs, R., Sverteczki, M., & Mészáros, E. (2008). Wakefulness-sleep transition: Emerging electroencephalographic similarities with the rapid eye movement phase. Available at http://www.sciencedirect.com/science/article/B6SYT-4RCN8CP-1/2 /eee96a80f27593096fdace6bb9fce440

Bower, B. (2007, September 15). Consciousness in the raw: The brain stem may orchestrate the basics of awareness [Online]. *Science News*.

Brugnoli, A. (2004). *Stato di coscienza totalizzante, alla ricerca del profondo Se*. Verona, Italy: La Grafica Editrice.

Brugnoli, A. (2005). *Stati di coscienza modificati neurofisiologici*. Verona, Italy: La Grafica Editrice.

Brugnoli, M. P. (2001). Neurofisiologia di realtà percepita e realtà rappresentata: quale relazione tra working memory e visualizzazione mentale in ipnosi. *Acta Hypnologica, 3,* 21–22.

Brugnoli, M. P. (2002). Rilassamento ed ipnosi in età evolutiva. *Acta Hypnologica, 1,* 8–14.

Brugnoli, M. P. (2004). Tecniche di rilassamento e ipnosi nel controllo della sofferenza del paziente terminale. *Acta Hypnologica, 7*(1-2), 3–14.

Brugnoli, M. P. (2009). *Tecniche di rilassamento e ipnosi clinica in terapia del dolore e cure palliative* [*Clinical hypnosis, spirituality and palliation: The way of inner peace*]. Verona, Italy: Del Miglio Editore.

Brugnoli, M. P., Brugnoli, A., & Norsa, A. (2009). *Nonpharmacological and noninvasive management in pain: Physical and psychological modalities*. Verona, Italy: La Grafica Editrice.

Brugnoli, M. P., & Shivchandra Parolini, M. (2009). *La via della pace interiore: tecniche di rilassamento e di meditazione per il benessere dell'anima*. Verona, Italy: Del Miglio Editore.

Buswell, R. E. (Ed.). (2003). *Encyclopedia of Buddhism*. New York: Macmillan Reference Books.

Cahn, B. R., & Polich, J. (2006). Meditation states and traits: EEG, ERP, and neuroimaging studies. *Psychological Bulletin, 132*(2), 180–211.

Charon, J. E. (2004). *The spirit: That stranger inside us*. Califormula Publishing.

Cheyne, J. A. (2003). Sleep paralysis and the structure of waking-nightmare hallucinations. *Dreaming, 13*(3), 163–179.

Cohen, A., & Rafal, R. D. (1991). Attention and feature integration. *American Psychological Society, 2*(2), 106–110.

Cohen, M. X. (2011, January). It's about time. *Frontiers in Human Neurosciences, 19*(5), 2.

Coogan, M. D. (Ed.). (2003). *The illustrated guide to world religions.* New York: Oxford University Press.

Coren, S., Ward, L. M., & Enns, J. T. (1999). *Sensation and perception.* New York: Harcourt Brace.

Cowan, N. (1995). *Attention and memory: An integrated framework.* New York: Oxford University Press.

Cowan, N. (2005). *Working memory capacity.* New York: Psychology Press.

Crosley, R. O. (2004). *Alternative medicine and miracles: A grand unified theory.* Lanham, MD: University Press of America.

De Zazzo, J., & Tully, T. (1995). Dissection of memory formation. From behavioural pharmacology to molecular genetics. *Trends in Neurosciences, 18,* 212–218.

Deiber, M. P., Rodriguez, C., Jaques, D., Missonnier, P., Emch, J., Millet, P., ..., & Ibañez, V. (2010). Aging effects on selective attention-related EEG patterns during face encoding. *Neuroscience, 171*(1), 173–186.

Dietrich, A., & Kanso, R. (2010). A review of EEG, ERP, and neuroimaging studies of creativity and insight. *Psychological Bulletin, 136*(5), 822–848.

Dossey, L. (2001). *Il potere curativo della mente.* Red, Italy.

Drummond, S. P. A., Gillin, J. C., & Brown, G. G. (2001). Increased cerebral response during a divided attention task following sleep deprivation. *European Sleep Research Society, 10,* 85–92.

Ellis, H. (1897). A note on hypnagogic paramnesia. *Mind, New Series, 6*(22), 283–287.

Erickson, M. (1983). *La mia voce ti accompagnerà.* Rome, Italy: Casa Editrice Astrolabio.

Ferrari, M., & Sternberg, R. J. (Eds.). (1998). *Self-awareness: Its nature and development.* New York: Guilford Press.

Feuerstein, G. (1996). *The Shambhala guide to yoga.* Boston: Shambhala Publications.

Flood, G. (1996). *An introduction to Hinduism.* Cambridge: Cambridge University Press.

Freeman, W. J. (2000). La fisiologia della percezione. *Le Scienze, 101,* 32–39.

Freud, S. (1969). *Saggi sull'arte la letteratura e il linguaggio.* Boringhieri.

Freud S. *Opere* (Vol. 2). Torino, Italy: Boringhieri.

Frost, S. E. (1989). *Basic teachings of the great philosophers.* New York: Anchor Books.

Fuller, R. C. (1996). Holistic health practices. In P. H. Van Ness (Ed.), *Spirituality and the secular quest* (pp. 230–234). New York: Crossroad Publishing Company.

Fuster, J. M. (2000). Reti di memoria. *Le Scienze, 101,* 66-75.

Gerrow, K., & Triller, A. (2010, October). Synaptic stability and plasticity in a floating world. *Current Opinion in Neurobiology, 20*(5), 631–639.

Gobet, F. (2000). Some shortcomings of long-term working memory. *British Journal of Psychology, 91,* 551–570.

Goldstein, J. (1983). *The experience of insight.* Boston: Shambhala.

Gombrich, R. F. (1988). *Theravāda Buddhism: A Social History from Ancient Benares to Modern Colombo.* London: Routledge.

Grof, S. (2000). *Il gioco cosmico della mente.* Red Edizioni.

Grun, A. (1995). *Autostima ed accettazione dell'ombra.* Edizioni San Paolo.

Guidano, V. F., & Liotti, G. (1983). *Cognitive processes and emotional disorders.* New York: Guilford Press.

Gunaratana, B. H. (2002). *Mindfulness in plain English.* Somerville, MA: Wisdom Publishers.

Gurstelle, E. B., & Oliveira, J. L. (2004). Daytime parahypnagogia: A state of consciousness that occurs when we almost fall asleep. *Medical Hypotheses, 62*(2), 166–168.

Harner, R., & Naquet, R. (1975). *Clinical EEG, II: Altered states of consciousness, coma, cerebral death.* Hempstead, NY: Coma Recovery Association.

Hefner, A. G. (2008). The MYSTICA™. Copyright (c) 1997. Alan G. Hefner. http://www.law.cornell.edu/uscode/17/107.shtml.

Hinnells, J. R. (1998). *The new penguin handbook of living religions.* London: Penguin Books.

James, W. (1902). Lectures 16 & 17: Mysticism. In *The varieties of religious experience: A study in nature* (pp. 206–234). Huntington, MA: Seven Treasures Publications.

Jevning, R., Wallace, R. K., & Beidebach, M. (1992). The physiology of meditation: A review. A wakeful hypometabolic integrated response. *Neuroscience and Biobehavioral Reviews, 16*(3), 415–424.

Jonas, H. (1997). *Tecnica, medicina ed etica.* Biblioteca Einaudi.

Juergensmeyer, M. (Ed.). (2006). *The Oxford handbook of global religions.* Oxford: Oxford University Press.

Jung, C. G. (1989). *La psicologia dell'inconscio.* Newton Compton Editori.

Jung, C. G. (1991). *Opere* (Vol. 11.). Torino, Italy, Boringhieri.

Kearney, M. (1996). *Mortally wounded: Stories of soul pain, eeath, and healing.* New Orleans, LA: Spring Journal, Inc.

Kennet, W. M. (1953). *The religion of the Hindus.* New York: The Ronald Press Co.

King, R., & Brownstone, A. (1999). Neurophysiology of yoga meditation. *International Journal of Yoga Therapy, 9*(1).

Koch, C. (2004). *The quest for consciousness: A neurobiological approach.* Englewood, CO: Roberts & Company Publishers.

Kosslyn, S. M. (1999). *Le immagini della mente.* Barbera, Italy: Giunti.

Kubler Ross, E. (2005). *La morte e il morire.* Cittadella Editrice.

Lamotte, É. (1976). *Teaching of Vimalakirti* (Sara Boin, Trans.). London: Pali Text Society.

Laufs, H., Kleinschmidt, A., Beyerle, A., Eger, E., Salek-Haddadi, A., Preibisch, C., & Krakow, K. (2003). EEG-correlated fMRI of human alpha activity. *NeuroImage, 19*(4), 1463–1476.

Lehmann, D., Grass, P., & Meier, B. (1995). Spontaneous conscious covert cognition states and brain electric spectral states in canonical correlations. *International Journal of Psychophysiology, 19*, 41–52.

Lindtner, C. (1997). *Master of wisdom.* Berkeley, CA: Dharma Publishing.

Longhi Paripurna, M. (2001). *Bhagavad Gita.* Demetra.

Lopez, J. J. (1972). Masked depression. *British Journal of Psychiatry, 124,* 35–40.

Lu K'uan Yu. (1978). *The Surangama Sutra.* Bombay: B.I. Publications.

McMaster University. (2011). *Discover psychology attention and memory.* Toronto, Ontario: Nelson Education Ltd.

Melzack, R., & Wall, P. D. (2003). *Pain management.* London: Churchill Livingstone.

Miller, G. A., Galanter, E., & Pribram, K. H. (1960). *Plans and the structure of behavior.* New York: Holt, Rinehart & Winston.

Morin, A. (2004). Possible links between self-awareness and inner speech: Theoretical background, underlying mechanisms, and empirical evidence. Unpublished journal.

Muller, A. C. (1999). *The sutra of perfect enlightenment.* Albany, NY: State University Press of New York.

Myers, D. G. (2008). *Psychology* (9th ed.). New York: Worth Publishers.

Nagel, E. (1961). *The structure of science.* London: Routledge.

Namkai, N. (1983). *Il libro tibetano dei morti.* Newton Compton Editori.

Nattier, J. (2003). *A few good men: The Bodhisattva path according to the inquiry of Ugra (Ugrapariprccha).* Honolulu, HA: University of Hawaii Press.

Oberauer, K. (2002). Access to information in working memory: Exploring the focus of attention. *Journal of Experimental Psychology: Learning, Memory, and Cognition, 28,* 411–421.

Oswald, I. (1959). Sudden bodily jerks on falling asleep. *Brain, 82*(1), 92–103.

Oswald, I. (1962). *Sleeping and waking: Physiology and psychology.* Amsterdam: Elsevier.

Pancheri, P., & Biondi, M. (1987). *Stress, emozioni e cancro.* Il Pensiero Scientifico Editore.

Parker, J. J., & Blackmore, S. J. (2002). Comparing the content of sleep paralysis and dream reports. *Dreaming, 12*(1), 45–59.

Penrose, R. (1989). *The emperor's new mind.* Oxford: Oxford University Press.

Petersen, R. (1997). *Out of body experiences.* Charlottesville, VA: Hampton Roads Publishing Company, Inc.

Radhakrishnan, S. (1977). *The Bhagavadgita.* New Delhi, India: Blackie and Son.

Rammurti, S. M. (1973). *Yoga sutras.* Garden City, NY: Doubleday.

Rinpoche, S. (1994). *The Tibetan book of living and dying.* London: Rider.

Runco, M. A., & Pritzker, S. R. (1999). *Encyclopedia of creativity.* New York: Academic Press.

Sadaghiani, S., Scheeringa, R., Lehongre, K., Morillon, B., Giraud, A. L., & Kleinschmidt, A. (2010). Intrinsic connectivity networks, alpha oscillations, and tonic alertness: A simultaneous electroencephalography /functional magnetic resonance imaging study. *Journal of Neuroscience, 30*(30), 10243–10250.

Schiff, N. D. (2004). The neurology of impaired consciousness: Challenges for cognitive neuroscience. In M.S. Gazzaniga (Ed.), *The cognitive neurosciences* (3rd ed.). Cambridge, MA: MIT Press.

Schmeichel, B. J., Volokhov, R., & Demaree, H. A. (2008). Working memory capacity and the self-regulation of emotional expression and experience. *Journal of Personality and Social Psychology, 95,* 1526–1540.

Silberer, H. (1909). Report on a method of eliciting and observing certain symbolic hallucination phenomena. In D. Rapaport (Ed. & Trans.), *Organization and pathology of thought* (1951, pp. 195–207). New York: Columbia University Press.

Singer, J. L., & Pope, K. S. (1981). Daydreaming and imagery skills as predisposing capacities for self-hypnosis. *International Journal of Clinical and Experimental Hypnosis, 29*(3), 271–281.

Sinha, H. P. (1993). Bhāratīya Darshan kī rūprekhā [*Features of Indian philosophy*]. New Delhi, India: Motilal Banarasidas Publishers.

Smith, E. E., & Jonides, J. (1999). Storage and executive processes in the frontal lobes. *Science, 283*, 1657–1661.

Spanos, N. P., McNulty, S. A., DuBreuil, S. C., & Pires, M. (1995). The frequency and correlates of sleep paralysis in a university sample. *Journal of Research in Personality, 29*(3), 285–305.

Squire, L. R. (2008). *Fundamental neuroscience* (3rd ed.). New York: Academic Press.

Staal, F. (1975). *Exploring mysticism.* London: Penguin.

Stickgold, R., Malia, A., Maguire, D., Roddenberry, D., & O'Connor, M. (2000). Replaying the game: Hypnagogic images in normals and amnesics. *Science, 290*(5490), 350–353.

Stickgold, R. (1998). Sleep: Off-line memory reprocessing. *Trends in Cognitive Sciences, 2*(12), 484–492.

Tart, C. T. (1970). Transpersonal potentialities of deep hypnosis. University of California, Davis. Reprinted from *Journal of Transpersonal Psychology, 1970, 2,* 27–40. Copyright (c) 1970 American Transpersonal Association.

Tart, C. T. (1977). *Stati di coscienza.* Rome, Italy: Casa Editrice Astrolabio.

Tart, C. T. (1990). *Altered states of consciousness* (3rd ed.). San Francisco, CA: Harper.

Thera, P. (1999). *Dhammacakkappavattana Sutta* [*The book of protection*]. Kandy, Sri Lanka: Buddhist Publication Society.

Thompson, M. (1997/2003). *Philosophy of religion.* Columbus, OH: McGraw-Hill Companies.

Thorpy, M. J. (Ed.). (1990). Sleep paralysis. *International classification of sleep disorders: Diagnostic and coding manual.* Rochester, MN: American Sleep Disorders Association.

Thurman, R. A. F. (Trans.). (1976). *Holy teaching of Vimalakirti: Mahayana scripture.* State College, PA: Pennsylvania State University Press.

Tolle, E. (1999). *The power of now: A guide to spiritual enlightenment.* Vancouver, BC, Canada: Namaste Publishing.

Tononi, G. (2004). An information integration theory of consciousness. *BMC Neuroscience, 5,* 42–72.

Upanishad. (2001). *La via della liberazione.* Italy: Demetra.

Veith, I. (1976). Huang Ti Nei Ching Su Wen, *Canone di Medicina Interna dell'Imperatore Giallo.* Edizioni Mediterranee Roma.

Vertes, R. E., & Eastman, K. E. (2000). The case against memory consolidation in REM sleep. *Behavioral and Brain Sciences, 23,* 867–876.

Visuddhimagga. (Nyanamoli, Trans.) London: Shambhala. The path of purification, appeared originally in the fifth century AD.

Vlug, A. (1993). *Balanceren op de rand van de rede,* with contributions of D. R. Hofstadter, H. P. Barendregt, H. B. G. Casimir and G. Zukav, Lemniscaat, Rotterdam.

Vogels, T. P., Rajan, K., & Abbott, L. F. (2005). Neural network dynamics. *Annual Review of Neurosciences, 28,* 357–376.

Wackermann, J., Pütz, P., Büchi, S., Strauch, I., & Lehmann, D. (2000). A comparison of Ganzfeld and hypnagogic state in terms of electrophysiological measures and subjective experience. Proceedings of the 43rd Annual Convention of the Parapsychological Association, pp. 302–315.

Wall, P. D. (1979). *Advances in pain research and therapy.* New York: Raven Press.

White, K. (2005). The role of Bodhicitta in Buddhist enlightenment including a translation into English of Bodhicitta-sastra, Benkemmitsu-nikyoron, and Sammaya-kaijo. The Edwin Mellen Press.

Chapter IV

CLINICAL HYPNOSIS TECHNIQUES IN PAIN AND PALLIATIVE CARE

1. THE TECHNIQUES OF PAIN ANALGESIA WITH CLINICAL HYPNOSIS

A. The Benefits of Hypnosis in Pain

In the previous chapter, we learned many different techniques of relaxation, hypnosis, and mindfulness in the modified states of consciousness. Many people worldwide, have learned these very important techniques, people of all ages, cultures, philosophies, and religions. The mindfulness and hypnosis techniques allow your mind to settle inward beyond thought to experience the source of thought, pure awareness, also known as transcendental consciousness or higher consciousness. This is the most silent and peaceful level of consciousness, the awareness of your innermost self (Samraj, 2005). In this state of restful alertness, your brain functions with significantly greater coherence and your body gains deep rest (Austin, 1999).

The aim of mindfulness is to bring inner peace within ourselves and the world in a positive mental and spiritual way. Research has shown clinical hypnosis and mindfulness to be helpful for acute and chronic pain.

Pain is the major problem in the treatment of patients with chronic diseases and cancer. During prolonged illnesses, the best way that we can change our suffering is to modify our thoughts from being negative to bring positive. The positive discovery about meditation and clinical hypnosis, is that we are focusing within ourselves and becoming free of negativity.

Clinical hypnosis improves psychological resilience. It helps an individual's tendency to cope with stress and adversity. This coping may result in the individual's "bouncing back" to a previous state of normal functioning or simply not showing negative effects. In all these instances, resilience is best understood as a process. It is often assumed to be a trait of the individual, an idea more typically referred to as "resiliency." Most research now shows that resilience is the result of individuals being able to interact with their environments and the processes that either promote well-being or protect them against the overwhelming influence of risk factors. These processes can be individual coping strategies or may be helped by clinical hypnosis (Casula, 2001).

Meditation and hypnosis techniques simply involve a process of transforming ourselves and our thoughts and recognizing the negative thoughts and changing them into beneficial and peaceful thoughts (A. Brugnoli, 2005; Brugnoli, Brugnoli & Norsa, 2006; Casula, 2001; De Sousa, 1987; Erickson, 1959; Linden, 1999).

The best attitude toward mindfulness and hypnosis is to be very patient, because the mind does not always want to focus. Having a sense of expectation toward positive results can create uncomfortable pressure and thus take away the enjoyment of the experience. By practicing mindfulness and hypnosis regularly, the person gains a wonderful sense of the inner self. Meditation and hypnosis are self-healing processes; any form of pain is a sign of our negative thinking and unease within our mind. If we don't attend to unase in the mind, we may find that chronic suffering can lead to disease of the body.

The human mind and body are intrinsically linked, something that mystics from time immemorial have been indicating. The state of the mind, to a great extent, controls the well-being of the body. This is something that has recently been proven by scientific researchers (Fourie, 1997; Handel, 2001; Patterson, 2010).

In Chapter III, we saw that there are various methods of practicing relaxation, hypnosis, and mindfulness. Each method depends on our objective in practicing it. One of the common objectives of these practices is to acquire a tension-free, relaxed, happy, and peaceful state of mind, so that we can face the day-to-day challenges of life and relationships, healing inwardly in a more creative, balanced, and objective manner.

In this chapter, we improve the knowledge of some specific hypnosis techniques to relieve acute and chronic pain. Pain management (also called pain medicine or algiatry) is a branch of medicine employing an interdisciplinary approach for easing the suffering, and improving the quality of life of those living with pain.

Pain management (also called pain medicine or algiatry) is a branch of medicine employing an interdisciplinary approach for easing suffering and improving the quality of life of those living with pain. Medicine treats injury and pathology to support and speed healing and manages distressing symptoms, such as pain, to relieve suffering during treatment and healing. When a distressful injury or pathology is resistant to treatment and persists after the injury or the pathology has healed, and when medical science cannot identify the cause of pain, the task of medicine is to relieve suffering.

We have studied in detail the neurophysiological and behavioral assessment of pain and suffering (*see* Chapter II). WHO has developed a three-step pharmacological "ladder" for pain relief. If pain occurs, there should be prompt oral administration of drugs in the following order:

1. nonopioids (aspirin and paracetamol);
2. mild opioids (codeine), as necessary;
3. strong opioids, such as morphine, until the patient is free of pain

To calm fears and anxiety, additional adjuvant drugs should be used. To maintain freedom from pain, drugs should be given "by the clock"; that is every 3 to 6 hours, rather than "on demand." This three-step approach of administering the right drug, in the right dose, at the right time, is inexpensive and 80 to 90 percent effective. Surgical or anesthesiological interventions on appropriate nerves may provide further pain relief, if drugs are not wholly effective.

Treatment approaches to chronic pain include pharmacological measures, such as analgesics, tricyclic antidepressants and anticonvulsants; interventional and anesthesiological procedures; physical therapy; and psychological measures, such as cognitive behavioral therapy, clinical hypnosis, and mindfulness. Clinical hypnosis can be considered a nonpharmacological intervention as adjuvant in pain therapy.

Nonpharmacological interventions adjuvant in pain therapy can be classified as either cognitive behavioral interventions or physical agents. Cognitive and behavioral approaches include several ways to help patients understand more about their pain and take an active part in its assessment and control. The goals of interventions, classified as cognitive behavioral therapies, are to change patients' perceptions of pain, alter pain behavior, and provide patients with a greater sense of control over pain. The goals of interventions classified as physical agents or modalities are to provide comfort, correct physical dysfunction, alter physiological responses, and reduce fears associated with pain-related immobility or activity restriction.

Nonpharmacological approaches and hypnosis are intended to supplement, not substitute for, the pharmacologic or invasive techniques described. Nonpharmacological interventions are appropriate in chronic diseases, in cancer patients and in palliative care for the patient who

1. finds such interventions appealing
2. expresses anxiety or fear, as long as the anxiety is not incapacitating or due to a medical or psychiatric condition that has a nonspecific treatment
3. may benefit from avoiding or reducing drug therapy (e.g., history of adverse reactions, fear of or physiological reason to avoid oversedation)
4. is likely to experience, and needs to cope with, a prolonged interval of postoperative pain, particularly if punctuated by recurrent episodes of intense treatment or procedure-related pain
5. has incomplete pain relief following appropriate pharmacological interventions
6. needs physical and psychological suffering relief, and in palliative care at the end of life

Cognitive behavioral approaches include preparatory information, simple relaxation, imagery, and hypnosis. Physical therapeutic agents and modalities include application of superficial heat or cold, massage, exercise, immobility, and electroanalgesia such as transcutaneous electrical nerve stimulator (TENS) therapy or electroacupuncture.

The conitive behavioral stratgies require greater professional involvement; these include complex imagery, hypnosis, biofeedback, mindfulness, and combined therapies. Such strategies can be commonly applied when patients have acute or chronic pain.

I have worked for 15 years as an anesthetist in surgical rooms and in critical care, and now I work as a pain therapist. Since 1985, I have been interested in and have studied clinical hypnosis to help the relief of pain and suffering. In this chapter I explain the use of clinical hyponosis techniques in pain therapy. The techniques of hypnosis in pain therapy have two objectives:

1. physical pain relief (Patterson & Jensen 2005; Patterson, 2010)
2. psychological and spiritual suffering relief (Casula, Preti & Portaluri, 2005; Linden, Bhardwaj & Anbar, 2006; Perez-De-Albeniz & Jeremy, 2000)

B. What is Hypnosis?

Hypnosis is a state of inner absorption, concentration, or focused attention that assists a client in altering some aspects of thought, emotion, behavior, or perception. "Hypnosis is a procedure during which a health professional or researcher suggests that a client, patient, or subject experience changes in sensations, perceptions, thoughts, feelings or behavior. The hypnotic context is generally established by an induction procedure most include suggestions for relaxation, calmness and well-being" (APA, Div. 30, Kirsch, 1994).

Hypnosis typically involves an introduction to the procedure during which the subject is told that suggestions for imaginative experiences will be presented. The hypnotic induction is an extended initial suggestion for using one's imagination and may contain further elaborations of the introduction. A hypnotic procedure is used to encourage and evaluate responses to suggestions. When using hypnosis, one person (the subject) is guided by another (the hypnotist) to respond to suggestions for changes in subjective experience and alterations in perception, sensation, emotion, thoughts, or behavior. Persons can also learn self-hypnosis, which is the act of administering hypnotic procedures on one's own. If the subject responds to hypnotic suggestions, it is generally inferred that hypnosis has been induced. Many believe that hypnotic response and experiences are characteristic of a hypnotic state. Whereas some think that it is not necessary to use the word hypnosis as part of the hypnotic induction, others view it as essential.

During my work in critical care, I was always very touched by pain, suffering, and sometimes the death of young people, and now that I work on the pain relief therapy, I happen to deal with many cancer patients. The suffering of these patients is not only physical but also psychological and spiritual, and in my experience, hypnosis can help all of these types of sufferings, in chronic diseases and in the last stage of the dying patient.

During hypnosis, your body relaxes and your thoughts become more focused. Like other relaxation techniques, hypnosis lowers blood pressure and heart rate and changes certain types of brain wave activity. In this relaxed state, you will feel at ease physically yet be fully awake mentally and may be highly responsive to a suggestion.

There are several stages of hypnosis in pain therapy:

- Reframing the problem (pain and suffering)
- Becoming relaxed, then absorbed (deeply engaged in the words or images presented by a hypnotherapist)
- Dissociating (letting go of critical thoughts)
- Responding (complying with a hypnotherapist's suggestions)
- Returning to usual awareness
- Reflecting on the experience

C. What Happens During the First Visit of the Hypnotherapist?

During the first visit, you will be asked about your medical history and what brought you in and what condition you would like to address. The hypnotherapist may explain to you what hypnosis is and how it works. You will then be directed through relaxation techniques, using a series of mental images and suggestions intended to change behaviors and relieve symptoms. The hypnotherapist will also teach you the basics of self-hypnosis and, sometimes, give you a CD to use at home so you can reinforce what you learn during the session.

Each session lasts about an hour, and most people start to see results within two to five sessions. You and your hypnotherapist will monitor and evaluate your progress over time. Children are easily hypnotized and may respond after only one or two sessions (Linden, Bhardwaj & Anbar, 2006).

Hypnosis is used in a variety of pain therapy settings: from emergency rooms, to critical care to anesthesiology to anesthesiological procedures to chronic diseases to palliative care (Accardi & Milling, 2009; Patterson & Jensen, 2003; Patterson, 2010).

Clinical studies suggest that hypnosis may improve immune function, increase relaxation, decrease stress, and ease pain and feelings of anxiety. Hypnotherapy can reduce the fear and anxiety that some people feel before medical or surgical procedures. For example, hypnosis may improve recovery time and reduce anxiety as well as pain following surgery. Clinical trials on burn patients suggest that hypnosis decreases pain (enough to replace pain medication) and speeds healing. Generally, clinical studies show that using hypnosis may reduce your need for medication, improve your mental and physical condition before an operation, and reduce the time it takes to recover.

A hypnotherapist can teach you self-regulation skills. For instance, someone with arthritis or cancer pain may learn to turn down pain like the volume on a radio. Hypnotherapy can be used to help manage chronic illness. Self-hypnosis can enhance a sense of control and improve pain and suffering relief, which is often lacking when someone has a chronic illness. Clinical studies on children in emergency treatment centers show that hypnotherapy reduces fear, anxiety, and discomfort.

Pain management distills down to a very simple endpoint: patients' relief and comfort. If patients feel better, feel comforted, feel less stressed and more functional in life, and their practice poses no health risk, then supporting complementary and alternative therapies creates a true holistic partnership in health care.

In my profession, pain, suffering, and death are always very close, and when I started to experiment on the process of clinical hypnosis in its deepest way, I discovered not only pain relief but also the awakening of the spiritual experience in palliative care. I discovered that in chronic suffering relief, hypnosis can be an experience similar to what the patient faces in the predeath state. As was explained by people who survived a cardiopulmonary resuscitation, they felt a state between life and death, and they say it was a state of psychological and spiritual well-being.

At the beginning, I use the classic techniques of physical and psychological relaxation until the finalized hypnosis aimed to the pain therapy. In helping patients with chronic diseases, the first step is to take away the physical pain. Besides the different drugs available and the anesthetics, there are several methods of hypnosis that help the patient not only in physical pain but also in need of controlling anxiety. What follows are some hypnosis methods to be used as pain relief suitable for all patients.

D. The Techniques of Pain Analgesia With Hypnosis

- Technique of a different interpretation of the symptoms
- Technique of the transferred symptoms
- Technique of the transport of the symptoms
- Technique of positive and negative visualizations
- Technique of partial or total hypnotic amnesia
- Technique of the activation of a type of conditioned reflex
- Technique of switching attention
- Hypnosis technique of the self-training of Shultz
- Technique of self-hypnosis in pain relief
- Schedule of relaxation with hypnosis for acute pain

Technique of a Different Interpretation of the Symptoms

When a state of a lighter or deeper relaxation is achieved through different techniques, the patient is trained how to interpret the feeling of chronic pain coming from a specific place in the body and to transform it slowly from a feeling of pain to a feeling of a different nature, for example, light or medium tension, moderate pressure, beneficial warmth, or cold sensation of an anesthetizing nature.

EXAMPLE OF ANESTHESIA TO ONE HAND

While in a state of relaxation, you can imagine immersing your hand in a container of melting ice cubes and from the wrist up to the tip of your fingers the ice acts on your hand like a very powerful anesthesia . . . making it feel more and more insensitive. You will feel your hand becoming increasingly insensitive . . . and the anesthesia will increase. You will also know that the anesthesia will last until you repeat to yourself for three times "Everything is normal."

Exercise "Warm Hands"

During this exercise you will repeat to yourself:
"My hands are warm"
During the period of "deep relaxation," you will imagine you are keeping your hand in front of the flames of an open fire under a solar lamp (UVB lamp), or immersed in hot water, or any other thought of this kind that might come easy to you.
Duration: 5 (or also only 3) minutes.

Exercises With Different Types of Pain Relief Feelings

During this training, imagine finding yourself in the circumstances corresponding to the situation indicated here:

• My feet are warm.
Duration: (5 or also only 3) minutes.

During this exercise, repeat to yourself:
• My feet are warm.
• My feet are cold.
• My hands are cold.
• My hands are warm.

Technique of the Transferred Symptoms

After achieving relatively strong analgesia in a certain part of the body with the techniques just described, you aim to mentally transfer the analgesia to another part of the body (for instance, from the hands to the abdomen or to the back), obtaining this way a gradual and progressive reduction of the global suffering.

Technique of the Transport of the Symptom

When the patient has achieved a medium or, better, a deeper state of relaxation, you do an intense analgesia on one hand, preferably the one that is most used. You then proceed by moving the analgetic hand on to the painful side of the body or wherever the patient wants to direct the analgesia. In this way, with repeated procedures, you lessen the suffering, especially if this pain has not been there for a very long time.

Technique of the Positive and Negative Visualizations

When the patient remains in a state of relaxation or in medium hypnosis status, introduce particular visualizations that will cause, after a certain time, major feeling visualization that is capable of modifying the painful information in the CNS and, therefore, reduce the pain to the patient. What follows is an example.

THE SCHEDULE FOR THE DESENSITIZATION OF PAIN. Since 1800, certain methods have been used in the Western world to induce the modification of the pain threshold through hypnotic techniques in the field of surgery analgesia. During the deep hypnotic state, the patient does not seem to react to the surrounding environment and usually seems to have a reduced sensitivity to painful stimulation. This happens even if you can have some or all of the reflexive or vegetative signs of the painful stimulation. Therefore, the best use for this technique is to induce deep relaxation up until the unconscious can register and activate through hypnotic suggestion a minor sensitivity to pain for a longer time even in a state of normal awakening,

The use of this technique is to diminish the anxiety connected with pain, in the case of headaches, for example, when besides the body pain, a great emotional dysfunction arises; in the case of phantom arm or leg pain after an amputation; or in the chronic pain of cancer patients.

The methods most used during the state of deep relaxation or hypnosis are

- Direct instructions for the reduction of pain
- The use of metaphors
- The transportation of the painful symptom
- The detachment of pain through imagination

Technique of Partial or Total Hypnotic Amnesia

For this technique, you need the patient to be in a medium or deep hypnotic state. It is possible to achieve a better result by taking the patient back to the state of well-being and healthy status from before the illness started through specific questions. In this way, the patient will eventually forget the memories of the bad experiences, which are related to his or her pain, and in some cases also forget the memories of the anxiety related to the pain in chronic diseases.

Technique of the Activation of a Type of Conditioned Reflex

This technique, called the "non painful pain," uses the same methods that Pavlov applied to dogs. He created a typical conditioned reflex for dogs by showing them the food together with or soon after a painful stimulation. After a certain number of tests, depending also on the breed and the sex of the dog, the painful stimulation was not felt thanks to the gratification of the food.

Almost the same thing happens with human beings thanks to a mechanism of emotional restructuring in the perception of painful stimulation at the level of the brain areas. During a deep state of relaxation, it is possible to activate a conditioned reflex through images and music preferred by the patient so that the pain is reduced.

EXERCISE BASED ON THE "CHOSEN IMAGE"

Train yourself to accept your favorite image for 5 minutes . . .
Then you look at the image for 4 minutes . . .
Then 3 minutes of your favorite image . . .
Then 2 minutes of you favorite image . . .
Then 1 minute of your favorite image . . .
Obviously this exercise will last about 15 minutes.
Every "entrance" of the favorite image will be preceded by a countdown from twenty to one . . .
Think that by counting down your pain also decreases . . . progressively.

The patient can train herself or himself to do this exercise.

Technique of Switching Attention

This method used by Kroger can be very useful for chronic pain by training the patient to move his or her attention to those parts of the body that are not affected by pain.

Using gratifying visualization, you train the patient to move his or her attention to another pleasant sensation of his or her body that is past or present. This method is also useful in chronic pain when it is not too strong, but it is understood that the patient must participate actively in the visualization.

Sometimes this is easier than the previous systems, especially by suggesting gratifying visualization. If the patient cannot do the self-training you can use the following method:

METHOD OF THE CD. This consists of simply recording the desired suggestion on a CD and then listening to it when you are relaxing. This will be very effective for people who have difficulty visualizing.

Hypnosis Technique of the Self-Training of Shultz

When the patient has been well-trained to practice the easier exercises of the self-training of Shultz, we can use these exercises during the hypnotic state to obtain good relief of pain. The simple exercises of the self-training of Shultz are as follows:

- Exercise of feeling heavy
- Exercise of heat
- Exercise of the heart
- Exercise of the breath
- Exercise of the abdomen
- Exercise of the cool forehead

All of these exercises are suitable for pain therapy, but we will consider only a few examples.

The Technique of the Heat

My body . . . in the time passing by . . . is becoming more and more
pleasantly warm . . .
Even more pleasantly warm . . . and a feeling of great well-being . . .
Great calm . . . great tranquility . . . it becomes part of me . . . the time goes by
I feel well . . . I feel well . . . I feel really well . . .
and everything else does not bother me anymore . . .

For this exercise, please repeat the sentences slowly with calm at least ten times.

EXERCISE OF THE COOL FOREHEAD. "My forehead is pleasantly cool." This can be another exercise for pain-relief therapy, depending on the patient's personality and character. It is also a very important exercise for controlling chronic headache and for different types of cancer as well. This is how to carry out the technique of the cool forehead:

Concentrating on your forehead please repeat . . .
My head is light . . . all the muscles of my face are rested . . .
I am calm . . . calm . . . perfectly calm.. in a state of great well-being . . .

My forehead is cool . . . pleasantly cool . . . even more pleasantly cool . . .
The coolness is all around me and gives me well-being . . .
Well-being of the body and wellbeing of the mind . . .

Repeat this formula between five and ten times.

Technique of the Self-Hypnosis in Pain Relief

This is one of the most efficient techniques and is carried out in three phases:

1. You are living a pleasant feeling in deep relaxation.
2. You connect this feeling mentally to your symptoms.
3. You are using it mentally to cancel your symptoms.

The most efficient way to achieve this feeling is to repeat this technique until you achieve your goal, and sometimes this will take quite a while.

Imagine that we are going to use this technique of posthypnotic state to achieve the following goal: "I can hear very soft music that helps my pain."

Phase 1. You are living this moment in a status of relaxation.
You relax for 5 minutes and concentrate on remembering the last time you could hear soft music.
You can hear the harmony of this music, and of all the other times that you heard soft music in your past.
You imagine hearing this music in the ears of your mind; after you have recaptured that moment, you go to phase 2.

Phase 2. You make the connection with the hypnosis.
Yet again in a state of relaxation, you can see yourself in different circumstances; use the key words:
"Let me hear the soft sound of the music," and at that point, you will be here.

Phase 3. You use this system to eliminate the pain.
Try to examine the result of your experiment and, if necessary, repeat the whole procedure again.

To achieve the best results in these techniques, it is important to learn, first of all, to relax and concentrate without being distracted by anything and take the focus of your attention within yourself. At the beginning, this can be difficult, but with the practice, you will achieve surprising results. Try to create within yourself the sentiment that what you wish is real and that it can be achieved through your will.

It is advisable to remember this willingness or condition that you want to achieve during your normal day so that this becomes part of your everyday life.

Schedule of Relaxation With Hypnosis for the Treatment of the Acute Pain

With this exercise, you will be under hypnosis for different lengths of time, measured in minutes or seconds (acute pain in emergency and in critical care).

> Before you count down from twenty to one always think:
> "Now I will sleep for *X* minutes; meanwhile, my pain will decrease."
> Then, begin to count down from twenty to one.
> While you are practicing this experiment, you must use the following suggestion:
> Every time faster and deeper.
> This means of course that every time you go to sleep your eyes will close faster, and you will sleep more deeply.
> Try this exercise for different lengths of time.
> Try to do self-inductions that last 10, 15, and 20 seconds.

This technique can be used in the acute pain relief.

2. DEEP HYPNOSIS IN RELIEF OF PAIN AND SUFFERING

Hypnosis is a form of deep mental and physical relaxation that allows you to access your inner emotions, memories, and inner self. Hypnotherapy uses this state of relaxation to enable you to tap into your inner resources and gain access to the root cause of a problem.

Have you ever caught yourself daydreaming? When you are daydreaming, it is as though you are not in the here and now. You are somewhere else, you are very calm and still, you are actually caught up in the moment, but you are perfectly aware of what is going on around you. We go into hypnotic states several times during our day and do not even know it is hypnosis.

This is exactly what it is like when you are hypnotized. You experience an overall feeling of calmness throughout your entire body and mind. At all times, you are totally aware of what is going on around you. You are in complete control, and you can communicate clearly and effectively with the hypnotherapists, with your inner self, and with you higher consciousness.

What is so important about the relationship between hypnosis and your subconscious mind? Deep hypnosis is the door to your mind, your inner self, and your higher consciousness. The subconscious is the part of the mind that is utilized in hypnosis, and your subconscious mind looks after every organ, muscle, and cell in your body 24 hours a day. It never sleeps. Your subconscious mind regulates all involuntary bodily functions, including your heart rate, breathing, blood pressure, hormone production, and elimination system (Vannoni & Brugnoli, 1971; Vaitl et al., 2005). Your subconscious mind is also the seat of your emotions, your feelings, and your sensations. It is also where your permanent memory is stored.

The brain and nervous system respond only to mental images. It does not matter whether the image is imagined or real. Like a computer, your subconscious mind holds good programs and "bad" ones. Hypnosis is like a virus scan for your computer, detecting the "bad" programs and upgrading your "software" (inner self).

A. Deep Self-Hypnosis and Deepening Techniques to Achieve Deeper Levels of Trance

Going into a trance is a skill. For many things, ultradeep trances are not necessary. If you are going to create anesthesia in pain therapy or have some need to create a deeper hypnotic phenomenon, having a deeper trance is helpful (Spiegel, 1985). You can do this for yourself or for your subjects.

The techniques should contain some types of suggestions:

- Deepening suggestions
- Suggestions that each time you are hypnotized, you more easily and quickly go into a much deeper and relaxing state of hypnosis.
- Suggestions that you enjoy the hypnosis state.

Deepening Suggestions

The deepening suggestions that are easiest to use in this situation are suggestions that relate to breathing, escalators, elevators, and counting. Here are some examples.

BREATHING

And every single deep and natural breath you take allows you to deepen your relaxation.

COUNTING

In a moment, I'm going to count from ten down to one . . .
And in allowing each number to help your body grow more relaxed . . .
your mind go more relaxed . . .
so that certain thoughts just fade away . . .
like sand slipping through your fingers . . .
You can find that easy relaxation of mind and body . . .
because of these words... just happens now . . .
ten . . . easily relaxing all over again . . .
9 . . . then . . .
8 deeper still . . .
. . . feeling great
7 . . . 6 . . . 5 . . .
mind and body relaxed . . .
4 . . . relaxing more . . .
. . . 3 then
2 . . .
your deepening grew at
1 . . . derful deep levels
going deeper . . .
. . .That's right . . .

ELEVATORS AND ESCALATORS

In a moment, I'm going to ask you to imagine yourself at the top of an escalator. I'm going to count down from ten to one. As I say the number ten, in your
imagination step onto the escalator. Allow yourself to go deeper into relaxation
with each number I say. When I reach the number one, step off the escalator
into a state of relaxation deeper than you've ever felt before.
ten steps on the escalator and go much deeper . . .
nine relaxing more and more with each number . . .
eight allowing yourself to go deeper and deeper with each number . . .
seven, each number and each easy, natural breath you take helps you relax
more fully . . .
six . . .
five . . . doing deeper into relaxation . . .
four. . . . feeling relaxation flow and every area of your body . . .
three . . .
two . . . allowing your body to feel a wonderful . . . at the relaxation . . .
one . . . now more deeply relaxed than ever before . . .

Go Easily and Go Quickly Into a Much Deeper and Relaxing State of Hypnosis

And each time you relax yourself, you more easily and quickly go into a much deeper state of hypnosis.

And because you are learning . . . really learning what hypnosis is, the next time you are hypnotized you will easily and quickly, effortlessly and wonderfully enter a deep and profoundly useful trance.

Enjoy Going Into the Hypnosis State

You enjoy going easily and effortlessly achieving deeper and deeper levels of hypnosis.
In a nutshell, here it is . . .
Create your deepening hypnosis state.
Create a posthypnotic reinduction cue for yourself or your subject.
Sit or lie down, get comfortable and relaxed, and start the self-hypnosis.
Give yourself your posthypnotic re-induction cue.

The Instant Trance and Posthypnotic Reinduction Cues

A posthypnotic reinduction cue is simply a posthypnotic suggestion to enter a trance at a later time at some prearranged signal. This can save you from having to go through a lengthier induction process in chronic pain.

Posthypnotic reinduction may be what is happening when you see a stage hypnotist snap his fingers or say a word and have his subjects immediately go into trance. The subjects were first hypnotized and then given the cue. After that time, they respond to the cue. An example would be "And when I look at you directly in the eyes and snap my fingers like this (snap fingers), you'll instantaneously go to this level of trance or deeper."

. . . Good, now you've achieved a wonderful level of relaxation . . .
and I'd like to make sure that we can have this relaxation available to us any time we want it . . .
That way, we can get the maximum amount of good done in the time we have available . . .
From this day forward, in my office, any time I say the phrase "blue moon" . . .
instantaneously go to this level of trance or deeper . . .
"Blue moon" takes you deeper . . .
In a moment, I'm going to say that phrase again . . .
just feel how wonderfully you relax when I say it . . . "blue moon"
. . . that's right . . . even deeper.

Good . . . in a moment I'm going to count from one to three . . .
when I reach the number three allow your eyes to become open . . .
Then I'll say the phrase "blue moon" again . . . that's right . . .
When I do . . . close your eyes and go to this level of relaxation or deeper . . .
one . . .
two . . .
three . . . open your eyes . . . "blue moon" . . .
That's right . . . even deeper . . .
In a moment, I'm going to count from one to five . . .
When I reach the number five, be oriented to this room, this time, this place
feeling alert and refreshed and wonderful in every way.
• feeling good
• re-orienting more to this room, time and place
• in a moment your muscles will begin to stir
• on the next number open your eyes and feel great
• open you eyes and feel great.

After Hypnosis Induction Slowly Return to Being Awake

Now let's take a deep breath . . .
And slowly . . . return to being awake . . .

I regain my normal waking state.
I can start my first movements of my feet and hands, calm . . . without rushing
. . . slowly . . .
I can start to slowly open my eyes . . . slowly . . .
and regain . . . always slowly . . . my normal waking state,
moving my arms and my legs . . .
I move again . . . good.
I am awake.
. . . How are you?
How are you? Did you reach a calm state?
Good . . . very good.

3. CLINICAL HYPNOSIS IN PALLIATIVE CARE

When we allow death and awareness of life to occupy their natural position in our life, we are presented with many opportunities to open ourselves to the beauty of life, and we will never fear the unexpected but gain strength, love, and compassion when we understand that all this is a natural part of our life. It is a rewarding feeling to be able to sit with your dying friend and patient to make him or her understand the mystery of love. It is rewarding to be able to make him or her relax in the face of death, with peace and spir-

ituality, and to feel that this love is growing in his or her heart. It is rewarding to communicate that death is not the end but is "the natural way of life"
and is something much bigger and more divine than will ever be possible in
our physical life.

Studies of human evolution over the course of the centuries and millennia and of the neurophysiological development of the brain and the mind
can give us some help in providing medical therapy for the suffering of the
body but are of no help for emotional suffering; that is a therapy we can
learn through the path toward the spiritual consciousness (Jung, 1952; Kallio
& Revonsuo, 2003; Rinpoche, 1994; Sherman, 2004). It is, therefore, important also in the medical therapy and in palliative care, to study the expansion
of the conscience to take us toward new horizons.

There are a lot of studies these days connected with the latest physical
and neurophysiological theories that will help depressed individuals who are
tired and bored with the everyday life. Through these new studies and interests, this work might solve "life's struggle," "the obscure fear" that is the
cause of so many depressive diseases and often reaches an intensity when,
with death, we let go of all our life work (Assagioli, 1991; Brugnoli, 1974a,
1974b, 2004, 2005). Instead, this is the moment of most strength and awareness to face our life with more enthusiasm.

In truth, there is a slow path toward spiritual awareness, and even if it
does not cure all our illnesses, it will be certainly a good and valid help for
the conquest and the knowledge of ourselves, of the deepest self and the
internal personal world, and of all the hidden qualities that everyone has
within their rational and intuitive mind. We need to reflect more on the spiritual sides—"the vital spirit" or "vibration energy"—of the most advanced
physicians, mathematicians, cosmologists, and philosophers who are studying to understand the holistic conscience and global conscience of the human
being. We need to wake up our mind to the new wind of our spirit. We need
to wake up our mind to new important paths. We need to wake up our mind
and brain with the new discoveries in all the fields of the human being and
even the ones that are less observed and analyzed in all the moments of life.

We need to consider our soul as part of the whole being. We know
through our intuition that we are reaching a new stage of evolution that will
develop more during this century. We need to reflect more on the spiritual
sides of all the matters that concern and surround the microcosm and macrocosm from everything down to the smallest particle and the heaviest, the
most enormous galactic bodies that lie among the millions of stars where we
will find other beings more advanced than we are.

What we could call the superintelligence or cosmic superconscience or,
in other words, the spiritual awareness, is waiting for us, is observing us, so

that when we are ready, we will become part of it, and thereby we will understand the reason for our life and especially to give meaning to life (A. Brugnoli, 2004, 2005).

At least, we can agree that the only material life, as we see it today, has no reason to exist just on its own. We are aware that there exists an entropic relationship among all of us because we know that together we can go through the path of spiritual awareness. We are aware that the energy we receive is transformed into further information that then transforms itself into knowledge, consciousness and awareness.

Therefore, every moment in our life becomes of interest about who we are and where we are, becomes a joy of living and participating to the whole universe of life, and becomes minute by minute a moment of life in a "continuum time and space" that will adapt and expand to the infinite within ourselves and in the macrocosms.

When we experience the awareness, we will feel it for sure because we will experience a wave of happy emotions. We can call this a mystic experience, and this is described in all religions and cultures throughout the history of humanity. This means we have arrived. We have understood and discovered the basis of existence where the physic and metaphysic level have become one.

Everybody can feel this sooner or later, maybe by watching a wonderful sunset, or looking at a work of art, or by listening to the words of someone you love. If we could muster the courage, we would call it a divine experience or a spiritual experience. This entrance to the state of consciousness can be compared to what someone might call illumination, samadhi, ecstasy, or nirvana.

We need to understand that our mind allows us to have two lives, one that is the everyday life, which we can call the exterior life; the other one is the internal life that continuously searches, sometimes spasmodically, for the truth of the eternal image of our life after death.

The philosopher Jidd Krishnamurti was quite clear in his thesis at the beginning of the century. He said, "every being is the world." Again, we have not yet reached the point where everyone contains the whole world, we contain the whole cosmos, and therefore, it contains the "path to the spiritual awareness" or the "spiritual awareness" (A. Brugnoli, 2004, 2005). We can call this by several different names depending on our culture, from our awareness in understanding the life within and outside ourselves and also depending on our religion and beliefs and faith.

So the names we can give to this path to spiritual awareness or spiritual awareness are varied. The absolute power, the infinite power, the spiritual conscience, God, but no matter what we call it, we all mean the same thing, the arrival point of the personal and collective evolution and the cosmic and planetary evolution.

Through this path, we will find the presence of happiness and calm at the end of our life's journey, when all mystic people consider it to be the darkest time of our soul and all philosophers consider it to be a night of depression. In reality, this will be the moment of the "light," the light that will never blind and never end, the light of the spirit that will envelop our heart and soul until the fusion of all matter.

This is a journey of the deepest analysis within ourselves and of all the possibilities of the vital spirit of all the beings; it isthe search of the direct presence of the unknown being, that the philosophers talk about. Thomas Merton, the Trappist monk and author, who died in 1968, he offered a marvelous description of his experiences in his mystic state within half a minute in his book *Dialogues with Silence.*

> What can I say about the void and the freedom I experienced when I passed the threshold of that half a minute. This experience was enough for a whole life because it was a completely new life? There is nothing that I can compare this with. I could call it the void, but it is an infinite freedom, to be able not to have any needs nor to feel myself and be in the pure joy which lies beyond all beings. Do not let me build walls around it otherwise I will be forever locked outside. (A. Brugnoli, 2004, 2005)

Let us now look at a technique for inducing the awakening of spiritual awareness, or for the awakening of our deepest self, or for the awakening of the "internal world"; the objective is one of personal achievement, but it also should be therapeutic.

4. THE TECHNIQUE OF HYPNOSIS FOR THE ACTIVATION OF SPIRITUAL AWARENESS

I would like to express my immense gratitude to my father Dr. Angelico Brugnoli for improving my knowledge and studies in clinical hypnosis and stages of consciousness. He wrote this technique, and together we studied the meaning of every particular word, in Italian and in English, to make entering the state of spiritual well-being in palliative care better (A. Brugnoli, 2004, 2005; M. P. Brugnoli, 2004, 2009a, 2009b).

I would like to point out that for this type of induction I will, during my verbal instructions with the patient, use the word us, so that the patient feels reassured, as if I am going with him or her, hand in hand, toward something that at first can be unknown. You can also reassure your patient that in self-deep hypnosis, he or she can enter the state of sleep.

Let us start with a physical relaxation, which can be achieved fairly quickly, then we will go on to a visualization of a natural, relaxing place that will help with the mental relaxation, and then we will go on to the technique of activating of our spiritual awareness, our inner light, and well-being.

You, my colleagues and friends, may try this just relaxing in your seat, if you wish.

Technique of Hypnosis for the Activation of Spiritual Awareness

Let's dedicate a little time only for ourselves . . .
outside of all the things we must do . . .
away from all our thoughts . . .
to find our energy . . .
our well-being . . .
our serenity . . .
let's find the most comfortable position possible . . .
with eyes open or closed . . .
whichever way we like . . .
as time passes serenely . . .
as time passes slowly . . .
as time passes . . . very slowly
we enter in a state of well-being . . .
great serenity . . . great tranquility . . . great well-being . . . serenity . . .
tranquility . . .
nothing else matters
we take a deep breath . . .
and exhaling we slowly let go of all our thoughts . . .
we let go . . .
we let ourselves go . . .
in this great serenity . . . great calm . . .
great well-being . . .
relaxing . . . great relaxing of our body and mind . . .
relaxing muscles . . .relaxing tendons . . .
relaxing nerves . . . as time passes . . .
nothing bothers us any more . . .
our hearts contemplate this peace
outside noises slowly . . . slowly disappear . . .
and as time passes . . .
and as time passes slowly . . . nothing bothers us any more . . .
this sweet well-being cradles us
our heart cradles us in this peace
immersed in this serenity

we let go . . . we let go serenely . . .
in this particular state of relaxation . . .
which is not awake . . . not sleep
a great sense of well-being . . . relaxing . . .
great calm . . . tranquility . . . great serenity . . . and well-being . . . physical well-
being . . . well-being of the mind . . .
and calm . . . at every level . . .
with great relaxing of the tendons . . .
relaxing of the muscles . . . and relaxing of the nerves . . .
as time passes serenely . . .
everything else does not matter anymore
good . . . we let go completely . . . we let go . . .
within this state which is not awake . . .
and not sleep . . . while we feel our well-being . . .
the calm . . . the tranquility . . . and relaxing . . .
we feel much better this time in this particular state of relaxation and well-being
. . .
while the outside noises disappear . . .
disappear slowly . . .
good . . .
we are enjoying this particular state of the relaxation of our body . . . of our muscles . . . of our tendons . . .
and of our nerves . . .
and for some moment . . . while time passes . . .
and everything around us . . . everything within us . . .
is at great calm . . .
is at great tranquility . . . well-being . . . relaxing . . . relaxing . . .
relaxing the body . . . relaxing of the muscles . . .
relaxing of the tendons . . .
relaxing of the nerves . . .
all our body is relaxed . . . relaxing . . .
well-being . . . tranquility . . . relaxing . . .
while time goes by . . . and everything is calm . . . serene
. . . again great well being of the body . . .
well being of the mind . . . great calm . . .
great tranquility . . . at all levels . . .
of the tendons . . . of the muscles...of the nerves . . .
while time passes . . .
we are relaxing even more and even better . . .
this is a moment only for us . . .
beyond all that can disturb us . . . only serenity . . .
well being . . . peace . . . we are relaxing . . .
we are relaxing . . .
we are relaxing even more and even better . . .
only calm . . . only serenity . . .

muscular relaxation . . . peace . . . tranquility
our body is relaxing . . .
our heart is cradled by this peace
and our thoughts pass . . . without stopping calmly . . .
our body relaxes . . .
our heart is at peace . . .
we let our body relax . . . our muscles relax . . .
our tendons relax . . . our nerves relax slowly . . .
submerged in this peace . . . in this serenity
Let's imagine now, we are walking towards the sun . . . on a wonderful clear day
. . .
with a pleasant temperature . . .
a light breeze is caressing and relaxing us . . .
a beautiful blue sky . . .
with a few white clouds on the horizon . . .
we are walking on a path of small white pebbles . . .
we are waling in the midst of this green natural place . . .
while this breeze is caressing our body . . .
and is giving us such a pleasant feeling . . .
the temperature and the landscape are so sublime . . .
and relaxing . . . very relaxing . . .
we walk down this path very slowly . . .
and in the distance . . .
we see a great beach of white sand and the sea
the sea is the color of emeralds . . .
some sailboats are on the horizon . . .
slowly we arrive at the sea . . .
and we dive into the waves . . .
while our body . . . and our mind are perfectly relaxed . . .
in this serene atmosphere of peace . . .
and tranquility . . .
we are relaxing . . . relaxing . . . relaxing . . .
deeply and completely . . . deeply and completely . . . deeply and completely .
. . deeply . . . deeply . . . deeply . . . deeply . . . deeply . . . deeply and completely
. . .
even more deeply . . . even more completely . . .
we are immersing ourselves in a sea of tranquility . . . of relaxation . . . of calm
. . . calm . . .
of pleasant feelings . . .
at all levels . . .
at all levels . . .
at physical level . . . at physical level . . .
at mental level . . . at mental level . . .
at spiritual level . . . at spiritual level . . .
we immerse ourselves again in a sea of tranquility . . . of tranquility . . . of relax-

ation . . . of relaxation . . . of calm . . . of calm . . .
of pleasant feeling . . . of pleasant feeling . . .
at all levels . . . at all levels
physical level . . . physical level . . .
mental leve . . . mental level . . .
spiritual level . . . spiritual level . . .
and now that we are immersed
in this welcoming and cool sea . . .
welcoming and cool sea . . .
slowly we go towards the light . . .
towards the light of our conscience . . .
the light of our deepest self . . .
the light of the cosmos . . .
the light of the cosmos . . .
the light that never goes out
the light that never goes out
the light that never goes out . . .
and now that we are immersed
in this welcoming cooling sea . . .
welcoming cooling sea . . .
slowly we go towards the light . . .
the light of our conscience . . .
the light of our deepest self . . .
the light of the cosmos . . .
the light of the cosmos . . .
the light that never goes out
the light that never goes out
the light that never goes out . . .
every moment is a step forward towards the light . . .
a step forward towards the light . . .
a very important step towards the light of the infinite . . .
towards the light that shows us the way . . .
the light that shows us the way
in the unknown path . . . never explored . . .
where our soul is resting . . .
where our soul is resting cradling in the light . . .
where our soul cradles us in this sea of light . . . of light . . .
of light that never goes out . . .
and the spirit is enjoying the infinite . . .
is enjoying the infinite . . . is enjoying the infinite . . .
all of our being is immersing
like in the welcoming cooling sea . . .
like in the welcoming cooling sea . . .
in the same way in this great sea of light, great sea of light, which is bringing a
great physical . . . mental . . . and spiritual well-being . . .

a well-being all over our body . . .
a great well-being in the soul and in the spirit . . .
a great well-being in the soul and in the spirit . . .
everything is taking us towards the light . . .
the light that surround us . . . the light that embraces us . . .
the light that is around us in this sea of well-being . . . sea of tranquility, . . .
sea of tranquility . . .
a sea of intense and continuous spiritual feeling
a sea of intense and continuous spiritual feeling
intense and continuous . . .
intense and continuous . . .
everything takes us towards the light . . . the light that surround us . . . the light
that embraces us . . .
the light that makes us feeling this sea of well-being . . . within a sea of well-being
. . . a sea of tranquility . . . a sea of tranquility . . .
the light of intense and continuous spiritual feeling
the light of intense and continuous spiritual feeling . . .
intense and continuous...intense and continuous . . .
the light is all around us . . .
and it send us more towards friendly untouched places . . .
towards places which are unknown but where there is love . . .
towards places which are unknown but exciting . . .
towards unknown and untouched places . . .
unknown and untouched places . . .
the light is all around us . . .
and it send us more towards friendly untouched places . . .
towards places which are unknown
but where there is love . . .
towards places which are unknown but exciting . . .
towards unknown and untouched places . . .
towards unknown and untouched places . . .
every moment is used to strengthen our body and our spirit and enjoying the
light . . . the light . . .
the brightest light . . . the surreal light . . . the light that never goes out . . . the
light that never goes out . . . the light that never goes out . . .
we are here now to enjoy this moment
of immersion in the light . . . in the light of our soul . . .
in the light of our spirit . . .
which is slowly embracing us in its comforting way . . .
in its encouraging embrace . . .
in its welcoming embrace . . . in its infinite embrace . . .
in its infinite embrace . . . in its infinite embrace . . .
and all the rest is not important anymore . . .
nothing bothers us anymore . . .
only to live this moment . . .

only to appreciate this moment . . .
only to enjoy this moment . . .
a moment of great joy for the soul
and for the spirit . . .
this moment of great joy for the soul and for the spirit . . .
this moment of immersion in the light of the soul and the spirit . . .
the light that never goes out . . . the light of the cosmos . . . that never goes out
. . .
nothing bothers us anymore . . .
only to live this moment . . .
only to appreciate this moment . . .
only to enjoy this moment . . .
a moment of great joy for the soul and for the spirit . . .
this moment of immersion in the light of the soul and the spirit . . .
the light that never goes out . . .
the light of the cosmos . . .
that never goes out . . .
that never goes out . . .
in this very particular moment, feel the intense light,
the encouraging light, the comforting light,
the soul and the spirit have reached home . . .
the soul and the spirit are comfortable with each other . . .
. . . immersed in the light of the cosmos . . . in the light that embraces everything
. . .
the light that surrounds everything . . .
the light that covers everything . . .
the light that never goes out . . .
in the great light of the soul and the spirit . . .
beyond the time and space . . .
beyond time and space . . .
beyond time and space . . .
the time and the space . . .
towards the infinite . . .
towards the infinite . . .
within the infinite . . . within the infinite . . .
within the infinite . . .
now we immerse ourselves again in a sea of tranquility . . . of tranquility . . .
of relaxation . . . of relaxation . . . of calm . . . of calm . . .
a sea of tranquility . . . a sea of tranquility . . .
a sea of intense and continuous spiritual feeling
in a beautiful natural place . . . our favorite place . . .
our favorite place . . .
our hearts contemplate this peace
and now that we are immersed in this welcoming and cool sea . . . welcoming
and cool sea . . .

we look at the sky . . . look at the sky . . .
a beautiful blue sky, with a few white clouds . . .
they move slowly, almost rocking . . .
a beautiful blue sky, a light breeze which caresses our faces . . . and the bright
sun . . . which gives us new energy . . .
energy of the body and of the mind . . .
we are in our favorite place . . .
with beautiful blue sky and white clouds slowly moving . . .
the peaceful sky calming . . .
the serene sky calms my soul . . .
. . . on a wonderful clear day . . . with a pleasant temperature . . .
a light breeze is caressing and relaxing us . . . a beautiful blue sky . . . with a few
white clouds on the horizon . . .
the sea is the color of emeralds . . .
some sailboats are on the horizon . . .
in a beautiful natural place . . . our favorite place . . .
our favorite place . . .
and now we are walking again on a path of small white pebbles . . .
we are walking in the midst of this green natural place . . . while this breeze is
caressing our body . . . and is giving us such a pleasant feeling . . . the temperature and the landscape are so sublime . . . and relaxing . . . very relaxing . . .
while our body . . . and our mind are perfectly relaxed . . . in this serene atmosphere of peace . . . and tranquility . . .
we are relaxing . . . relaxing . . . relaxing . . . deeply and completely . . . deeply
and completely . . . deeply and completely . . . deeply. deeply . . . deeply . . .
deeply . . . deeply . . . deeply and completely . . . even more deeply . . . even
more completely . . .
. . . well-being is all around us . . . well-being surrounds us . . . and it gives us
new energy . . .
very good . . . very good . . .
we are living this moment so intensely . . .
charged with new energy . . .
this moment of great physical and psychic relaxation
and we are recharging all of our body . . .
and our mind . . . here, in our favorite place . . .
in our favorite place . . .
we are recharging our body and mind . . .
we are again recharging our body and mind . . .
and when we are going to restart our day,
after this relaxation . . .
all of our mind and body will be recharged . . .
all of our mind and body are recharged . . .
full of physical and mental energy . . . rich of mental and physical energy . . .
now let's take a deep breath . . .
and let's leave with our mind from this wonderful natural place . . .

let's start to feel where our body makes contact with what we lying . . .

. . . but still keep this feeling of well-being . . .

well-being of our mind and body . . .

and this feeling of wonderful new energy we have just experienced . . .

let's start slowly to return to our being awake,

but still keeping within ourselves this feeling of calm, tranquility and happiness that we have just experienced.

now let's take another deep breath.

and slowly . . . return to being awake.

we can also slowly start to move our feet and hands, very slowly . . . with no hurry . . . slowly . . .

while the time goes by . . . while the time goes by.

let's take another deep breath . . . and let's start to move slowly all our body . . . especially arms and legs . . .

and let's keep within ourselves just for a little longer . . . the calm . . . the tranquility . . . the relaxation and the happiness that we have just experienced at all levels . . .

. . . we can slowly open our eyes . . . slowly and

return to being awake . . . always slowly . . .

very slowly we awake . . . moving slowly our arms and legs . . .

let's start to move very slowly . . . good . . . very good . . . normal movements . . .

and still keep within ourselves just a little longer the calm . . . and tranquility . . . that we have achieved in this exercise.

we move again . . . good, we are awake.

how are you? how are you? . . . have you achieved the state of calm, tranquility, happiness, relaxation and concentration?

or may be is it still a little early?

good . . . very good . . .

we are awake.

The more you repeat this exercise the easier it will come and it will be also more spontaneous and more enjoyable for your well-being.

REFERENCES

Accardi, M. C., & Milling, L. S. (2009). The effectiveness of hypnosis for reducing procedure-related pain in children and adolescents: A comprehensive methodological review. *Journal of Behavioral Medicine, 32*(4), 328–339.

Assagioli, R. (1991). *Psicosintesi terapeutica.* Rome, Italy: Casa Editrice Astrolabio.

Austin, J. H. (1999). *Zen and the brain: Toward an understanding of meditation and consciousness.* Cambridge, MA: First MIT Press paperback edition.

Brugnoli, A. (1974a). Hypnotic therapeutic methods for pain. *Minerva Medica, 65*(47), 2637–2641.

Brugnoli, A. (1974b). Hypnotherapy of pain. *Minerva Medica, 65*(63), 3288–3295.

Brugnoli, A. (2004). *Stato di coscienza totalizzante, alla ricerca del profondo Se.* Verona, Italy: La Grafica Editrice.

Brugnoli, A. (2005). *Stati di coscienza modificati neurofisiologici.* Verona, Italy: La Grafica Editrice.

Brugnoli, M. P. (2004). Tecniche di rilassamento e ipnosi nel controllo della sofferenza del paziente terminale. *Acta Hypnologica, 7*(1-2), 3–14.

Brugnoli, M.P. (2009). *Clinical hypnosis, spirituality and palliation: The way of inner peace.* Verona, Italy: Del Miglio Editore.

Brugnoli, M. P., Brugnoli, A., & Norsa, A. (2006). *Nonpharmacological and noninvasive management in pain: Physical and psychological modalities.* Verona, Italy: La Grafica Editrice.

Casula, C. (2001). *La forza della vulnerabilità. Utilizzare la resilienza per superare le avversità.* Milan, Italy: Franco Angeli Editore.

Casula, C., Preti, M., & Portaluri, S. (2005). *7 meditazioni guidate. Per risvegliare l'energia dei chakra.* Con CD Audio. Red Edizioni, Italy.

De Sousa, R. (1987). *The rationality of emotion.* Cambridge, MA: MIT Press.

Erickson, M. H. (1959). Hypnosis in painful terminal illness. *American Journal of Clinical Hypnosis, 1,* 1117–1121.

Fourie, D. P. (1997). Indirect suggestion in hypnosis: Theoretical and experimental issues. *Psychological Report, 80*(3 Pt 2), 1255–1266.

Handel, D. L. (2001, February). Complementary therapies for cancer patients: What works, what doesn't, and how to know the difference. *Texas Medicine, 97*(2), 68–73.

Jensen, M. P., & Patterson, D. R. (2005, April). Control conditions in hypnotic-analgesia clinical trials: Challenges and recommendations. *International Journal of Clinical and Experimental Hypnosis, 53*(2), 170–197.

Jung, C. G. (2006). The undiscovered self: The problem of the individual. In *The collected works of C. G. Jung* (Bollingen series, Vol. 11, Psychology and Religion). Princeton, NJ: Princeton University Press. It was first published as "Antwort auf Hiob," Zürich, 1952, and translated into English in London, 1954.

Linden, J. H. (1999). Discussion of symposium. Enhancing healing: The contributions of hypnosis to women's health care. *American Journal of Clinical Hypnosis. 42*(2), 140–144.

Linden, J. H., Bhardwaj, A., & Anbar, R. D. (2006). Hypnotically enhanced dreaming to achieve symptom reduction: A case study of 11 children and adolescents. *American Journal of Clinical Hypnosis, 48*(4), 279–289.

Patterson, D. R. (2010). *Clinical hypnosis for pain control.* Washington, DC: APA Books.

Patterson, D. R., & Jensen, M. P. (2003). Hypnosis and clinical pain. *Psychological Bulletin, 129,* 495–521.

Perez-De-Albeniz, A., & Jeremy, H. (2000). Meditation: Concepts, effects and uses in therapy. *International Journal of Psychotherapy, 5*(1), 49–59.

Rinpoche, S. (1994). *The Tibetan book of living and dying.* London: Rider.

Samraj, A. D. (2005). *What is required to realize the non-dual truth?: The controversy between the "talking" school and the "practicing" school of advaitism (The Basket of Tolerance Booklet Series, Number 9).* Self-published.

Sherman, R. A. (2004). *Pain assessment and intervention from a psychophysiological perspective.* Wheat Ridge, CO: Association of Applied Psychophysiology and Biofeedback.

Spiegel, D. (1985). The use of hypnosis in controlled cancer pain. *CA: A Cancer Journal for Clinicians, 4,* 221–231.

Vaitl, D., Birbaumer, N., Gruzelier, J., Jamieson, G.A., Kotchoubey, B., Kübler, A., ..., & Weiss, T. (2005, January). Psychobiology of altered states of consciousness. *Psychological Bulletin, 131*(1), 98–127.

Vannoni, S., & Brugnoli, A. (1971). Hypnotherapy in orthopedics and traumatology. *Minerva Ortopedica, 22*(3), 77–83.

SUGGESTED READINGS

Alcock, J. E. (1979). Psychology and near-death experiences. *Skeptical Inquirer, 3(3):25-41.*

American Society of Clinical Oncology. (1998). *Policy on Cancer Care During the Last Phase of Life.* Available at http://www.asco.org/ac/1,1003,12-002174-00_18-0010346-00_19 0010351-00-20-001,00.asp

Anton, F. (2009). Chronic stress and pain—A plea for a concerted research program. *Pain, 143*(3), 163-164.

Arena, J. G., & Blanchard, E. B. (1996). Biofeedback and relaxation therapy for chronic pain disorders. In R. J. Gatchel & D. C. Turk (Eds.), *Psychological approaches to pain management* (pp. 179–230). New York: The Guilford Press.

Armstrong, D. M. (1978). Naturalism, materialism and first philosophy. *Philosophia, 8,* 261–276.

Arntz, A., Dreessen, L., & Merckelbach, H. (1991). Attention, not anxiety, influences pain. *Behaviour Research and Therapy, 29,* 41–50.

Bandura, A. (1977). Self-efficacy: Toward a unifying theory of behavioral change. *Psychological Review, 84*(2), 191–215.

Bartolomeo, P. (2002). The relationship between visual perception and visual mental imagery: A reappraisal of the neuropsychological evidence. *Cortex, 38,* 357–378.

Battino, R. (2002). *Metaphoria.* New York: Crown House Publishing Co.

Battino, R., & South, T. L. (2005). *Ericksonian approaches.* New York: Crown House Publishing Co.

Bechert, H., & Gombrich, R. (Eds.). (1984). *The world of Buddhism.* London: Thames & Hudson.

Benedetti, G. (1969). The unconscious from the neuropsychological viewpoint [Review]. *Der Nervenarzt, 40*(4), 149–155.

Bennett, M. V. L., & Zukin, R. S. (2004). Electrical coupling and neuronal synchronization in the mammalian brain. *Neuron, 41,* 495–511.

Benson, H. (1975). *The relaxation response.* New York: William Morrow.

Berman, M., & Brown, D. (2000). *The power of metaphor.* New York: Crown House Publishing Co.

Bickle, J. (2003). *Philosophy and neuroscience: A ruthlessly reductive account.* Norwell, MA: Kluwer Academic Press.

Blackmore, S. (2003). *Consciousness: An introduction.* London: Hodder & Stoughton.

Bloom, P. (2004). *Advances in Neuroscience Relevant to the Clinical Practice of Hypnosis: A Clinician's Perspective.* Keynote address to the 16th International Congress of Hypnosis and Hypnotherapy, Singapore.

Bob, P. (2008). Pain, dissociation and subliminal self-representations. *Consciousness and Cognition, 17*(1), 355–369.

Bonica, J. J. (Ed.). (1990). *The management of pain* (2nd ed.). Philadelphia: Lea & Febiger.

Bower, B. (2007, September 15). Consciousness in the raw: The brain stem may orchestrate the basics of awareness [Online]. *Science News.*

Brugnoli, M. P. (2001). Neurofisiologia di realtà percepita e realtà rappresentata: quale relazione tra working memory e visualizzazione mentale in ipnosi. *Acta Hypnologica, 3,* 21–22.

Brugnoli, M. P., & Shivchandra Parolini, M. (2009). *La via della pace interiore: tecniche di rilassamento e di meditazione per il benessere dell'anima.* Verona, Italy: Del Miglio Editore.

Capra, F. (2003). *The hidden connections: A science for sustainable living.* New York: Anchor Books.

Carrithers. M. (1986). The Buddha. In *Founders of faith* (pp. 13–14). Oxford, UK: Oxford University Press.

Carruthers, P. (2000). *Phenomenal consciousness.* Cambridge, UK: Cambridge University Press.

Charon, J. E. (2004). *The spirit: That stranger inside us.* Califormula Publishing.

Chochinov, H. M., Krisjanson, L. J., Hack, T. F., Hassard, T., McClement, S., & Harlos, M. (2006, June). Dignity in the terminally ill: Revisited. *Journal of Palliative Medicine, 9*(3), 666–672.

Churchland, P. (1986). *Neurophilosophy.* Cambridge, MA: MIT Press.

Cleeland, C. S. (1987). Nonpharmacologic management of cancer pain. *Journal of Pain and Symptom Control, 2,* 523–528.

Cleeland, C. S., & Syrjala, K. L. (1992). How to assess cancer pain. In D. C. Turk & R. Melzack (Eds.), *Handbook of pain assessment* (pp. 360–387). New York: Guilford Press.

Coslett, H. B., Medina, J., Kliot, D., & Burkey, A. (2010, April). Mental motor imagery and chronic pain: The foot laterality task. *Journal of the International Neuropsychological Society, 12,* 1–10.

Council on Scientific Affairs, American Medical Association. (1996). Good care of the dying patient. *Journal of the American Medical Association, 275,* 474–478.

Crick, F., & Koch C. (1995). Cortical areas in visual awareness [Reply]. *Nature, 377,* 294–295.

Crosley, R. O. (2004). *Alternative medicine and miracles: A grand unified theory.* Lanham, MD: University Press of America.

Dalai Lama. (1999). *The Dalai Lama's book of wisdom.* London: Thorsons.

Damasio, A. (1999). *The feeling of what happens: Body, emotion and the making of consciousness.* London: Heinemann.

Dennett, D. (1991). *Consciousness explained.* London: Penguin Books.

Ellis, H. (1897). A note on hypnagogic paramnesia. *Mind, New Series, 6*(22), 283–287.

Erickson, M. (1983). *La mia voce ti accompagnerà.* Rome, Italy: Casa Editrice Astrolabio.

Erickson M. H. (1978). *Le nuove vie dell'ipnosi.* Rome, Italy: Casa Editrice Astrolabio.

Erickson, M. H., & Rossi, E. L. (1976, January). Two level communication and the microdynamics of trance and suggestion. *American Journal of Clinical Hypnosis, 18*(3), 153–171.

Erickson, M. H., & Rossi, E. L. (1980). *The nature of hypnosis and suggestion* (Vol. 1). New York: Irvington Publishers.

Erickson, M. H., Rossi, E. L., & Rossi, S. I. (1976). *Hypnotic realities: The induction of clinical hypnosis and forms of indirect suggestion.* New York: Irvington Publishers.

Ewin, D. (1986). The effect of hypnosis and mind set on burns. *Psychiatric Annals, 16,* 115–118.

Fainsinger, R., Miller, M. J., Bruera, E., Hanson, J., & Maceachern, T. (1991). Symptom control during the last week of life on a palliative care unit. *Journal of Palliative Care, 7,* 5–11.

Farthing, G. W. (1992). *The psychology of consciousness.* Englewood Cliffs, NJ: Prentice-Hall.

Farthing, G. W., Venturino, M., & Brown, S. W. (1984). Suggestion and distraction in the control of pain: Test of two hypotheses. *Journal of Abnormal Psychology, 93,* 266–276.

Faymonville, M. E., Laureys, S., Degueldre, C., Del Fiore, G., Luxen, A., Franck, G., ..., & Maquet, P. (2000). Neural mechanisms of antinociceptive effects of hypnosis. *Anesthesiology, 92,* 1257–1267.

Ferioli, W. (1974). Hypnotherapy and psychosomatic disorders. *Minerva Medica, 65*(47), 2630–2632.

Ferrari, M., & Sternberg, R. J. (Eds.). (1998). *Self-awareness: Its nature and development.* New York: Guilford Press.

Field, M . J., & Cassel, C. K. (1997). *Approaching death: Improving care at the end of life.* Washington, DC: National Academy Press.

Fuller, R. C. (1996). Holistic health practices. In P. H. Van Ness (Ed.), *Spirituality and the secular quest* (pp. 230-234). New York: Crossroad Publishing Company.

Gheorghiu, V. A. (1972). On suggestion and suggestibility. *Scientia, 107.*

Goldstein, J. (1983). *The experience of insight.* Boston: Shambhala.

Graffam, S., & Johnson, A. (1987). A comparison of two relaxation strategies for the relief of pain and its distress. *Journal of Pain and Symptom Management, 2*(4), 229–231.

Grof, S. (2000). *Il gioco cosmico della mente.* Red Edizioni.

Grun, A. (1995). *Autostima ed accettazione dell'ombra.* Edizioni San Paolo.

Grun, A. (1995). *Autostima ed accettazione dell'ombra.* Edizioni San Paolo.

Haley, J. (1963). *Strategies of psychotherapy.* New York: Grune and Stratton.

Heal, J. (2001). On speaking thus: The semantics of indirect discourse. *Philosophical Quarterly, 51,* 433–454.

Hendler, C. S., & Redd, W. H. (1986). Fear of hypnosis: The role of labeling in patients' acceptance of behavioral interventions. *Behavioral Therapy, 17*(1), 2–13.

Hilgard, E. R, & Hilgard, J. R. (1994). *Hypnosis in the relief of pain.* New York: Brunner/Mazel.

His Divine Grace A. C. Bhaktivedanta Swami Prabhupada. (1972). *Bhagavad-Gita.* Krishna Store.

Hoffman, H. G., Doctor, J. N., Patterson, D. R., Carrougher, G. J., & Furness, T. A. (2000). Virtual reality as an adjunctive pain control during burn wound care in adolescent patients. *Pain, 85*(1-2), 305–309.

Honderich, T. (1995). Consciousness, neural functionalism, real subjectivity. *American Philosophical Quarterly, 32,* 369–381.

Hopkins, J. (2004). *Mind as metaphor: A physicalistic approach to the problem of consciousness.* Unpublished work in progress. http://www.kcl.ac.uk/kis/schools/hums /philosophy/staff/jimh.html

Hori, T., Hayashi, M., & Morikawa, T. (1993). Topographical EEG changes and hypnagogic experience. In R. D. Ogilvie & J. R. Harsh (Eds.), *Sleep onset: Normal and abnormal processes* (pp. 237–253). Washington, DC: American Psychological Association.

James, W. (1902). Lectures 16 & 17: Mysticism. In *The varieties of religious experience: A study in nature* (pp. 206–234). Huntington, MA: Seven Treasures Publications.

Jensen, M., & Patterson, D. R. (2006, February). Hypnotic treatment of chronic pain. *Journal of Behavioral Medicine, 29*(1), 95–124.

Jevning, R., Wallace, R. K., & Beidebach, M. (1992). The physiology of meditation: A review. A wakeful hypometabolic integrated response. *Neuroscience and Biobehavioral Reviews, 16*(3), 415–424.

Jung, C. G. (1942/1948). *Saggio d'interpretazione psicologica del dogma della Trinità.*

Jung, C. G. (1969). Psychology of transference. In *The collected works of C. G. Jung* (Vol. 16), Princeton, NJ: Princeton University Press.

Jung, C. G. (1989). *La psicologia dell'inconscio.* Newton Compton Editori.

Jung, C. G. (1991). *Opere.* (Vol. 11.). Torino, Italy, Boringhieri.

Kabat-Zinn, J., Lipworth, L., & Burney, R. (1985). The clinical use of mindfulness meditation for the self regulation of chronic pain. *Journal of Behavioral Medicine, 8*(2), 163–190.

Kallio, S., & Revonsuo, A. (2003). Hypnotic phenomena and altered states of consciousness: A multilevel framework of description and explanation. *Contemporary Hypnosis, 20*(3), 111–164.

Kearney, M. (1996). *Mortally wounded: Stories of soul pain, death, and healing.* New Orleans, LA: Spring Journal, Inc.

Kolcaba, K. Y., & Fisher, E. M. (1996, February). A holistic perspective on comfort care as an advance directive. *Critical Care Nursing Quarterly, 18*(4), 66–76.

Kosslyn, S. M. (1980). *Image and mind.* Cambridge, MA: Harvard University Press.

Kubler Ross, E. (2005). *La morte e il morire.* Cittadella Editrice.

Last Acts. (2003). *Care Beyond Cure-Palliative Care and Hospice.* Fact Sheet. Accessed February 24, at http://www.lastacts.org/scripts/la_res01.exe FNC=FactSheets __Ala_res_NewHome_html

Levitan, A. (1992). The use of hypnosis with cancer patients. *Psychiatry and Medicine, 10,* 119–131.

Lindtner, C. (1997). *Master of wisdom.* Berkeley, CA: Dharma Publishing.

Liossi, C., & Hatira, P. (2003). Clinical hypnosis in the alleviation of procedure-related pain in pediatric oncology patients. *The International Journal of Clinical and Experimental Hypnosis, 51,* 4–28.

Lo, B. (1995). Improving care near the end of life: Why is it so hard? *Journal of the American Medical Association, 274,* 1634–1636.

Luciano, M. C., Rodríguez, M., & Gutiérrez, O. (2004). A proposal for synthesizing verbal contexts in experiential avoidance disorder and acceptance and commitment therapy. *International Journal of Psychology and Psychological Therapy, 4,* 377–394.

Luthe, W., & Schultz, J. H. (2001). Autogenic Therapy. London: The British Autogenic Society. (Original work published in 1969 by Grune and Stratton.)

Lynn, S. J., Neufeld, V., & Matyi, C. L. (1987). Inductions versus suggestions: Effects of direct and indirect wording on hypnotic responding and experience. *Journal of Abnormal Psychology, 96*(1), 76–79.

Manzoni, G. M., Pagnini, F., Castelnuovo, G., & Molinari, E. (2008). Relaxation training for anxiety: A ten-years systematic review with meta-analysis. *BMC Psychiatry, 8,* 41.

Manzotti, R., & Gozzano, S. (2004). Verso una scienza della coscienza. *Networks –:* i-iii. Available at http://www.swif.uniba.it/lei/ai/networks/

Matthews, W. J., & Langdell, S. (1989). What do clients think about the metaphors they receive? An initial inquiry. *American Journal of Clinical Hypnosis, 31*(4), 242–251.

McCaul, K. D., & Malott, J. M. (1984). Distraction and coping with pain. *Psychology Bulletin, 95*(3), 516–533.

McFarlane, T. J. (1995). *The meaning of sunyata in Nagarjuna's philosophy.* Available at http://www.integralscience.org/sacredscience/SS_sunyata.html

McGlashan, T. H., Evans, F. J., & Orne, M. T. (1969). The nature of hypnotic analgesia and placebo response to experimental pain. *Psychosomatic Medicine, 31,* 227–246.

Melzack, R. (1998). Pain and stress: Clues toward understanding chronic pain. In M. Sabourin, F. Craik & M. Robert (Eds.), *Advances in psychological science* (Vol. 2, Biological and Cognitive Aspects, pp. 63–85). London: Psychology Press.

Melzack, R. (1999). Pain and stress a new perspective. In R. J. Gatchel & D. C. Turk (Eds.), *Psychosocial factors in pain* (pp. 89–106). New York: Guilford Press.

Melzack, R. (2001). Pain and the neuromatrix in the brain. *Journal of Dental Education, 65,* 1378–1382.

Melzack, R. (2002). Evolution of Pain Theories. *Program and Abstracts of the 21st Annual Scientific Meeting of the American Pain Society,* March 14–17, Baltimore, Maryland. Abstract 102.

Merker, B. (2007, September). Consciousness in the raw. *Science News Online.* Available at http://www.sciencenews.org/articles/20070915/bob9.asp

Miaskowski, C., Cleary, J., Burney, R., Coyne, P., Finley, R., Foster, R., ..., & Zahrbock, C. (2005). *Guideline for the management of cancer pain in adults and children.* Glenview, IL: American Pain Society.

Miller, G. A., Galanter, E., & Pribram, K. H. (1960). *Plans and the structure of behavior.* New York: Holt, Rinehart &Winston.

Modern Society. New York: New American Library.

Morin, A. (2004). Possible links between self-awareness and inner speech: Theoretical background, underlying mechanisms, and empirical evidence. Unpublished journal.

Mosca, A. (2000). A review essay on Antonio Damasio's *The Feeling of What Happens: Body and Emotion in the Making of Consciousness. PSYCHE, 6*(10).

Muller, A. C. (1999). *The sutra of perfect enlightenment.* Albany, NY: State University Press of New York.

Murphy, T. M. (1986). Treatment of chronic pain. In R. D. Miller (Ed.), *Anesthesia.* New York: Churchill Livingstone.

Nattier, J. (2003). *A few good men: The Bodhisattva path according to the inquiry of Ugra* (Ugrapariprccha). Honolulu, HA: University of Hawaii Press.

Ospina, M. B., Bond, K., Karkhaneh, M., Tjosvold, L., Vandermeer, B., Liang, Y., ..., & Klassen, T. P. (2007). *Meditation practices for health: State of the research.* Evidence Report/Technology Assessment (Full Report), June (155), 1–263.

Paivio, A. (1986). *Mental representations: A dual coding approach.* New York: Oxford University Press.

Patterson, D. R., Wiechman, S. A., Jensen, M., & Sharar, S. R. (2006). Hypnosis delivered through immersive virtual reality for burn pain: A clinical case series. *International Journal of Clinical and Experimental Hypnosis, 54*(2), 130–142.

Power, D., Kelly, S., Gilsenan, J., Kearney, M., O'Mahony, D., Walsh, J. B., & Coakley, D. (1993). Suitable screening tests for cognitive impairment and depression in the terminally ill-a prospective prevalence study. *Palliative Medicine, 7,* 213–218.

Raz, A., Fan, J., & Posner, M. I. (2005, July 12). Hypnotic suggestion reduces conflict in the human brain. *Proceedings of the National Academy of Sciences of the United States of America, 102*(28), 9978–9983.

Ready, L. B., & Edwards, W. T. (Eds.). Task Force on Acute Pain. (1992). *Management of acute pain: A practical guide.* Seattle, WA: IASP Publications.

Reeves, J. L., Redd, W. H., Storm, F. K., & Minagawa, R. Y. (1983). Hypnosis in the control of pain during hyperthermia treatment of cancer. In J. J. Bonica, U. Lindblom, & A. Iggo (Eds.), *Proceedings of the Third World Congress on pain,*

Edinburgh. (Vol. 5, Advances in Pain Research and Therapy, pp. 857–861). New York: Raven Press.

Richardson, A. (1969). *Mental imagery*. London: Routledge & Kegan Paul.

Richardson, J. (1999). *Mental imagery*. Hove, UK: Psychology Press.

Richardson, J., Smith, J. E., McCall, G., & Pilkington, K. (2006). Hypnosis for procedure-related pain and distress in pediatric cancer patients: a systematic review of effectiveness and methodology related to hypnosis interventions. *Journal of Pain and Symptom Management, 31*(1), 70–84.

Schwartz, M. S. (Ed.). (1995). *Biofeedback: A practitioner's guide*. New York: The Guilford Press.

Searle, J. (1990). Consciousness, explanatory inversion and cognitive science. *Behavioral and Brain Sciences, 13*, 585–642.

Searle, J. (1992). *The rediscovery of the mind*. Cambridge, MA: MIT Press.

Shapiro, D. (1977). A biofeedback strategy in the study of consciousness. In N.E. Zinberg (Ed.), *Alternate states of consciousness* (pp. 145–37). New York: The Free Press.

Sharar, S. R., Miller, W., Teeley, A., Soltani, M., Hoffman, H. G., Jensen, M. P., & Patterson, D. R. (2008). Applications of virtual reality for pain management in burn-injured patients. *Expert Reviews of Neurotherapeutics, 8*(11), 1667–1674.

Shepard, R. N., & Cooper, L. (1982). *Mental images and their transformations*. Cambridge, MA: The MIT Press.

Shor, R. E. (1979). The fundamental problem in hypnosis research as viewed from historic perspectives. In E. Fromm & R. E. Shor (Eds.), *Hypnosis: Developments in research and new perspectives*. New York: Aldine Publ. Co.

Staal, F. (1975). *Exploring mysticism*. London: Penguin.

Stoelb, B. L., Molton, I. R., Jensen, M. P., & Patterson, D. R. (2009, March 1). The efficacy of hypnotic analgesia in adults: A review of the literature. *Contemporary Hypnosis, 26*(1), 24–39.

Sugarmann, L. I. (1996). Hypnosis in a primary care practice: Developing skills for the "new morbidities." *Journal of Developmental and Behavioral Pediatrics, 17*(5), 300–305.

Sutcher, H. (2008). Hypnosis, hypnotizability and treatment. *American Journal of Clinical Hypnosis, 51*(1), 57–67.

Syrjala, K. L. (1990). Relaxation techniques. In J. J. Bonica (Ed.), *The management of pain* (2nd ed., pp. 1742–1750). Philadelphia: Lea & Febiger.

Tart, C. T. (1970). Transpersonal potentialities of deep hypnosis. University of California, Davis. Reprinted from *Journal of Transpersonal Psychology, 1970, 2*, 27–40. Copyright © 1970 American Transpersonal Association.

Tart, C. T. (1972). States of consciousness and state-specific sciences. *Science, 176*, 1203–1210.

Tart, C. T. (1977). *Stati di coscienza*. Rome, Italy: Casa Editrice Astrolabio.

Tart, C. T. (1990). *Altered states of consciousness* (3rd ed.). San Francisco, CA: Harper.

Taylor, J. (2000, February). The enchanting subject of consciousness (or is it a black hole?). *PSYCHE, 6*(2).

Thurman, R. A. F. (Trans.). (1976). Holy Teaching of Vimalakirti: Mahayana Scripture. State College, PA: Pennsylvania State University Press.

Tolle, E. (1999). *The power of now: A guide to spiritual enlightenment.* Vancouver, BC, Canada: Namaste Publishing.

Travis, C. (2004). The silence of the senses. *Mind, 113,* 57–94.

Travis, F., Arenander, A., & DuBois, D. (2004). Psychological and physiological characteristics of a proposed object-referral/self-referral continuum of self-awareness. *Consciousness and Cognition, 13*(2), 401–420.

Upanishad. (2001). *La via della liberazione.* Italy: Demetra.

Valente, S. M. (2006, February). Hypnosis for pain management. *Journal of Psychosocial Nursing and Mental Health Services, 44*(2), 22–30.

Van Der Werf, Y. D., Witter, M. P., & Groenewegen, H. J. (2002).The intralaminar and midline nuclei of the thalamus. Anatomical and functional evidence for participation in processes of arousal and awareness. *Brain Research Reviews, 39,* 107–140.

Van Gulick, R. (2004). Higher-order global states HOGS: An alternative higher-order model of consciousness. In R. Gennaro (Ed.), *Higher-order theories of consciousness.* Philadelphia: John Benjamins.

Van Tilburg, M. A., Chitkara, D. K., Palsson, O. S., Turner, M., Blois-Martin, N., Ulshen, M., & Whitehead, W. E. (2009). Audio-recorded guided imagery treatment reduces functional abdominal pain in children: A pilot study. *Pediatrics, 124*(5), 890–897.

Vanhaudenhuyse, A., Boly, M., Balteau, E., Schnakers, C., Moonen, G., Luxen, A., ..., & Faymonville, M. E. (2009, September). Pain and non-pain processing during hypnosis: A thulium-YAG event-related fMRI study. *NeuroImage, 47*(3), 1047–1054.

Vincent, J. L. (2005). Give your patient a fast hug (at least) once a day. *Critical Care Medicine, 33*(6), 1225–1229.

Wallace, B. A. (2006). Vacuum states of consciousness: A Tibetan Buddhist view. In D. K. Nauriyal (Ed.), *Buddhist thought and applied psychology: Transcending the boundaries.* London: Routledge Curzon.

Weitzenhoffer, A. M. (1953). *Hypnotism: An objective study in suggestibility.* New York: Wiley.

Wenrich, M. D., Curtis, J. R., Shannon, S. E., Carline, J. D., Ambrozy, D. M., & Ramsey, P. G. (2001). Communicating with dying patients within the spectrum of medical care from terminal diagnosis to death. *Archives of Internal Medicine, 161,* 2623–2624.

Willmarth, E. K., & Willmarth, K. J. (2005). Biofeedback and hypnosis in pain management. *Biofeedback, 20,* Spring.

Wilson, K. G., & Luciano, M. C. (2002). *Terapia de aceptación y compromiso. Un tratamiento conductual orientado a los valores [Acceptance and commitment therapy. A behavioural treatment oriented towards values].* Madrid: Pirámide.

Zeltzer, L., & LeBaron, S. (1982). Hypnosis and nonhypnotic techniques for reduction of pain and anxiety during painful procedures in children and adolescents with cancer. *Journal of Pediatrics, 101*(6), 1032–1035.

Chapter V

MINDFULNESS AND MEDITATIVE STATES IN SPIRITUAL CARE: TYPES AND TECHNIQUES

Meditation is a powerful technique to help all of us make more of our own potential and to relate better to others at the workplace, at home, in the community, and in our lives generally.

Recent research by prominent neuroscientists in the United States has shown that for experienced meditators, activity in the area of the brain associated with happiness is more persistent. Moreover, it also appears that experienced meditators do not get nearly as flustered, shocked or surprised by unpredictable events as do nonmeditators (Flanagan, 2003).

Meditation and hypnosis can help us develop our potential, in ways that have a positive effect on our life, suffering, and general well-being. They can help individuals to

- Cultivate a better understanding of others, leading to increased harmony and shared sense of purpose
- Deal more calmly with potentially stressful circumstances
- Experience increased energy at work and at home
- Decrease pain and suffering
- Bring greater concentration and focus to the mind and inner self
- Develop the ability to see and respond to situations with clarity and creativity
- Develop higher consciousness and the knowledge of higher self
- Help suffering people in pain therapy
- Help dying people in palliative care

When we start practicing hypnosis and meditative states, we start feeling relaxed, peaceful, and happy. This is a kind of intergenerative process. You meditate, and you get the reward in the form of joy and happiness, which in

179

turn motivates you to meditate more. Over time, it becomes your automatic practice, a kind of "sanskar." You feel uneasy and think something is missing from your life if you do not meditate on any particular day. When you start your day with meditation, the peace and joy generated last the whole day. whatever the nature of your activities. It is like having a healthy and nourishing meal before the start of a strenuous and stressful routine during the day.

Hypnosis and meditative states enable you to become aware of your inner resources of joy and peace. You can tap them whenever you feel stressed and worried. You acquire a habit of detached observation. So, if something wrong and irritating happens during the course of your day, you can view it as a detached observer. You thus get an inner poise that ultimately percolates into your daily life.

Research shows that even skeptics cannot stifle the sense that there is something greater than the concrete world we see. As the brain processes sensory experiences, we naturally look for patterns and then seek out the meaning in those patterns.

In the world, there are many important religions and spiritual philosophies and groups. It is impossible to cover all of them in this chapter. Our apologies if your own religion or philosophy is not here. We have included those we were able to study. In this chapter, the philosophies of religions are in alphabetical order.

Spirituality means something different to everyone. For some, it is about participating in organized religion: going to church, a synagogue, a mosque, and so on. For others, it is more personal: some people remain in touch with their spiritual side through private prayer, yoga, meditation, quiet reflection, or even long walks. In palliative care, spirituality is very important to relieve suffering and help people to perceive higher consciousness.

In spirituality, I believe in

- Personal worth: The inner worth of every person. People are worthy of respect, support, and caring simply because they are human.
- Lack of discrimination: Working toward a culture that is relatively free of discrimination.
- Dignity: The dignity of the human person.
- Freedom of speech: The freedom to compare the beliefs of faith groups with each other and with the findings of science.

Spirituality is the concept of an ultimate or an alleged immaterial reality, an inner path enabling a person to discover the essence of his or her being, or the deepest values and meanings by which people live. Spiritual practices, including meditation and mindfulness, prayer and contemplation, are intended to develop an individual's inner life. Spiritual experiences can include being connected to a larger reality, yielding a more comprehensive self; and joining with other individuals or the human community, with nature or the cosmos, or with the divine realm.

1. BUDDHISM

Buddhists believe that they are temporary vessels in this world and that until they attain enlightenment or Buddhahood, they do not know their own self or soul. They believe that this world is an illusion and that, as a result, one cannot know one's true nature. Buddhism teaches its followers that in this life they are only temporary vessels of body, emotions, thoughts, tendencies, and knowledge. A fundamental concept of Buddhism is the notion that the goal of one's life is to break the cycles of death and birth. Reincarnation exists because of the individual's craving and desires to live in this world. The ultimate goal of a Buddhist is to achieve freedom from the cycle of reincarnation and attain nirvana.

Buddhism is a family of beliefs and practices considered by most to be a religion. Buddhism is based on the teachings attributed to Siddhartha Gautama, commonly known as "The Buddha" (the Awakened One), who lived in the northeastern region of the Indian subcontinent and likely died around 400 BCE. Buddhists recognize him as an awakened teacher who shared his insights to help sentient beings end their suffering, by understanding the true nature of phenomena, thereby escaping the cycle of suffering and rebirth, that is, achieving Nirvana.

Among the methods various schools of Buddhism apply toward this goal are ethical conduct and altruistic behavior, devotional practices, ceremonies and the invocation of bodhisattvas, renunciation of world matters, meditation, physical exercises, study, and the cultivation of wisdom. In the yoga meditation of the Himalayan tradition, one person systematically works with senses, body, breath, and the various levels of mind and then goes beyond, to the center of consciousness.

When dealing with the feelings and body, there is the emphasis on exploring and examining, being open to all the thoughts, emotions, and sensations. When attention goes further inward, there is the mind field itself. In this stage of practice, the perceptions have been withdrawn, and there is no longer any sensory awareness of the body, nor of the physical. One is now fully in the level of mind itself. Here is still another form of mindfulness, exclusive of bodily sensation, and once again, concentration is its companion.

Finally, one comes at the end of the mind and all of its associated thoughts, emotions, sensations, and impressions. Concentration is essential at this stage.

As Patanjali notes in the Yoga Sutras (4.31) there is then little to know because the experiences have been resolved into their causes. By working with both mindfulness and concentration, it is easy to see three skills in which the mind is trained and how these go together.

Focus. The mind is trained to be able to pay attention, to not be drawn here and there, whether due to the spontaneous rising of impressions in meditation or due to external stimuli.

Expansion. The ability to focus is accompanied by a willingness to expand the conscious field through that which is normally unconscious, including the center of consciousness.

Nonattachment. The ability to remain undisturbed, unaffected, and uninvolved with the thoughts and impressions upon the mind is the key ingredient that must go along with focus and expansion.

While speaking here of integrating the practices of mindfulness and concentration, it is useful to note that, in a sense, integrating is not quite the right word. The science of yoga meditation as taught by the Himalayan sages is already a whole, complete science that has been torn into smaller pieces over time. Individual parts have been cut out from the whole, given separate names, and then taught as unique systems of meditation. Mindfulness and concentration have both been part of the same, one process of meditation for a very long time.

Concentration. In this approach, one intentionally focuses the attention on only one object, such as the breath, a mantra, a chakra center, or an internally visualized image.

Mindfulness. In this approach, one does not focus the mind on one object but rather observes the whole range of passing thoughts, emotions, sensations, and images.

To the sages of the Himalayas, both methods are used in yoga meditation. In fact, they are not seen as different choices at all. Mindfulness and concentration are companions in the same one process that leads inward to the center of consciousness.

If you go deeper in meditation, you will find that both processes are essential. If one practices only mindfulness, the mind is trained to always have this surface level activity present. Having this activity constantly present may be seen as normal, and the attention simply does not go beyond the mind field. Attention can "back off" from experiencing deeper meditation and samadhi to remain in the fields of sensation and thoughts. If one practices only concentration, or one-pointedness, the mind is trained not to experience this activity of thoughts, sensations, emotions, and images. The activity is seen as something to be avoided, and the attention may not even be open to the existence of these experiences. Attention can back off from the deeper aspects of the mind field and thus prevent deeper meditation and samadhi.

By practicing both mindfulness and concentration, one can experience the vast impressions, learning the vital skill of nonattachment, while also using concentration to focus the mind in such a way as to be able to transcend the whole of the mind field, where there is only stillness and silence, beyond all the impressions. Finally, one can come to experience the center of consciousness, the absolute reality.

When exploring the mind, mindfulness may be emphasized while remaining focused. Then, if a particular thought pattern or samskara is to be examined to weaken its power over the mind, concentration is the tool with which this examination is done. This allows an increase in vairagya, nonattachment.

When settling the mind, trying to pierce the layers of our being, including senses, body, and breath, concentration carries the attention inward through the layers. When attention moves into that next deeper level of our being, then concentration and mindfulness once again work together to explore that layer, to once again move beyond, or deeper.

According to Tibetan medicine, the human microcosm, just as the macrocosm, is made of these five fundamental energies: Earth, Water, Fire, Air, and Ether, which monitor the vitality of the mind and the body. The whole world, the human body, but also illnesses and medicaments, are in communication with one another. The five elements are represented in us by the three body energies: Lung (the principle of motion), Tripa (the principle of warmth), and Beken (the stabilizing and cooling principle). In a healthy body, these three principles are balanced. This balance and, therefore health, depends on the mind because on the mental level disharmony leads to an imbalance of these energies that then manifest as illness in the physical body.

Ignorance is the cause of illness. Ignorance provokes the illusion of being separated from the environment. The perception of "I" and "Mine" creates the Three Interior Poisons: Hatred, Ignorance, and Desire.

A. The Experience of Enlightenment

The Four Noble Truths of Buddhism are about dukkha, a term usually translated as suffering. The Four Noble Truths are one of the most fundamental Buddhist teachings. In broad terms, these truths relate to suffering's (or dukkha's) nature, origin, cessation, and the path leading to the cessation.

They are among the truths Gautama Buddha is said to have realized during his experience of enlightenment.

The Four Noble Truths were the first teaching of Gautama Buddha after attaining nirvana. Life as we know it ultimately is or leads to suffering in one way or another. Suffering is caused by craving for or attachments to worldly pleasures of all kinds. This is often expressed as a deluded clinging to a certain sense of existence, to selfhood, or to the things or people that we consider the cause of happiness or unhappiness. This interpretation is followed closely by many modern Theravadins, described by early Western scholars, and taught as an introduction to Buddhism by some contemporary Mahayana teachers (e.g., the Dalai Lama).

According to other interpretations by Buddhist teachers and scholars and lately recognized by some Western non-Buddhist scholars, the "truths" do not represent mere statements, but are categories or aspects that most worldly phenomena fall into.

B. The Four Noble Truths of Buddhism

1. Life Means Suffering

To live means to suffer, because the human nature is not perfect and neither is life. During our lifetime, we inevitably have to endure physical suffering such as pain, sickness, injury, tiredness, old age, and death, and we have to endure psychological suffering such as sadness, fear, frustration, disappointment, and depression.

Although there are different degrees of suffering and there are also positive experiences in life that we perceive as the opposite of suffering, such as ease, comfort, and happiness, life in its totality is imperfect and incomplete because our world is subject to impermanence. This means we are never able to keep permanently what we strive for, and just as happy moments pass by, we ourselves and our loved ones will pass away one day, too.

2. The Origin of Suffering is Attachment

The origin of suffering is attachment to transient things and the ignorance thereof. Transient things include not only the physical objects that surround us, but also ideas and, in a greater sense, all objects of our perception. Ignorance is the lack of understanding of how our mind is attached to impermanent things. The reasons for suffering are desire, passion, pursuit of wealth and prestige, and striving for fame and popularity, or, in short, craving and clinging. Because the objects of our attachment are transient, their loss is inevitable, thus suffering will necessarily follow. Objects of attachment also include the idea of a "self," which is a delusion because there is no abiding self. What we call self is just an imagined entity, and we are merely a part of the ceaseless becoming of the universe.

Impermanence is one of the Three Marks of Existence. The term expresses the Buddhist notion that all compounded or conditioned phenomena (things and experiences) are inconstant, unsteady, and impermanent. Everything we can experience through our senses is made up of parts, and its existence depends on external conditions. Everything is in constant flux, and so conditions and the thing itself are constantly changing. Things are constantly coming into being, and ceasing to be. Nothing lasts.

According to the impermanence doctrine, human life embodies this flux in the aging process, the cycle of rebirth (samsara), and in any experience of loss. The doctrine further asserts that because things are impermanent, attachment to them is futile and leads to suffering.

According to Buddhism, life against death is a delusive way of thinking. It is dualistic: the denial of being dead is how the ego affirms itself as being alive, so it is the act by which the ego constitutes itself. To be self-conscious is to be conscious of oneself, to grasp oneself, as being alive. Then death terror is not something the ego has; it is what the ego is. This fits well with the Buddhist claim that the ego-self is not a thing, not what I really am, but a mental construction.

The aim of meditation is to bring inner peace within ourselves and the world in a positive and spiritual way. The world is not a peaceful place and within every soul, there is some form of tension and stress. It is therefore essential to create positive and peaceful thoughts to bring peace to our mind. Meditation is one of the best methods to bring about transformation and nurture the natural qualities within.

3. The Cessation of Suffering is Attainable

The cessation of suffering can be attained through nirodha. Nirodha means the unmaking of sensual craving and conceptual attachment. The third noble truth expresses the idea that suffering can be ended by attaining dispassion. Nirodha extinguishes all forms of clinging and attachment. This means that suffering can be overcome through human activity, simply by removing the cause of suffering. Attaining and perfecting to dispassion is a process of many levels that ultimately results in the state of nirvana. Nirvana means freedom from all worries, troubles, complexes, fabrications, and ideas. Nirvana is not comprehensible for those who have not attained it.

4. The Path to the Cessation of Suffering

There is a path at the end of suffering, a gradual path of self-improvement, which is described more detailed in the eightfold path. It is the middle way between the two extremes of excessive self-indulgence (hedonism) and extreme self-mortification (asceticism), and it leads at the end to the cycle of rebirth. The latter quality discerns it from other paths, which are merely "wandering on the wheel of becoming" because they do not have a final object. The path at the end of suffering can extend over many lifetimes, throughout which every individual rebirth is subject to karmic conditioning. Craving, ignorance, delusions, and their effects will disappear gradually, as progress is made along the path.

C. The Noble Eightfold Path

The eightfold path illustrates the moral principles in which all Buddhists should practice the way of enlightenment. It goes into detail about the basis of all Buddhist teachings: morality, meditation, and wisdom. This is the eightfold path.

1. Right Knowledge
2. Right Thinking
3. Right Speech
4. Right Conduct
5. Right Livelihood
6. Right Effort
7. Right Mindfulness
8. Right Concentration

Following The Noble Eightfold Path helps a person realize that greed and selfishness cause all earthly suffering. With this new understanding, one's suffering may end. The Noble Eightfold Path, the fourth of the Buddha's noble truths, is the way for the cessation of suffering. It has eight sections, each starting with the word samyak (Sanskrit, meaning correctly, properly, or well, frequently translated into English as right) and presented in three groups:

1. *Prajñā* is the wisdom that purifies the mind, allowing it to attain spiritual insight into the true nature of all things.
2. *Sila* is the ethics or morality.
3. *Samādhi* is the mental discipline required to develop mastery over one's own mind. This is done through the practice of various contem-

plative and meditative practices, and includes
- vyāyāma (vāyāma): making an effort to improve
- sati: awareness to see things for what they are with clear consciousness, being aware of the present reality within oneself, without any craving or aversion
- samādhi (samādhi): correct meditation or concentration, explained as the first four dhyānas.

The eighth principle of the path, right concentration, refers to the development of a mental force that occurs in natural consciousness, although at a relatively low level of intensity, namely concentration. Concentration in this context is described as one-pointedness of mind, meaning a state where all mental faculties are unified and directed onto one particular object. Right concentration on the purpose of the eightfold path means wholesome concentration, in other words, concentration on wholesome thoughts and actions. The Buddhist method of choice to develop right concentration is through the practice of meditation.

The meditating mind focuses on a selected object. It first directs itself onto it, then sustains concentration, and finally intensifies concentration step by step. Through this practice, it becomes natural to apply the elevated levels of concentration also in everyday situations.

The practice of the eightfold path is understood in two ways: as requiring either simultaneous development (all eight items practiced in parallel) or as a progressive series of stages through which the practitioner moves, the culmination of one leading to the beginning of another. Bodhi is both the Pali and Sanskrit word traditionally translated into English as "enlightenment." Bodhi is also frequently (and more accurately) translated as "awakening." Suffering ends when craving ends, when one is freed from desire. This is achieved by eliminating all delusion, thereby reaching a liberated state of enlightenment (bodhi).

D. The Four Noble Truths State

The nature of suffering, its cause, its cessation, and the way leading to its cessation, is The Noble Eightfold Path. Buddhism considers liberation from suffering as basic for leading a holy life and attaining nirvana.

In Shingon Buddhism, the state of bodhi is also seen as naturally inherent in the mind, the mind's natural and pure state (as in Dzogchen), and is viewed as the perceptual sphere of nonduality, where all false distinctions between a perceiving subject, and perceived objects are lifted and the true state of things (nonduality) is revealed.

E. Nondualism Is the Belief That Dualism and Dichotomy are Illusory Phenomena

Examples of dualisms include self/other, mind/body, male/female, good/evil, active/passive, and many others. A nondual philosophical or religious perspective or theory maintains that there is no fundamental distinction between mind and matter or that the entire phenomenological world is an illusion. The term nondual is a literal translation of the Sanskrit term advaita.

To the Nondualist, reality is ultimately neither physical nor mental. To achieve this vision of non-duality, it is necessary to recognize one's own mind. Nonduality means that reality is essentially unitive and that both unity and multiplicity are irreducible truths of our experience.

F. The Way to Enlightenment

Enlightenment is more than an intellectual understanding, however, it is also an intuitive knowing. It is a total transformation of the heart and mind.

When a person realizes enlightenment, the "Great Compassion" cannot but arise in his or her heart. This person is no longer able to view the world in the same way he or she did before Enlightenment. He or she can now see, feel, know, and understand. He or she views the world as an ocean and is directly connected to each being in the same way the ocean connects to every single wave. This person is most compassionate and most loving, knows the path, is expert in the path, is adept at the path. His or her disciples now keep following the path and afterwards become endowed with the path.

> Enlightenment, for a wave in the ocean, is the moment the wave realises it is water. (Thich Nhat Hanh, 1999)

G. The Seven Steps Buddhist Breath Meditation

BUDDHIST BREATH MEDITATION ONE. Start out with three or seven long in-and-out breaths.

BUDDHIST BREATH MEDITATION TWO. Be clearly aware of each in-and-out breath during this meditation.

BUDDHIST BREATH MEDITATION THREE. Observe the breath as it goes in and out, noticing whether it is comfortable or uncomfortable, broad or narrow, obstructed or free-flowing, fast or slow, short or long, warm or cool. If the breath does not feel comfortable, change it until it does. For instance, if breathing in long and out long is uncomfortable, try breathing in short and out short. As soon as you find that your breathing feels comfortable, let this comfortable breath sensation spread to the different parts of the body.

To begin with, inhale the breath sensation at the base of the skull and let it flow all the way down the spine. Then, if you are male, let it spread down your right leg to the sole of your foot, to the ends of your toes, and out into the air. Inhale the breath sensation at the base of the skull again and let it spread down your spine, down your left leg to the ends of your toes and out into the air. If you are female, begin with the left side first, because the male and female nervous systems are different.

Then let the breath from the base of the skull spread down over both shoulders, past your elbows and wrists, to the tips of your fingers and out into the air. Let the breath at the base of the throat spread down the central nerve to the front of the body, past the lungs and liver, all the way down to the bladder and colon. Inhale the breath right at the middle of the chest and let it go all the way down to your intestines. Let all these breath sensations spread so that they connect and flow together, and you will feel a greatly improved sense of well-being.

BUDDHIST BREATH MEDITATION FOUR. Learn four ways of adjusting the breath:

- in long and out long
- in short and out short
- in short and out long
- in long and out short

Breathe whichever way is most comfortable for you. Better yet, learn to breathe comfortably all four ways, because your physical condition and your breath are always changing.

BUDDHIST BREATH MEDITATION FIVE. Become acquainted with the bases or focal points of the mind, the resting spots of the breath, and center your awareness on whichever one seems most comfortable. A few of these bases are

- the tip of the nose
- the middle of the head
- the palate
- the base of the throat
- the breastbone (the tip of the sternum)
- the navel (or a point just above it)

If you suffer from frequent headaches or nervous problems, do not focus on any spot above the base of the throat. Do not try to force the breath or put yourself into a trance. Breathe freely and naturally. Let the mind be at ease with the breath, but not to the point where it slips away.

BUDDHIST BREATH MEDITATION SIX. Spread your awareness, your sense of conscious feeling, throughout the entire body.

BUDDHIST BREATH MEDITATION SEVEN. Coordinate the breath sensations throughout the body, letting them flow together comfortably, keeping your awareness as broad as possible. May your meditation bring you inner peace and harmony.

One of the fundamental statements of Buddhism is that our consciousness is selfless. Our feeling of self is seen to be a form of attachment that has to be overcome in order to eliminate suffering. It is remarkable that in order to obtain this insight, one has to overcome a strong emotional resistance, the so-called attachment to self: that we are manipulated by our emotions because these consist of several components that diligently reinforce each other.

Both Spinoza and Freud have remarked that our behavior is determined only partially by our conscious will but much more by something else. For Spinoza this something is our feeling, for Freud it is our unconscious.

Often these distinct forces (conscious will versus feeling/unconscious) cause conflicts. Buddhism holds that if we are no longer attached to our feeling, then we are free.

2. ZEN BUDDHISM

Zazen is a particular kind of meditation, unique to Zen, that functions centrally as the very heart of the practice. In fact, Zen Buddhists are generally known as the "meditation Buddhists." Basically, zazen is the study of the self.

The great Master Dogen said, "To study the Buddha Way is to study the self, to study the self is to forget the self, and to forget the self is to be enlightened by the ten thousand things." To be enlightened by the 10,000 things is to recognize the unity with the self and the 10,000 things.

Upon his own enlightenment, Buddha was in sitting meditation; Zen's practice returns to the same sitting meditation repeatedly. For 2500 years that meditation has continued, from generation to generation; it is the most important thing that has been passed on. It spread from India to China, to Japan, to other parts of Asia, and then finally to the West. It is a very simple practice. It is extremely easy to describe and very comfortable to follow. Like all other practices, however, it takes doing in order for it to happen.

We tend to see body, breath, and mind separately, but in zazen they come together as one reality. The first thing to pay attention to is the position of the body in zazen. The body has a way of communicating outwardly to the world and inwardly to oneself. How you position your body has a lot to do with what happens with your mind and your breath.

Either in isolation or as a spiritual belief, Zen is a tradition or philosophy that is nondual. It can be considered a religion, a philosophy, or simply a practice depending on one's perspective. It has also been described as a way of life and work and an art form.

A. Zen Meditation

If you have never meditated before, it is suggested that you follow your breaths or count your breaths. Let all thoughts pass. If thoughts arise, treat them as clouds passing by. Acknowledge them, and let them pass. Focus your attention on your breath or on the counting. If you count breaths, you can count from one to ten, either as you inhale and exhale, or on the inhalations or exhalations. The more common method is to count as you exhale. However, find the method that suits you. Count from one to ten, then start the sequence over and continue this cycle. If you follow your breaths, simply put your attention on your breath, as you inhale and exhale. When your mind wanders, return your attention to the breath, or to the counting. Do not chastise yourself if your attention wanders.

The purpose of the mind is to produce thoughts; they are with us always. The idea is to keep returning our attention to our breath, or our counting, and our thoughts will settle down naturally.

Zen teachers suggest that we sit for short periods in the beginning. Ten minutes is a good goal to start with. Later, as you gain experience and confidence, you can extend the periods up to 20 or 30 minutes.

It is a good idea to take a break after 25 or 30 minutes of sitting. The right hand is made into a fist, with the thumb tucked in, and held to the chest, palm down. The left hand is placed, palm down, on top of the right. The arms are held level, with elbows projecting at the side. Walk slowly and deliberately, placing one foot in front of the other.

Your attention is placed on the feeling of walking; notice how your feet touch the floor, how your muscles contract and relax as you take each step. If you make a misstep, simply experience that and let it pass. If your mind wanders, return your attention to the slow, deliberate movement of just walking. After a few minutes, you may return to sitting meditation.

The point of Zen's meditation is to open our eyes to our true nature, to enable us to live a truly awakened life. Simply put, it gets us in touch with our pure being. In Buddhist terms, it opens us to the realization of emptiness. (The Heart Sutra)

The seemingly nonsensical Zen practice of "thinking about not thinking" could help free the mind of distractions, new brain scans reveal. This suggests Zen meditation could help treat attention-deficit-hyperactivity disorder (ADHD), obsessive-compulsive disorder, anxiety disorder, major depression, and suffering in pain therapy and palliative care.

Zen meditation vigorously discourages mental withdrawal from the world and dreaminess and instead asks one to keep fully aware with a vigilant attitude. It typically asks one to silently focus on breathing and one's posture with eyes open in a quiet place and to calmly dismiss any thoughts as they pop up, essentially thinking nothing. Over time, one can learn how to keep one's mind from wandering, become aware of otherwise unconscious behaviors and preconceived notions, and hopefully gain insights into oneself, others, and the world.

Imaging of the brain's conventional working people who meditate regularly revealed increased thickness in cortical regions related to sensory, auditory, and visual perception, as well as internal perception, the automatic monitoring of heart rate or breathing, for example.

B. The Zen Meditation Technique

Zen meditation allows the mind to relax. Please follow these easy instructions.

Sit on the forward third of a chair or a cushion on the floor.

Arrange your legs in a position you can maintain comfortably. If they are in the half-lotus position, place your right leg on your left thigh. In the full lotus position, put your feet on opposite thighs. You may also sit simply with your legs tucked in close to your body, but be sure that your weight is distributed on three points: both of your knees on the ground and your buttocks on the round cushion. On a chair, keep your knees apart about the width of your shoulders, feet firmly planted on the floor.

Take a deep breath, exhale fully, and take another deep breath, exhaling fully.

With proper physical posture, your breathing will flow naturally into your lower abdomen. Breathe naturally, without judgment or trying to breathe a certain way.

KEEP YOUR ATTENTION ON YOUR BREATH eracticing this Zen meditation. When your attention wanders, bring it back to the breath again and again (as many times as necessary). Remain as still as possible, following your breath and returning to it whenever thoughts arise.

BE FULLY, VITALLY PRESENT WITH YOURSELF. Simply do your very best.

At the end of your sitting period, gently swing your body from right to left in increasing arcs. Stretch out your legs, and be sure they have feeling before standing.

PRACTICE EASY ZEN MEDITATION EVERY DAY for at least 10 to 15 minutes (or longer), and you will discover for yourself the treasure house of the timeless life of zazen, your very life itself.

In the process of working with the breath, the thoughts that come up, for the most part, will be just noise, just random thoughts. Sometimes, however, when you are in a crisis or involved in something important in your life, you will find that the thought, when you let it go, will recur. You let it go again but it comes back, you let it go and it still comes back. Sometimes that needs to happen. Do not treat that as a failure; treat it as another way of practicing. This is the time to let the thought happen, engage it, let it run its full course. Watch it, however, and be aware of it. Allow it to do what it has got to do, let it exhaust itself. Then release it, let it go. Come back again to the breath. Start at one and continue the process.

Do not use zazen to suppress thoughts or issues that need to come up.

Scattered mental activity and energy keep us separated from each other, from our environment, and from ourselves. In the process of sitting, the surface activity of our minds begins to slow down. The mind is like the surface of a pond: when the wind is blowing, the surface is disturbed and there are ripples. Nothing can be seen clearly because of the ripples; the reflected image of the sun or the moon is broken up into many fragments. Out of that stillness, our whole life arises. If we do not get in touch with it at some time in our life, we will never get the opportunity to come to a point of rest.

In deep zazen, deep samadhi, a person breathes at a rate of only two or three breaths a minute. Normally, at rest, a person will breathe about fifteen breaths a minute, even when we are relaxing, we do not quite relax. The more completely your mind is at rest, the more deeply your body is at rest.

Respiration, heart rate, circulation, and metabolism slow down in deep zazen. The whole body comes to a point of stillness that it does not reach even in deep sleep. This is a very important and very natural aspect of being human. It is not something particularly unusual. All creatures of the earth have learned this and practice this.

It is a very important part of being alive and staying alive: the ability to be completely awake.

The model of suffering and its purification explains well an important incident in the history of Chinese Buddhism. At the time that Hung Jen, the fifth patriarch of Zen Buddhism in China, felt that he wanted to appoint his successor, he asked his disciples to write a poem expressing their understanding of the teachings. Then the head monk Shen Hsiu wrote the following poem.

> The body is like the bodhi [enlightenment] tree,
> the mind is like a mirror bright.
> Constantly we should wipe them clean,
> Not allowing any dust to align. (Shen Hsiu)

Monks at the monastery were impressed and expected that the head monk would become the successor of the fifth patriarch. There was, however, a novice named Hui Neng that could not read or write. When he heard the verse of the head monk he asked a friend to write down the following poem.

> There is no body,
> there is no mind.
> Since fundamentally nothing exists
> where is the dust to align? (Hui Neng)

It was Hui Neng who was chosen as sixth patriarch.

How can we understand this? The head monk was describing the state of mysticism, in which one has to keep working to keep the volume of feeling at level. Hui Neng described the state of nirvana, in which no work needs to be done.

3. CHRISTIAN MEDITATION

The practice of Christian meditation dates back to the beginning of Christianity; its objective is to empty the self daily to experience the fullness of God. It is consonant with Jesus's invitation to his disciples to take up their cross daily and follow him. It is central to Christian celebrations, dying to rise to a new life.

Jesus taught a way of life based on love that would unite all people in the common bonds of brotherhood and orient them to a more exalted state of consciousness in which they would have communion with God the Father. He called humanity back toward the primordial state described in Genesis in which Adam and Eve lived in harmony with each other and with nature in the original state of paradise.

The Christian doctrine of the Trinity defines God as three divine persons or hypostases: the Father (God), the Son (Jesus Christ), and the Holy Spirit. The three persons are distinct, yet are one substance, essence or nature. A nature is what one is, whereas a person is who one is. The Trinity is considered to be a mystery of Christian faith. According to this doctrine, there is only one God in three persons. Each person is God, whole and entire. For the large majority of Christians, the Holy Spirit (or Holy Ghost, from Old English gast, "spirit") is the third divine person of the Holy Trinity.

The theology of spirits is called pneumatology. The Holy Spirit is the creator spirit, present before the creation of the universe, and through his power everything was made in Jesus Christ, by God the Father. Christian hymns such as *Veni Creator Spiritus* reflect this belief.

In early Christianity, the concept of salvation was closely related to the invocation of the Father, Son, and Holy Spirit. Since the first century, Christians have called upon God with the name Father, Son, and Holy Spirit in prayer, baptism, communion, exorcism, hymn singing, preaching, confession, absolution and benediction. This is reflected in the saying, "Before there was a 'doctrine' of the Trinity, Christian prayer invoked the Holy Trinity."

Jesus of Nazareth is the central figure of Christianity, and most Christian denominations hold him to be the Son of God. He is regarded as a major Prophet in Islam and in the Hindu religion. Christians hold Jesus to be the awaited Messiah of the Old Testament and refer to him as Jesus Christ or simply as Christ, a name that is also used secularly. Most Christians believe that Jesus was conceived by the Holy Spirit, born of a virgin, performed miracles, founded the church, died sacrificially by crucifixion to achieve atonement, rose from the dead, and ascended into heaven, from which he did or will return. Most Christians worship Jesus as the incarnation of God the Son, and the second person of the Holy Trinity.

Christian traditions have various practices that can be identified as forms of meditation. Monastic traditions are the basis for many of these practices. Practices of **repetitive prayers** such as the rosary, the Adoration (focusing on the Eucharist) in Catholicism, or the Hesychast tradition in Eastern Orthodoxy may be compared to forms of Eastern meditation that focus on an individual object. Christian meditation is considered a form of prayer.

A. St. Francis of Assisi's Vocation Prayer

There is probably no saint more revered and well-known in all of Christian history than St. Francis of Assisi. Today, Christians, and many non-Christians alike, celebrate the life and legacy of this medieval Italian man, who is known the world over for his exemplary life of holiness and the model of peaceable living he leaves to us nearly 800 years after his death.

The most well-known writing of St. Francis is probably the Canticle of the Creatures, in which the saint from Assisi poetically praises God in and through various elements of the created order. The fundamental spiritual insight of the Canticle is that each aspect of God's creation gives glory and praise to God by being what it was created to be. The sun praises God by giving the world light; the wind praises God by bringing every kind of weather; and the earth praises God by sustaining us through producing fruits, flowers and herbs. All of God's creation perfectly praises God because each element does what it was intended to do. Near the end of the Canticle, St. Francis finally introduces humans. He writes,

> Praised be You, my Lord, through those who give pardon for Your love,
> and bear infirmity and tribulation.
> Blessed are those who endure in peace,
> for by You, Most High, shall they be crowned.

In this sense, the so-called "Prayer of St. Francis" reflects the spirit and outlook of the man for whom it is named. To be most authentically human is to be an instrument of peace or, to put it in the sense of the prayer's following lines, one who sows love, pardon, faith, hope, light, and joy in our world.

> Most High, Glorious God, enlighten the darkness of our minds. Give us a right faith, a firm hope and a perfect charity, so that we may always and in all things act according to Your Holy Will. Amen. (Prayer of St. Francis)

Psalm 19:14 states, "Let the words of my mouth, and the meditation of my heart, be acceptable in Thy sight. . . ." The psalmist asks that his words and thoughts be equal. Words of the mouth are a sham if they are not backed up by meditation of the heart.

Christian meditation is an active thought (thinking, resolving) process whereby you give yourself to study of the Word, praying over it, asking God to give you understanding by the Spirit, putting it into practice in daily life, and allowing it (the Scriptures) to become the rule for life and practice as you go about your daily activities. This causes spiritual growth and maturing in the things of God, as taught you by His Holy Spirit dwelling within you as a believer.

B. Mystical Experiences and Unconscious Mind

St. Teresa of Avila wrote in *The Interior Castle* that in the orison of union,

> the soul is utterly dead to the things of the world, and lives solely in God . . . I do not know whether in this state she has enough life left to breathe. It seems to me she has not; or at least that if she does breathe, she is unaware of it.

Interior Castle is one of the most celebrated books on mystical theology in existence. It is the most sublime and mature of Teresa of Avila's works and expresses the full flowering of her deep experience in guiding souls toward spiritual perfection. In addition to its profound mystical content, it is also a treasury of unforgettable maxims on such ascetic subjects as self-knowledge, humility, detachment, and suffering. Above all, this account of a soul's progress in virtue and grace is the record of a life, of the interior life of Teresa of Avila, whose courageous soul, luminous mind, and endearingly human temperament hold so deep an attraction for the modern mind.

In its central image and style, *Interior Castle,* like so many works of genius, is extremely simple. Teresa envisioned the soul as "a castle made of a single diamond . . . in which there are many rooms, just as in Heaven there are many mansions." She describes the various rooms of this castle (the degrees of purgation and continual strife), through which the soul in its quest for perfection must pass before reaching the innermost chamber, the place of complete transfiguration and communion with God. Teresa was an incredibly gifted teacher whose devotion to the sublimest task–the guidance of others toward spiritual perfection–has resulted in the widespread fame of her writings. There is no life more real than the interior life, and few persons have had such an extraordinarily rich experience of that reality as has Teresa. In *Interior Castle,* she exhorts and inspires her readers to participate in the search for this ultimate spiritual reality, the source of her own profound joy.

In *Interior Castle,* Teresa is entering more deeply into the psyche, into the unconscious part of the psyche. Teresa experienced the transpersonal layer of the psyche, the layer Jung called collective unconscious. "Religion is obedience to awareness," said Jung. Teresa wrote, "the gate to entry to this castle is prayer and reflection." The *Interior Castle* is the document in which both psyche and soul relate the story that emerged as one Christian prayerfully attended to depth experiences.

In the prayer of quiet, ego activity is minimal, and we can encourage letting the intellect go. There is an outer and inner stillness with a loving openness to God. It is a time of healing contact with depth of the self, and the absorption in God brings peace to the soul. The individual's personal identification has cracked, and ego consciousness no longer has the total control of the psyche. A new, more powerful center, is emerging.

C. The Way of Meditation is the Way of Silence

Silencing the ceaseless chatter of a mind buzzing with thoughts is not easy. The way to silence and to the inner self of prayer is how.

> I began to think of the soul
> as if it were a castle
> made of a single diamond . . . (St. Teresa D'Avila)

> The Lord appears in this center of the soul,
> Not in an imaginative vision,
> But in an intellectual One. (St. Teresa D'Avila)

The result of this meditative state is an identification in Christ. This reality is experienced as graced by a divine presence. The movement into personhood, in the *Interior Castle,* is a response to a divine call. The free, autonomous person emerges as the relationship in God deepens. The sign of the union in God does not lie in an ecstatic phenomenon but in the quality of reflective awareness that characterizes a Christian.

In the Hesychastic practice, the recitation of the Jesus Prayer is used:

> "through the grace of God and one's own effort, to concentrate the nouns in the heart."

Prayer as a form of meditation of the heart is described in the Philokalia, a practice that leads towards. In 1975, the Benedictine monk John Main introduced a form of meditation based on repetitive recitation of a prayer-phrase, traditionally the Aramaic phrase "Maranatha," meaning "come, Lord," as quoted at the end of both Corinthians and Revelation.

The World Community for Christian Meditation was founded in 1991 to continue Main's work, which the Community describes as "teaching Christian meditation as part of the great work of our time of restoring the contemplative dimension of Christian faith in the life of the church."

The Old Testament book of Joshua, sets out a form of meditation based on scriptures:

> Do not let this Book of the Law depart from your mouth; meditate on it day and night, so that you may be careful to do everything written in it, then you will be prosperous and successful. (Joshua 1:8)

This is one of the reasons why Bible verse memorization is a practice among many evangelical Christians. The predominant form of worship among Quakers, or the Religious Society of Friends, has historically been communal silent prayer or meditation that consists of focusing on the Inner Light of Christ, listening for and awaiting the movement of the "still, small voice within," which may or may not result in being moved to spoken ministry.

Thomas Merton was a Catholic monk who lived from 1915 to 1968. Having studied Eastern meditation techniques, he is credited with reviving an interest in Christian meditation and contemplative prayer. He wrote:

> Some people may have a spontaneous gift for meditative prayer, but this is unusual. Most people have to learn how to meditate. And meditation is sometimes quite difficult. But if we bear with it and wait patiently for the time of grace, we may well discover that meditation is a joyful experience. Contemplative prayer raises the question: Is there something we can do to prepare ourselves, instead of waiting for God to do everything? In my experience, there is. We can use Centring Prayer to calm the mind, and to cultivate interior silence. (Thomas Merton)

Speaking to fellow monks, Merton recommended silent contemplation, writing,

> Contemplative prayer has to be always very simple, confined to the simplest of acts and using no words or thoughts. This prayer of the heart introduces us into deep interior silence so that we learn to experience its power. We seek the deepest ground of our identity with God, a direct experiential grasp just like St. Augustine sought when he prayed, "May I know you, may I know myself." (Thomas Merton)

Thomas Merton loved the contemplative life, the quiet, the wondrous ways of nature that are provided free of charge by the Holy Spirit. In *New Seeds of Contemplation,* he has some inspiring thoughts about meditation.

> Learn to meditate on paper. Drawing are writing are forms of meditation. Learn how to contemplate works of art. Learn how to pray in the streets or in the country. Know how to meditate not only when you have a book in your hand but when you are waiting for a bus or riding the train. (Thomas Merton)

In other words, meditate when there is quiet, but also meditate when there is not or when you are doing some other task. What a novel idea, one that permits us to find the contemplative life even during the hustle and bustle of daily life. Do you meditate? Do you simply call it prayer, as I do. No matter, finding the time to be one with God, with the Holy Spirit, or with any higher spirit that is calling you is one of the most exciting things about life.

The Thomas Merton "Magical" Methods

In meditation we should not look for a method or a system but cultivate an attitude, an outlook: faith, openness, attention, reverence, expectation, supplication, trust, joy. All these finally permeate our being with love in so far as our living faith tells us we are in the presence of God, that we live in Christ, that in the Sprit of God we "see" God our Father without "seeing." We know Him in "unknowing." Faith is the bond that unites us to Him in the Spirit who gives us light and love.

D. The Lectio Divina

The Lectio Divina is a Christian form of meditation aimed at allowing the individual to experience the presence of the triune God, the God of the Christian trinity, who comprises of the Father, the Son (Jesus), and the Holy Spirit.

The practice of the Lectio Divina (meaning holy reading) was first documented in the early third century. Lectio Divina involves concentrated study of Biblical scripture and the subsequent meditation upon the facets of the particular area of scripture upon which you have focused.

E. Practicing Holy Reading, Lectio Divina

Holy reading is much like meditation and involves first clearing the mind in a quiet setting, preferably dedicated for the purpose of reading and contemplation. Once you have calmed yourself and are ready to dedicate yourself to reading, you may wish to pray first for guidance from God before proceeding.

Following this there are four stages to the Lectio Divina.

- First, the lectio involves reading the passage diligently, slowly, and several times over.
- Second, meditation involves a considered and slow contemplation of the text, akin to meditation yet more, in which any area of the text that stands out, if only one word, is to be focused upon.
- Third, oratio involves intuitively opening your heart to God in order to feel the meaning of the text and to invite a dialogue with God.
- Fourth, contemplatio involves listening to God. This stage involves completely clearing the mind and noting the impressions that arise

and is most akin to meditation in the sense that it is practiced in other spiritual disciplines, where the aim might be to listen to the essence of the universe or to attain a oneness with all things.

Although clear parallels can be seen between this form of contemplation and meditation, it must be noted that this form depends on a deep held belief in God and Christianity. The Lectio Divina does not entail entering literally into a discussion with God, however, in which his voice is audible to us, and can rather be seen as a discussion with our own inner calm in the form of an acknowledgment that it exists as more truthful than the complex lives we erect around us.

4. HINDUISM

Contemporary Hindu culture originated primarily with the Aryans who invaded India about 1500 BC bringing with them the Sanskrit language and the Vedic religion. For at least 1000 years prior to this invasion, however, there existed a culture in India about which we know very little. From some fragmentary evidence that does remain, scholars conclude this early culture contained within it many elements that were later incorporated into the Hindu religion.

A. The Language of Consciousness

The exploration of consciousness has developed to a remarkable degree in the Hindu culture. In fact, the Sanskrit language has shown itself to be sufficiently precise in describing the subtleties of consciousness exploration, and many Sanskrit words, with no adequate English equivalents, have become commonplace in our own contemporary culture. Consider, for example, these terms:

akasha: The ether; primordial substance that pervades the entire universe; the substratum of both mind and matter. All thoughts, feelings, or actions are recorded within it.

asanas: postures used to stimulate flow of life force through the body and to aid meditation.

atman: The human soul or spirit, the essence of the inner being.

Brahman: Hindu god who represents the highest principle in the universe; the essence that permeates all existence. Brahman is the same as atman in the philosophy of the Upanishads.

dharma: One's personal path in life, the fulfillment of which leads to a higher state of consciousness.

dhyana: The focusing of attention on a particular spiritual idea in continuous meditation.

Ishwara: Personal manifestation of the supreme; the cosmic self; cosmic consciousness.

karma: The principle by which all of our actions will effect our future circumstances, either in the present or in future lifetimes.

mandala: Images used to meditate.

mantras: Syllables, inaudible or vocalized, that are repeated during meditation.

maya: The illusions the physical world generates to ensnare our consciousness.

nirvana: The transcendental state that is beyond the possibility of full comprehension or expression by the ordinary being enmeshed in the concept of selfhood.

prana: Life energy that permeates the atmosphere, enters the human being through the breath, and can be directed by thought.

pranayama: Yogic exercises for the regulation of the breath flow.

samadhi: State of enlightenment of higher consciousness. The union of the individual consciousness with cosmic consciousness.

yoga: Sanskrit word meaning union; refers to various practices designed to attain a state of perfect union between the self and the infinite.

The capacity for awareness and experience, for logical analysis and joyful interaction, constitutes the intangible component in the fleeting persistence of Homo sapiens. This is the essence of what we call the human spirit. Just as there is more to a flower than soil and tree branch, the spirit is more than neural network, heartbeat, and vital breath, although these are what create and sustain it here below.

How are we to explain these extraordinary features of human consciousness in relation to its temporal and spatial insignificance? How can we comprehend the fact that to none but the human brain the universe is comprehensible? Science's suggestion that evolution led to this extraordinarily powerful complexity is one persuasive hypothesis, and it has found ample observational support. The sage-poets of Hinduism, who probed into the ultimate nature and roots of consciousness, arrived at a startlingly different conclusion.

If the splendor of the perceived world and the pattern in its functioning can result in the grand experiences of life and thought, then even prior to the advent of humans, there must have been a consciousness of a vastly superior order, an Experiencer who spanned the range in space and time. This undergirding cosmic principle is the Brahman in Hindu vision. Moreover, our consciousness is but an echo of something of far grander dimensions. Expressed through the pithy Upanishadic aphorism, tat tvam asi: [Thou art

That], the Hindu vision is that every conscious entity is a spark from an underlying effulgence and flashes its radiance as its source alone can.

Just as the expanse of water in the seas is scattered all over land in ponds, lakes, and rivers, all-embracing Brahman finds expression in countless life forms. We are miniature lights, one and all. We have emanated from that primordial effulgence like photons from a glorious galactic core, destined for the terrestrial experience for a brief span on the eternal time line, only to remerge with that from which we sprang.

Brahman, the ground-stuff, subdivides itself into purusha, the cosmic consciousness, and prakriti or nature. These are the experiencer and the experienced, not unlike the *res cogens* and the *res extensa* of Descartes. Prakriti is now bifurcated into animate and the inanimate realms with only a fuzzy dividing line separating them. On the other hand, purusha separates out into countless jîvâtmans or individual units of consciousness that fuse into the mind and body of the animate branch of prakriti. The conscious jîvatman endeavors to recognize its source, namely purusha, through religion and spirituality and tries to understand prakriti through science.

B. The Yoga Sutras of Patanjali

The *Yoga Sutras of Patanjali* prescribe a system of eight stages, or limbs for one's higher development of the consciousness. In The Yoga Sutras of Patanjali, which is a 2000-year-old collection of the oral teachings on yogic philosophy, there are 195 statements that are a kind of philosophical guidebook for dealing with the challenges of being human. *The Yoga Sutras* provide an eightfold path called ashtanga, which literally means "eight limbs." These eight steps are basic guidelines on how to live a meaningful and purposeful life. They are a prescription for moral and ethical conduct. They direct attention toward one's health, and they help us to acknowledge the spiritual aspects of our nature.

The first four steps or stages concentrate on refining our personalities, gaining mastery over our body, and developing an energetic awareness of ourselves, all of which prepare us for the second half of the journey, which deals with the senses, the mind, and attaining a higher state of consciousness.

1. Yama

The first step deals with one's moral or ethical standards and sense of integrity, focusing on our behavior and how we conduct ourselves in our interpersonal life. These are, literally, the *controls* or "don'ts" of life. They include areas where we must learn to control tendencies that, if allowed expression, would end up causing us disharmony and pain. They are the same moral virtues that you find in all the world's great religious traditions. The five yamas are

Nonviolence: Refrain from harming or demeaning any living thing, including yourself, by action, word, or thought.
Not lying: Control any tendency to say anything that is not truthful, including not being truthful to yourself.
Not stealing: Curb the tendency to take anything that does not belong to you, which includes not only material objects but also things such as praise or position.
Not sensuality: Learn the art of self-control; to control the tremendous energy expended in seeking and thinking about sensual pleasure and to abstain from inappropriate sexual behavior.
Not greedy: Learn not to be attached to or desirous of "things"; to learn to discriminate between "needs" and "wants."

2. Niyama

Niyama, the second step, comprises individual practices having to do with self-descipline, self-development, and spiritual observances. These are the *non-controls* or the "dos" of the path. The five niyamas are

Purity: Strive for purity or cleanliness of body, mind, and environment.
Contentment: Seek contentment and acceptance with what you have and with things as they are right now, but, also, seek ways to improve things in the future.
Self-control: Learn to have control over your actions and to have the strength and determination to do what you decide to do; to replace negative habits with positive ones.
Self-study: This requires introspection; studying our actions, words, and thoughts to determine if we are behaving in a harmonious and positive manner in order to achieve the happiness and satisfaction we strive for.
Devotion: Devotion is the turning of the natural love of the heart toward the Divine rather than toward the objects of the world.

3. Asana

Asana, the postures practiced in yoga, are the third step. In the yogic view, the body is a temple of the spirit, the care of which is an important stage of our spiritual growth. Through the practice of asana, we develop the habit of discipline and the ability to concentrate, both of which are necessary for meditation. If the body is in proper working order and comfortable in one position for a long time, it can ultimately become a vehicle for spiritual powers, instead of preventing progress by bothering its owner with physical distress.

4. Pranayama

Generally translated as breath control, this fourth step consists of techniques designed to gain mastery over the respiratory process while recognizing the connection between the breath, the mind, and the emotions. The literal translation of pranayama is "life force." Yogis believe that it not only rejuvenates the body but actually extends life itself. You can practice pranayama as an isolated technique (simply sitting and performing a number of breathing exercises) or integrate it into your daily Hatha Yoga routine.

5. Pratyahara

Pratyahara, the fifth step, means withdrawal or sensory transcendence. It is during this stage that we make the conscious effort to draw our awareness away from the external world and outside stimuli. We direct our attention internally. The practice of pratyahara provides us with an opportunity to step back and take a look at ourselves. This can happen during breathing exercises, during meditation, during the practice of yoga postures, or during any activity requiring concentration. Detachment is a great technique for pain control and an excellent way to deal with uncomfortable symptoms or chronic conditions.

6. Dharana

The practice of pratyahara creates the setting for dharana, or concentration. Having relieved ourselves of outside distractions, we can now deal with the distractions of the mind itself. In the practice of concentration, which precedes meditation, we learn how to slow down the thinking process by concentrating on a single mental object. The goal is to become aware of nothing but the object on which you are concentrating, whether it is a candle flame, a flower, a mantra you repeat to yourself, a specific energetic center in the body, or an image of a deity. The purpose is to train the mind to eliminate all the extra, unnecessary junk floating around, to learn to gently push away superfluous thought. Extended periods of concentration naturally lead to meditation.

7. *Dhyana*

Meditation or contemplation, the seventh step of ashtanga, is the uninterrupted flow of concentration. Although concentration (dharana) and meditation (dhyana) may appear to be one and the same, a fine line of distinction exists between these two stages. Where dharana practices one-pointed attention, dhyana is ultimately a state of being keenly aware without focus. At this stage, the mind has been quieted, and in the stillness it produces few or no thoughts at all. Meditation occurs when you have actually become linked to the object of your concentration so that nothing else exists. It is a keen heightened awareness, not nothingness. Your mind is completely focused and quiet but awake and aware of truth. Many methods exist to bring you to this state, but oneness with the object of your meditation, and subsequently, oneness with the entire universe, is the objective. It is quite a difficult task to reach this state of stillness, but it is not impossible. This state is a goal to keep striving for, and, even if it is never attained, there is benefit from each stage of progress.

8. *Samadhi*

Patanjali describes this eighth and final step of ashtanga as a state of ecstasy. All the paths of yoga lead to this stage. This stage is one which most of us are unlikely to attain in this lifetime. At this stage, the meditator merges with his or her point of focus and transcends the self altogether. When in this state, you understand not only that you and the object of your meditation are one, but also that you and the universe are one. There is no difference between you and everything else. The meditator comes to realize a profound connection to the Divine, an interconnectedness with all living things. What Patanjali has described as the completion of the yogic path is what, deep down, all human beings aspire to: joy, fulfillment, freedom, and peace

The first two limbs are known as yama and niyama. They involve a highly ethical and disciplined lifestyle: control, indifference, detachment, renunciation, charity, celibacy, vegetarianism, cleanliness, and nonviolence. The third step involves the development and care of the body through the use of exercises and postures called asanas. The fourth stage involves pranayama breathing exercises. The next stage, pratyahara, involves meditation, by means of which one withdraws consciousness from the senses. The next limb of yoga is called dharana, which means concentration. An object of contemplation is held fixedly in the mind; it must not be allowed to waver or change its form or color, as it will have a tendency to do. Often the yogi will concentrate on different chakras, or focal points, within the body. Self-analysis is used to observe breaks in concentration. Often he will carry a string of beads and one is pulled over the finger every time a break begins. The next stage of dhyana occurs when the sense of separateness of the self from the object of concentration disappears and one experiences a union or oneness with that object. In the final stage, samadhi, one experiences an absolute, ecstatic, cosmic consciousness. This does not, as some suppose, entail a loss of individuality. "The drop is not poured into the Ocean; the Ocean is poured into the Drop." The self and the entire universe are simultaneously experienced.

In past decades, Western scientists have begun to study the abilities yogi practitioners can achieved. Body functions such as heartbeat, temperature, and brainwaves, which had been previously thought of as totally autonomic, have been shown to be under the conscious control of some yogis. This research has paved the way for the newly emerging science of consciousness.

C. The Nonduality

In Hindu religion, the basic cause of human suffering, pain, conflicts, and unhappiness is dualism, as distinct from duality. The core of this difference needs to be thoroughly analyzed and clearly understood. In fact, such a clear understanding could itself be the solution of human unhappiness because it would relieve people from the double bind in which they find themselves in their relentless pursuit of unalloyed happiness.

> That which is free from duality; which is infinite and indestructible; distinct from the universe and Maya, supreme, eternal; which is undying Bliss; taintless, that Brahman art thou, meditate on this in thy mind. (Vivekacudamani 261)

No philosophy, sermon, or concept will help relieve that suffering immediately. It is useful, however, to remember that at the core of any pain-causing conflict there is duality. We are part of a cycle that contains both pain and pleasure, creating a split between mind and body, delaying the healing process.

Duality is all pervasive; it is present in everything around us. Every one of our daily actions is preceded by a struggle, to come to a decision on this or that, pain or pleasure, day or night, north or south pole, hot or cold, left or right. All through life we keep on playing this game of duality. Duality is our own creation. We describe breathing as something that involves inhalation and exhalation, but actually there is only one breath.

In reality, however, there is no duality. There is only an all-pervasive Oneness. There is no day and night, since the sun never sets. There is no beginning and no end, no birth and no death. In that space there is total silence. This silence emanates not from the mind but from the very depth of the heart, wherein only one thing remains: that is love emerging from the very source, the *atman,* the consciousness that exists in every being.

We are all part of that same cosmic force. Despite being a part of it, every one of us is as complete as the whole universe. The body will die but the soul or atman is eternal; it never dies. It is only in the stillness of deep silence that thoughts are not active, they get dissolved. Those are the moments when body and mind are one and duality is absent. The silence of meditation or yoga dissolves the senses and the mind transcends to a higher level of consciousness. There emerges immense energy and compassion—the moment of creativity when you become one with nature.

Nature has bestowed on us abundant power or *atmashakti* to overcome any amount of pain. We seldom leave the task of alleviating pain to nature; rather, we want instant solutions. Pain and suffering, however, give us the opportunity to look within and experience that oneness or wholeness where no duality is present.

In order to get to your real self, you have to go inward, where there is no past and no future, but there is only the present. In this state of meditation, you may get in touch with your inner being, the nondual state. Once this insight is gained, one is awakened. This is nirvana or enlightenment, where there is no duality; there is only completeness.

The fact of the matter is that duality is polarized, interrelated, and, therefore, not really separate, whereas dualism is opposition, separation, and, therefore, conflict. Phenomenal manifestation is a process of objectification that basically requires a dichotomy into two elements: a subject that perceives and an object that is perceived. This is the process that is known as duality: all phenomena that are sensorially perceivable are the correlation of a subject (object-cognizer) and the object (the object cognized). This process of duality makes it evidently clear that without such a process there cannot exist any phenomena and that neither of the two phenomenal objects (neither the cognizer subject nor the cognized object) has any independent existence of its own. The existence of one depends on the existence of the other.

When the basis of duality is clearly apperceived, there is no question of either any *samsara* (phenomenal day-to-day living) or any bondage for any conceptual individual for the simple reason that the individual concerned is merely the psychosomatic apparatus, the instrument through which the process of perceiving and cognizing takes place. Our unhappiness, our conflict, our bondage arises as the effect of the identification of What We Are (consciousness) with the object-cognizer element in the dichotomy of the whole-mind (Consciousness) into subject and object in the process of duality. This identification or entitification as a separate independent entity (as the pseudo-subject) is the dualism, the maya, which results as the practical application in day-to-day living of the original principle of duality, that is polarized, interrelated and, therefore, not separate. *It is this illusory identification that causes all the conflict,* all the suffering, all the unhappiness that is collectively termed bondage. The instantaneous apperception of this very fact of the illusoriness of the pseudosubject as an independent doer-entity means the freedom from the bondage.

Holds that suffering follows naturally from personal negative behaviors in your current life or in a past life (*see* karma). People must accept suffering as a just consequence and as an opportunity for spiritual progress. Thus, the soul or true self, which is eternally free of any suffering, may come to manifest itself in the person, who then achieves liberation (moksha). Abstinence from causing pain or harm to other beings (ahimsa) is a central tenet of Hinduism.

Advaita (nonduality) simply means that the source, by whatever name known—primal energy, consciousness, awareness, plenitude, God—is uniqeness, oneness, nonduality. The manifestation that arises or emerges from the source is based on duality, the inevitable existence of interconnected opposites: male and female, beauty and ugliness.

> Fear not, O learned one, there is no death for thee; there is a means of crossing this sea of relative existence; that very way by which sages have gone beyond it, I shall inculcate to thee. (Vivekacudamani 43)

> By which this universe is pervaded, but which nothing pervades, which shining, all this [universe] shines as Its reflection. This is That. (Vivekacudamani 128)

The bodily pain of physical illness and deterioration is part of this suffering. Hindu belief is, however, that the physical body wears out, like our clothes do. The soul, which is immortal, lives on when the body perishes. Like a person changes worn out clothes, the soul changes deteriorated bodies. Hindus cremate their dead so that the elements of the body return to nature, from whence they came. Then there is rebirth. The cycle continues.

Anger, hate, guilt, insecurity, and fear are the weaknesses and limitations of people. When we overcome these limitations and weaknesses, we will be able to accomplish our goals and perform our duties

The central theme of Bhagavad Gita, one of the holy books of Hinduism, is to overcome reluctance (not necessarily fear) to do our duty (do what is right). The scriptures tell us that we do our duty, without regard to its consequences (and without expecting anything in return). If we do good things, we have nothing to fear. We are asked not to be afraid of our limitations and weaknesses. The Bhagavad Gita is considered by Eastern and Western scholars alike to be among the greatest spiritual books the world has ever known.

In a very clear and wonderful way the Supreme Lord Krishna describes the science of self-realization and the exact process by which a human being can establish his or her eternal relationship with God.

Bhagavad Gita is a part of the *Mahabharata,* comprising 700 verses. The teacher of the Bhagavad Gita is Sri Krishna, who is regarded by the Hindus as the supreme manifestation of the Lord Himself and is referred to as Bhagavan, the divine one. The Bhagavad Gita is commonly referred to as the Gita for short. In order to clarify his point, Krishna expounds the various yoga processes and understanding of the true nature of the universe. Krishna describes the yogic paths of devotional service, action, meditation, and knowledge. Fundamentally, the Bhagavad Gita proposes that true enlightenment comes from growing beyond identification with the temporal ego, the False Self, the ephemeral world, so that one identifies with the truth of the immortal self, the absolute soul, or atman. Through detachment from the material sense of ego, the yogi, or follower of a particular path of yoga, is able to transcend his or her illusory mortality and attachment to the material world and enter the realm of the Supreme.

Only God is Truth (ultimate reality) The world is an illusion. It is the veil that masks the Truth. Unless one can break free from the bonds of the world (human bondage) we cannot see the Truth.

D. The Vedas

The Vedas (Sanskrit; knowledge), the most sacred books of Hinduism and the oldest literature of India, represent the religious thought and activity of the Indo-European speaking peoples who entered South Asia in the second millennium BC, although they probably also reflect the influence of the indigenous people of the area. The Vedic texts presumably date from between 1500 and 500 BC. This literature was preserved for centuries by an oral tradition in which particular families were entrusted with portions of the text for preservation. As a result, some parts of the texts are known by the names of the families they were assigned to.

In its narrowest sense, the term Veda applies to four collections of hymns (samhita): *Rig Veda, Sama Veda, Yajur Veda, and Atharva Veda.* These hymns and verses, addressed to various deities, were chanted during sacrificial rituals. The *Upanishads* are Hindu scriptures that constitute the core teachings of Vedanta.

In the Darsana Mala (a Garland of Visions of the Absolute) (VIII. Bhakti Darsanam, Vision by Contemplation), we can read,

1. Meditation of the Self is contemplation,
Because the Self consists of bliss,
A knower of the Self meditates by the Self,
Upon the Self, for ever.
It is the Self alone that contemplates the Absolute;
The knower of the Self
Meditates on the Self, and not on any other.
That which is meditation on the Self
Is said to be contemplation.

It is because a wise man is a knower of the Self that he meditates on the Self. Not only does he meditate on the Self, but he meditates on nothing other than the Absolute, consisting of existence, subsistence, and value (i.e. bliss). He does not meditate on the inert and unreal non-Self, which is the cause of suffering. He does not (even) meditate on the world. Because of meditating on the Self, it is called bhakti or contemplation. So, the man who meditates on the Self is the real contemplative.

The Self is the Absolute, and the knower of the Self is the same as the knower of the Absolute. This is the same as saying he is a true contemplative.

> Similarly, discarding the body, the Buddhi and the reflection of the Chit in it, and realising the Witness, the Self, the Knowledge Absolute, the cause of the manifestation of everything, which is hidden in the recesses of the Buddhi, is distinct from the gross and subtle, eternal, omnipresent, all-pervading and extremely subtle, and which has neither interior nor exterior and is identical with one self fully realising this true nature of oneself, one becomes free from sin, taint, death and grief, and becomes the embodiment of Bliss. Illumined himself, he is afraid of none. For a seeker after Liberation there is no other way to the breaking of the bonds of transmigration than the realisation of the truth of one's own Self. (Vivekacudamani 220-222)

Sankara called his work on the Vedantic Absolute the *Vivekacudamani* (the Crest-Jewel of Discriminative Wisdom). Narayana Guru continues the same tradition, after him and thinks of not one ornament for the head but of a whole garland in which no vision of any religious or philosophical school would be neglected or left out. Each would be kept in mind by him, as the architect of the total integrated edifice. Thus would be commemorated the dignity and wisdom possible for humanity, from which alone should be derived the legitimate ornament to enhance his human quality as homo sapiens.

The garland further represents, in the symbolic gesture language of India, the whole of one's precious wealth. It is implied as when a bride gives herself to the bridegroom at the time of marriage. It represents the Sarv-asvam (total good) that one surrenders to God or the Absolute or submits to Humanity itself, in an extended sense of the analogy. When this epistemo-logical secret has been understood, in all its bearings and applications in sci-ence or philosophy, a man becomes able to see clearly through mazes of per-cepts and concepts. He can then organize them into ramified hierarchies rep-resenting values ranging from the actual to the nominal, with the perceptual and the conceptual, fitted between these extremes. The structure of the series of visions in Narayana Guru's Darsana Mala conforms broadly to the scheme that we have just referred to.

The Avadhuta Gita is a text of extreme Advaita-Vedanta. People like Nisargadatta, who speak in ways not different than what Advaita-Vedanta teaches, may come from distant backgrounds, even within Hinduism. They are not formally Advaita-Vedantists, yet speak as one. Nondualism is the same as Advaita-Vedanta. Only contexts differ.

The universe, the macrocosm, is in apparent chaos, and the individual body, the microcosm, is in apparent order. Energy in each atom is chaotic. In that chaos there is order. Chaos with order is cosmic intelligence. The stars and planets move in order, with no apparent regulatory authority. Nature is not just matter and power, it is also intelligence. Believing that the universe is just matter is what causes conflict. If we believe that the universe is intelligent energy, that it is compassionate, and that it responds to us then peace prevails. When you experience the order in cosmic chaos, you expe-rience bliss; when you realize the chaos within you as order, you exude com-passion; that compassion then leads you to enlightenment.

The Hindu spiritual vision paints individual consciousness on a cosmic canvas. It recognizes the transience of us all as separate entities yet incorpo-rates us into the infinity that encompasses us. It does not rule out the possi-bility of other manifestations of Brahman, sublime and subtle, carbon- or sil-icon-based, elsewhere amid the stellar billions. It recognizes the role of mat-ter and the limits of the mind but sees subtle spirit at the core of everything. It does not speak of rewards and punishments in anthropocentric terms or of a He-God communicating in local languages. Yet, it regards the religious expressions of humanity as echoes of the universal spirit, even as volcanic outbursts reveal submerged forces of far greater magnitude.

E. Raja Yoga Meditation

The basis for attaining an experience in Raja Yoga meditation is to un-derstand the self and the mind. The human mind is the most creative, pow-erful, and wonderful instrument we possess. Using this energy called mind we have been able to search the deepest oceans, send humans to the moon, and scan the molecular fabric of the building blocks of nature, but have we found our true self? We have become the most educated and civilized society in our history, but are we civil toward each other?

The soul has three main faculties; the mind or consciousness, the intellect, and the subconscious. Thoughts flow from the subconscious mind to the conscious mind. Feelings and emotions form in accordance with the montage of thoughts flowing in the mind. Therefore, our state of mind at any given moment is determined by the thoughts in our consciousness and also with the feelings that we associate with those thoughts. Because our subconsciousness contains all our previous thoughts and experiences, it is necessary to selectively control the flow of thoughts that emerges from the subconscious mind.

The intellect is the controller that is used to discriminate so that only positive and benevolent thoughts flow into our mind. With meditation or deep contemplation, the individual is able to strengthen and sharpen the intellect. The end result is a constant state of well-being. If we are able to understand the self as the source of energy that creates our feelings, then the following will become our aims.

- Become aware of our state of mind and of the thoughts that flow into the mind from our subconscious.
- Strengthen the intellect so that the individual can discriminate and thereby only allow positive and peaceful thoughts to flow into the mind.

Through this process of self-development, the individual develops more control over the mind.

The act of Raja Yoga meditation for at least 15 minutes in the early morning will have a positive effect during the entire day. Upon waking have the thought: I am a peaceful soul, my aim today is to radiate peace to every person that I come into contact with. Try to experience the stillness of mind of being a peaceful soul as other thoughts emerge in the mind do not judge or focus on them but repeat

I am a peaceful soul . . .
I am a peaceful soul . . .
My mind is filled with peace . . .
I radiate peace to the world . . .
I feel the gentle waves of peace flowing across my mind . . .
As these peaceful thoughts emerge in my mind . . .

I feel the stillness and silence envelopes my mind . . .
I am the peaceful soul . . . I am a peaceful loving soul . . .
My mind feels light and free from worries . . .
I realize my real nature is peace . . .
Peaceful thoughts flow through the mind . . .
and I feel the self becoming light . . .
I am a being of light shining like a star . . .
I radiate peace and light to the world . . .
The light and peace envelopes me . . .
and the waves of peace and light shine like a lighthouse . . .
This is the wonderful journey of self-discovery . . .

F. Kriya Yoga Meditation

Kriya Yoga meditation refers to actions designed to get rid of obstructions involving body and mind. Kriya Yoga meditation is a complete system covering a wide range of techniques, including mantras and techniques of meditation for control of the life force, bringing calmness and control of both body and mind. The goal is to unite with pure Awareness. Since pure Awareness is our original condition, it is also referred to as self-awareness.

Around 1920, Paramahansa Yogananda introduced Kriya Yoga meditation to the West and founded the Self-Realization Fellowship. Preparing the mind, Kriya Yoga is said to be a combination of the more useful yoga techniques. Like Raja Yoga, Kriya teaches the laws of general conduct, including harmlessness, truthfulness, and not stealing:

1. Life-force control (pranayama). At this point the difference from other systems, like Raja Yoga meditation, becomes quite obvious. Kriya pranayama is not as much about increasing the time of retention of breath as it is about magnetizing the spine and directing life force to the brain, with the effect of refining the brain and nervous system.
2. Initiation and shaktipat (transfer of energy). The seeker is initiated in the proper use of Kriya pranayama. When the seeker is ready, a transfer of energy might occur either from the outside or from within. To experience Kundalini (energy) on its way up the spine is an event powerful enough to change the way we think and function.
3. Higher Kriyas. For advanced students, there are still a few higher Kriya meditation techniques. Full self-realization may be achieved by practicing faithfully the mantras given for regular meditation.

G. Vipassana Meditation

Vipassana, one of the oldest techniques of meditation practiced in India, was rediscovered by Gautama the Buddha around 2500 years ago. The knowledge of the technique of Vipassana, however, disappeared from India nearly five centuries after Buddha. The torch lit by the Buddha was kept alive by some of his devoted disciples in other countries, particularly Burma. The teachings of Vipassana were preserved by a chain of devoted teachers, and they were transferred to the dedicated lineage of successive generations in their pristine purity. Vipassana is a simple and practical way to achieve real and lasting peace of mind and happiness by seeing things as they really are. This process of self-observation leads to mental and physical purification. It eliminates the frustration and disharmony from our life. This technique librates us from suffering and its deep-seated causes and takes us to our highest spiritual goal through a step-by-step approach. The liberation from fear helps the practitioners attain high levels of achievements in all the spheres of human activity.

What follows is a daily meditation to attain peace of mind.

> The act of meditation for at least 15 minutes in the early morning will have a positive effect on your mind during the entire day.
> Upon waking have these positive thoughts:
> I am a peaceful soul. My aim today is to have a peaceful mind and radiate peace to every person that I come into contact with.
> Try to experience the stillness of mind of being a peaceful soul.

This technique aims for the total eradication of mental impurities and the resultant highest happiness of full liberation. Healing, not merely curing diseases, but the essential healing of human suffering, is its purpose.

Vipassana is a way of self-transformation through self-observation. It focuses on the deep interconnection between mind and body, which can be experienced directly by disciplined attention to the physical sensations that form the life of the body and that continuously interconnect and condition the life of the mind. It is this observation-based, self-exploratory journey to the common root of mind and body that dissolves mental impurity, resulting in a balanced mind full of love and compassion.

The scientific laws that operate one's thoughts, feelings, judgments, and sensations become clear. Through direct experience, the nature of how one grows or regresses, how one produces suffering or frees oneself from suffering, is understood. Life becomes characterized by increased awareness, non-delusion, self-control, and peace.

H. Yoga-nidra

Yoga relaxation reduces tension and anxiety. The autonomic symptoms of high anxiety such as headache, giddiness, chest pain, palpitations, sweating, and abdominal pain respond well. It has been used to help soldiers from war cope with posttraumatic stress disorder (PTSD). Yoga-nidra or "yogi sleep" is a sleeplike state that yogis have reported experiencing during their meditations. It is the conscious awareness of the deep sleep state referred to as "prajna" in *Mandukya Upanishad* (Rama, 1982) and was experienced by Swami Satyananda Saraswati (1974), when he was living with his guru Swami Sivananda in Rishikesh. He began studying the tantric scriptures and, after practice, constructed a system of relaxation that he began popularizing in the mid-twentieth century. He explained yoga-nidra as a state of mind between wakefulness and sleep that opened deep phases of the mind, suggesting a connection with the ancient tantric practice called nyasa, whereby Sanskrit mantras are mentally placed within specific body parts while meditating on each part (of the body-mind). The form of practice taught by Swami Satyananda includes eight stages (internalisation, sankalpa, rotation of consciousness, breath awareness, manifestation of opposites, creative visualization, sankalpa, and externalization).

Teachers such as Osho and Anandmurti Gurumaa, define yoga-nidra as a state of conscious deep sleep. One appears to be sleeping, but the unconscious mind is functioning at a deeper level: it is sleep with a trace of deep awareness. In normal sleep, we lose track of our self, but in yoga-nidra, although consciousness of the world is dim and relaxation is deep, there remains an inward lucidity and experiences may be absorbed to be recalled later. Because yoga-nidra involves an aimless and effortless relaxation it is often held to be best practiced with an experienced yoga teacher who verbally delivers instructions.

Anandmurti Gurumaa taught two techniques based on creative visualization. Yoga-nidra as Yoga of Clear Light is proposed as a spiritual path (sadhana) in its own right, held to prepare and refine a seeker (sadhaka) spiritually, emotionally, mentally, and physically for consciousness and awareness. The yogi may work through the consequences of deeds (karma), cleansing the stored consciousness and purifying the unconscious mind. The state may lead to realization (samādhi) and being-awareness-bliss (satchitananda). The yogi is held to be in communion with the divine. A tantrika engaged in this sadhana may become aware of past or future lives or experience the astral planes (Saraswati, 1974).

Experimental evidence of the existence of a fourth state of unified, transcendental consciousness that lies in the yoga-nidra state at the transition between sensory and sleep consciousness was first recorded in 1971 in the United States at the Menninger Foundation in Kansas. Under the direction of Dr. Elmer Green, researchers used an electroencephalograph to record the brainwave activity of an Indian yogi, Swami Rama, while he progressively relaxed his entire physical, mental and emotional structure through the practice of yoga-nidra. What they recorded was a revelation to the scientific community. The swami demonstrated the capacity to enter the various states of consciousness at will, as evidenced by remarkable changes in the electrical activity of his brain. Upon relaxing himself in the laboratory, he first entered the yoga-nidra state, producing 70 percent alpha wave discharge for a predetermined 5-minute period, simply by imagining an empty blue sky with occasional drifting clouds. Next, Swami Rama entered a state of dreaming sleep that was accompanied by slower theta waves for 75 percent of the subsequent 5-minute test period. This state, which he later described as being "noisy and unpleasant," was attained by "stilling the conscious mind and bringing forth the subconscious." In this state he had the internal experience of desires, ambitions, memories, and past images in archetypal form rising sequentially from the subconscious and unconscious with a rush, each archetype occupying his whole awareness.

Finally, the swami entered the state of (unconscious) deep sleep, as verified by the emergence of the characteristic pattern of slow rhythm delta waves. He remained perfectly aware throughout the entire experimental period, however. He later recalled the various events that had occurred in the laboratory during the experiment, including all the questions that one of the scientists had asked him during the period of deep delta wave sleep, while his body lay snoring quietly.

Such remarkable mastery over the fluctuating patterns of consciousness had not been demonstrated under strict laboratory conditions previously. The capacity to remain consciously aware while producing delta waves and experiencing deep sleep is one of the indications of the superconscious state (turiya). This is the ultimate state of yoga-nidra in which the conventional barriers between waking, dreaming, and deep sleep are lifted, revealing the simultaneous operation of the conscious, subconscious, and unconscious mind. The result is a single, enlightened state of consciousness and a perfectly integrated and relaxed personality (Green, 1972).

Yoga nidra is the same as deep hypnosis. One looks to be sleeping, but the unconscious mind is functioning at a deeper level. It is sleep with a discover of deep awareness. In normal sleep, we lose track of ourselves, but in yoga nidra, and in deep hypnosis, while consciousness throughout the world is dim and relaxation is deep, there remains an inward lucidity, and experiences may be absorbed to be recalled later.

In the Hindu religion and philosophy, yoga and meditative states are the way to overcome pain and suffering. The word yoga can describe either a state of consciousness or an effort to attain that state. The state of consciousness is characterized by transcendental knowledge and bliss.

> Mistaking the body or not-I for the Self or I, is the cause of all misery, that is, of bondage. That bondage comes through ignorance of the cause of birth and death, for it is through ignorance that men regard these insentient bodies as real, mistaking them for the Self and sustaining them with sense objects and finally getting destroyed by them. (Vivekacudamani)

> Prana is born of the Self. Like a man and his shadow the Self and Prana are inseparable. Prana enters the body at birth, that the desires of the mind, continuing from past lives, may be fulfilled. (Prasna Upanisad)

> There are two causes of the activities of the mind; (1) Vâsana (desires) and (2) the respiration (the Prana). Of these, the destruction of the one is the destruction of both. Breathing is lessened when the mind becomes absorbed, and the mind becomes absorbed when the Prana is restrained. (Hatha Yoga Pradipika)

> For those who are afflicted, in the way of the world, by the burning pain due to the (scorching) sunshine of threefold misery, and who through delusion wander about in a desert in search of water—for them here is the triumphant message of Shankara pointing out, within easy reach, the soothing ocean of nectar, Brahman, the One without a second—to lead them on to Liberation. (Vivekacudamani 580)

5. ISLAM MEDITATION

Prayer is one of the most important aspects of a successful Islamic lifestyle. When we consciously adopt Islam for ourselves, we do so through recognition and cognizance of the Oneness of God. We contemplate and recognize that Allah is worthy of worship and that nothing else is. We recognize truth in His words and in the guides He sent to us for our benefit. None of this is possible without contemplation, reflection, concentration, observation, and presence of mind.

> Allah said, Remember Me and I will remember you. (Surat al-Baqara, 2:152)

The word dhikr means remembrance, and in the Islamic context, it is used in the sense of remembrance of Allah. On the journey to the Divine

Presence the seed of remembrance is planted in the heart and nourished with the water of praise and the food of glorification, until the tree of dhikr becomes deeply rooted and bears its fruit. It is the power of all journeying and the foundation of all success. It is the reviver from the sleep of heedlessness, the bridge to the one remembered.

The shaikhs strive to remember their Lord with every breath, as the angels are always in the state of dhikr, praising Allah. One of our shaikhs said, "I remembered You because I forgot You for a moment, and the easiest way for me is to remember You on my tongue." If the seeker will mention his Lord in every moment, he will find peace and satisfaction in his heart, he will uplift his spirit and his soul, and he will sit in the presence of his Lord. The Prophet(s) said in an authentic hadith mentioned in Ahmad's Musnad, "The people of Dhikr are the people of My presence." So the gnostic is the one who keeps the dhikr in his heart and leaves behind the attachments of the lower worldly life. A good Muslim has to pray at least five times a day:

1. once before dawn
2. at noon
3. once in the afternoon
4. at sunset
5. and once at night.

During prayer he or she is to focus and meditate on God by reciting the Qur'an and engaging in dhikr in order to reaffirm and strengthen the bond between creator and creation. This has the effect of guiding the soul to truth. Such meditation is intended to help maintain a feeling of spiritual peace in the face of whatever challenges work, social, or family life may present. The five daily acts of peaceful prayer are to serve as a template and inspiration for conduct during the rest of the day, transforming it, ideally, into one single and sustained meditation. Even sleep is to be regarded as but another phase of that sustained meditation.

Meditative quiescence is said to have a quality of healing and of enhancing, as contemporary terminology would have it, creativity. The prophet Muhammad, whose deeds and devotions Muslims are to emulate, is reported to have spent sustained periods in contemplation and meditation. It was during one such period that the Prophet began to receive the revelations of the Qur'an.

Tafakkur or tadabbur means *reflection upon the universe;* this is considered to permit access to a form of cognitive and emotional development that can emanate only from the higher level, in other words, from God. The sensation of receiving divine inspiration awakens and liberates both heart and intellect, permitting such inner growth that the apparently mundane actually takes on the quality of the infinite. Muslim teachings embrace life as a test of one's submission to, and one's *acceptance,* the literal meaning of the word Islam, of Allah, the unconditioned, the one God beyond all mere human imaginings.

A. Meditation in the Sufi Traditions

Largely based on a spectrum of mystical exercises, meditation in the Sufi traditions varies from one lineage to another. Numerous Sufi traditions place emphasis on a meditative procedure similar in its cognitive aspect to one of the two principal approaches to be found in the Buddhist traditions: that of the concentration technique, involving high-intensity and sharply focused introspection. In the Oveyssi-Shahmaghsoudi Sufi order, for example, this is particularly evident, where muraqaba takes the form of tamarkoz, the latter being a Persian term, that means concentration.

The goal and purpose of Sufi meditation is to manifest perpetual presence in the reality. The more people keep to this vital practice, the more its benefit will manifest in their daily lives to the point that they reach the state of annihilation.

When people sit for Sufi meditation and close their eyes, they focus their mind on one single point. The point in this case is usually the concept of their spiritual mentor; that is, they focus all their witnessing abilities concentratively in thinking about their spiritual teacher in order to get the image of their mentor on the mental screen, as long as they remain in the state of meditation. The properties, characteristics, and potentialities related to an image also transfer on the screen of the mind when the image is formed on the mental screen, and the mind perceives them accordingly. For instance, a person is looking at fire. When the image of fire transfers onto the mental screen, the warmth and heat of the fire are perceived by the mind. A person who is present in a garden enjoys the freshness and coolness of trees and plants present in the garden to create their image on her mental screen. Similarly when image of the spiritual mentor transfers on the screen of mind, the presented knowledge, which is operative in the spiritual teacher, also transfers with it and the mind of the student gradually assimilates the same.

B. Annihilation, the State of Oneness With the Holy Prophet

In the state of "Oneness with the Holy Prophet" a spiritual associate because of his passion, longing and love gradually, step by step, assimilates and cognizes the knowledge of the Holy Prophet. Then comes that auspicious moment when the knowledge and learning is transferred to him according to his capacity from the Holy Prophet. To be a thing nonexistent, a crystal clear vessel for whomever wishes to fill your being from Allah's Divine Kingdom, this affinity, in Sufism, is called "Annilation in Allah Love."

6. JAINISM: JAIN SADHVIS MEDITATING

Jainism is an ancient religion with its origins in India. Pacifism and compassion are central tenets of the Jain following, and it is these elements that have greatly influenced Eastern mysticism for several millennia. The Jainists believe that divine truth is communicated on Earth by Tirthankars, who communicate otherworldly knowledge to other humans. Tirthankars appear in groups of twenty-four, their lives following in succession. The twenty-fourth Tirthankar to have existed in our realm, Lord Vardhaman Mahavira, died in 527 BC. However, the Jains believe that there will be an ongoing succession of Tirthankars across time and space. For this reason, they do not worship Lord Vardhaman or any of the twenty-three Tirthankars that preceded him, as such, but rather follow the virtues that they taught through example.

The Jainists believe that all humans have an eternal soul (or Jina) that is capable of reaching spiritual Enlightenment or Moksha, by living a spiritual life that is strict and based principally around the virtue of respect for all living forms. Like Buddhists and Hindus, Jainists believe in karma, the notion that all your actions will come back to you; hence their desire to lead a life that is humble and free of aggression toward others. Jainists follow a strict ethical code prohibiting violence, dishonesty, stealing, promiscuousness, and possessiveness.

A. The Navkar Mantra

Jains pray daily, reciting the Navkar Mantra which reinforces the true path to becoming a Siddha, or Enlightened person, via the principles outlined earlier, and through an official commitment to the Jainist way of life by becoming a nun or monk. This Navkar Mantra is undoubtedly similar in form to other forms of meditation and can be recited by Jainists at any point of the day for as long as they wish.

Although there are clear parallels between Jainists and Buddhists, including their desire for spiritual Enlightenment and their teaching of compassion for all beings, Jainism is principally an ascetic religion that believes in attaining Enlightenment through self-denial.

Jainist meditation focuses on emptying the mind in order to better realize truth and is often also focused around denial. Mahavira often meditated outside with no clothes for warmth and sometimes meditated standing up. This kind of meditation is subject to leading the practitioner down an unhelpful path because the pain associated with asceticism can be sought as an end in itself and is quite at odds with the prevailing instinct in our society. Jainism may well suit some individuals, the path to Enlightenment being a personal road; however, due to its severity and strictness, most of what can be gleaned from it may be best found elsewhere. Specific Jainist mantras can be easily recited where they are felt to be helpful.

The Jains use the word Samayika, a word in the Prakrit language derived from the word samay (time), to denote the practice of meditation. The aim of Samayika is to transcend the daily experiences of being a "constantly changing" human being, Jiva, and allow for the identification with the changeless reality in the practitioner, the Atma. The practice of Samayika begins by achieving a balance in time. If the present moment of time is taken to be a point between the past and the future, Samayika means being fully aware, alert, and conscious in that very moment, experiencing one's true nature, Atma, which is considered common to all living beings. The Samayika takes on special significance during Paryushana, a special eight-day period practiced by the Jains.

Jain meditation techniques were available in ancient Jain scriptures that have been forgotten with time. A practice called preksha meditation is said to have been rediscovered by the tenth Head of Jain Swetamber Terapanth sect Acharya Mahaprajna and consists of the perception of the body, the psychic centers, breath and of contemplation processes that will initiate the process of personal transformation. It aims at reaching and purifying the deeper levels of existence. Regular practice is believed to strengthen the immune system and build up stamina to resist against aging, pollution, chemical toxins, viruses, diseases, and food adulteration.

Meditation practice is an important part of the daily lives of the religion's monks. Acharya Mahaprajna says,

> Soul is my god.
> Renunciation is my prayer.
> Amity is my devotion.
> Self-restraint is my strength.
> Non-violence is my religion.

7. JUDAISM AND KABBALAH MEDITATION

There is evidence that Judaism has meditative practices that go back thousands of years For instance, in the Torah, the patriarch Isaac is described as going lasuach in the field, a term understood by all commentators as some type of meditative practice (Genesis 24:63), probably prayer. Similarly, there are indications throughout the Tanach (the Hebrew Bible) that meditation was central to the prophets. In the Old Testament, there are two Hebrew words for meditation: hāgâ which means to sigh or murmur, but also to meditate, which means to muse or rehearse in one's mind.

In modern Jewish practice, one of the best known meditative practices is called hitbodedut or hisbodedus iand s explained in Kabbalah and Hassidic philosophy. The word hisbodedut, which derives from the Hebrew word "boded" (a state of being alone), means the process of making oneself understand a concept well through analytical study.

Kabbalah is inherently a meditative field of study. Kabbalistic meditative practices construct a supernal realm that the soul navigates through in order to achieve certain ends. One of the most well-known types of meditation is merkabah, from the consontal root r-k-b, meaning to ride.

A. What is Kabbalah?

Kabbalah is an ancient Jewish mystical system of meditation that teaches the profoundest insights into the essence of God, how He interacts with the world, and the purpose of creation. Kabbalah and its teachings are an integral part of the Torah, the entire body of Jewish wisdom and teachings, both the oral law, and the written law. Some Jewish scholars suggest that the Torah is the hand-written scroll of the Divine Law or the Five Books of Moses.

In the evolutionary chain of forms, we humans are the first form in that evolving chain to have self-consciousness added to the subconscious forms of the mineral, plant, and animal realms. A creature with upright posture, opposing thumbs for manipulating physical things, and a separate sense of "I"-ness or individuality. The "lower" three kingdoms evolve through physical adaptation to changing physical conditions, such as heat, cold, moisture, dryness, availability of food, and changes in predators. Humans differ in that our transformations are brought about by resolving differences between other individuals and groups. In time, such experiences assist us to realize our unity or oneness.

One of the foremost purposes of human existence is to create and maintain a bridge between subconscious life (the animal, vegetable, mineral realms) and superconscious existence and expression. Self-consciousness, the awareness of the divinity within each one of us and all of creation is that bridge. This acknowledges and celebrates both, The One in the all and the all in The One.

When spelled with the letter "Q," the word Qabalah refers to the Universal Qabalah. The Universal Qabalah is a body of esoteric and practical wisdom that encompasses both Judeo-Christian mysticism and the teachings of other traditions such as yoga, Buddhism, Sufism, Hermetics (tarot, astrology, alchemy, numerology, and sacred geometry) among them. Qabalah is a Western tradition that serves as a bridge between the inner traditions of the East and West. Study and practical application of the teachings of the Qabalah, Tree of Life, and Tarot may be used to enhance and augment the teachings of all spiritual disciplines.

Kabbalah meditations were devised by the Jewish mystics over 2000 years ago to *enhance the awareness and access higher planes of consciousness.* The Qabalah uses the Tree of Life as its major symbolic representation of the processes of evolutionary unfoldment. By studying and meditating on the Tree of Life, which is a pictorial representation of the descent of consciousness, into deepest matter, and its ascent back into the highest level of consciousness, the student can use the processes of evolutionary unfoldment to journey back to the highest levels of consciousness and simultaneously manifest these higher levels in deepest matter.

B. The Aim of Kabbalah Meditation

The aim of Kabbalah mditation is to make the practitioners the true carriers of the light of God. Kabbalah meditation continues to flourish in the oral tradition and rises above the written word. This system will enable you to attain peace and happiness through the union with God. The objective of Kabbalah meditation transcends the need for relaxation and quieting the mind. Kabbalah meditation enables the seekers to directly interact with the higher worlds and bring about positive changes in life. It wipes off the negative influences from both your body and your mind and establishes the power of mind over the matter. The essence of Kabbalah meditation is to bring new resources of joy, love, and understanding to everything you do.

Kabbalah meditation explores the complex character of the divine reality, particularly the inability of the human thought to grasp Him. It uses various techniques, including meditations on Hebrew letter permutations and combinations and the ways in which sefirot or the supernatural forces harmonize and interact with each other. These meditative techniques produce visionary experiences of the angels and their residential chambers.

Another important objective of Kabbalah is to rectify the imperfections of the soul rather than to create spiritual knowledge.

Kabbalah explains that all events in the universe are connected. Two fundamental concepts influence these connections:

1. There is a spectrum of space running through the universe, from absolute largeness, containing everything, to absolute smallness or nothingness at the other end. The largeness is referred to as Ein Sof (allness, without end); nothingness is known as Ayin. This spectrum of space is encountered in many religions.
2. This in turn vivifies the second major concept, which is that all events within this spectrum are manifestations of the workings of the ten Sephirot.

Sephirot, meaning "enumerations," are the ten attributes or emanations in Kabbalah through which God (who is referred to as Ein Sof, The Infinite) reveals himself or herself and continuously creates both the physical realm and the chain of higher metaphysical realms. The sephirot are related to the structure of the body and are reformed into Partsufim (personas). Underlying the structural purpose of each sephirah is a hidden motivational force that is understood best by comparison with a corresponding psychological state in human spiritual experience. The ten Sephirot are a step-by-step process illuminating the Divine plan, as it unfolds itself in Creation.

Because all levels of Creation are constructed around the ten Sephirot, their names in Kabbalah describe the particular role each plays in forming reality. These are the external dimensions of the Sephirot, describing their functional roles in channelling the Divine, creative Ohr (Light) to all levels. Because the sephirot are viewed to comprise both metaphorical "lights" and "vessels," their structural role describes the particular identity each Sephirah possesses from its characteristic vessel. Underlying this functional structure of the Sephirot, each one possesses a hidden, inner spiritual motivation that inspires its activity. This forms the particular characteristic of inner light within each Sephirah.

Identifying the essential spiritual properties of the soul, gives the best insight into their Divine source, and in the process reveals the spiritual beauty of the soul.

THE 10 SEPHIROT

Category	Sephirah
Above-consciousness	1 Keter "Crown"
Conscious intellect	2 Chokhmah "Wisdom" 3 Binah "Understanding"
Conscious emotions	Primary emotions 4 Chesed "Kindness" 5 Gevurah "Severity" 6 Tiferet "Beauty" Secondary emotions 7 Netzach "Eternity" 8 Hod "Splendour" 9 Yesod "Foundation" Vessel to bring action 10 Malkuth "Kingship"

In Hasidic philosophy these inner dimensions of the Sephirot are called the Powers of the Soul (Weiser S., 1997).

Two alternative spiritual arrangements for describing the Sephirot are given, metaphorically described as "Circles" and "Upright." Their origins come from Medieval Kabbalah and the Zohar. In later sixteenth-century Lurianic Kabbalah, they become systemized as two successive stages in the evolution of the Sephirot during the primordial cosmic evolution of Creation. This evolution is central to the metaphysical process of tikkun (fixing) in the doctrines of Isaac Luria.

8. NATIVE AMERICANS SPIRITUALITY AND PRAYERS

The Native American attitude is that everything is animated by divinity. Therefore, ordinary people, animals, and places are divine. Among all tribes there is a strong sense that behind all individual spirits and personifications of the divine, there is a single creative life force, sometimes called the Great Mystery, which expresses itself throughout the universe, in every human, animal, tree and grain of sand. Every story, too, is a working out of this life force.

An aspect of this outlook is the major role played in the stories by animals, who often speak to humans and assist them. Most tribes thought of individual members of a species as expressions of the spiritual archetype of that species, which in turn embodied a particular spirit power.

Another key feature of the Native American spiritual outlook is found in the powers ascribed to the Four Directions, which occur either literally or in symbolic form throughout the stories. These are often represented by particular colors, or by animals. The Four Directions have to be in balance for all to be well with the world, and often a central point of balance is identified as a fifth direction. For example, four brothers represent the outer directions, and their sister the center.

The Medicine Wheel is often representative of Native American Spirituality. The Medicine Wheel symbolizes the individual journey we each must take to find our own path. Within the Medicine Wheel are The Four Cardinal Directions and the Four Sacred Colors.

A. The Circle of Life

The Circle represents the Circle of Life, and the Center of the Circle, the Eternal Fire. The Eagle, flying toward the East, is a symbol of strength, endurance, and vision. East signifies the renewal of life.

- East = Red = success; triumph
- North = Blue = defeat; trouble
- West = Black = death
- South = White = peace; happiness

There are three additional sacred directions:

- Up Above = Yellow
- Down Below = Brown
- Here in the Center = Green

WINTER: The color for North is blue, which represents sadness, defeat. It is a season of survival and waiting.

SPRING: The color for East is red, which represents victory, power. Spring is the reawakening after a long sleep, victory over winter, the power of new life.

SUMMER: The color for South is white for peace, happiness, and serenity. Summer is a time of plenty.

AUTUMN: The color for West is black, which represents death. Autumn is the final harvest; the end of Life's Cycle.

Red was symbolic of success. Red beads were used to conjure the red spirit to ensure long life, recovery from sickness, success in love and ball play or any other undertaking where the benefit of the magic spell was wrought.

Black was always typical of death. The soul of the enemy was continual-ly beaten about by black war clubs and enveloped in a black fog. In conjur-ing to destroy an enemy, the priest used black beads and invoked the black spirits, which always lived in the West, bidding them to tear out the man's soul and carry it to the West and put it into the black coffin deep in the black mud with a black serpent coiled above it.

Blue symbolized failure, disappointment, or unsatisfied desire. To say "they shall never become blue" expressed the belief that they would never fail in anything they undertook. In love charms, the lover figuratively cov-ered himself with red and prayed that his rival would become entirely blue and walk in a blue path. He is entirely blue approximates the meaning of the common English phrase "He feels blue." The blue spirits lived in the North.

White denoted peace and happiness. In ceremonial addresses, as the Green Corn Dance and ball play, the people symbolically partook of white food and, after the dance or game, returned along the white trail to their white houses. In love charms, the man, to induce the woman to cast her lot with his, boasted, "I am a white man," implying that all was happiness where he was. White beads had the same meaning in bead conjuring, and white was the color of the stone pipe anciently used in ratifying peace treaties. The White spirits lived in the South.

Two numbers are sacred to these traditions. Four is one number; it rep-resented the four primary directions. At the center of their paths is the sacred fire. Seven is the other and most sacred number. Seven is represented in the seven directions: north, south, east, west, above, below, and here in the cen-ter. the place of the sacred fire. Seven also represented the seven ancient cer-emonies that formed the yearly religious cycle. The medicine wheel is a sym-bol for the wheel of life, which is forever evolving and bringing new lessons and truths to the walking of the path. The Earthwalk is based on the under-standing that each one of us must stand on every spoke of the great wheel of life many times and that every direction is to be honored.

The medicine wheel teaches us that all lessons are equal, as are all talents and abilities. Every living creature will one day see and experience each spoke of the wheel and know those truths. It is a pathway to truth, peace, and harmony. The circle is never ending, life without end.

In experiencing the Good Red Road, one learns the lessons of physical life, or of being human. This road runs South to North in the circle of the med-icine wheel. After the graduation experience of death, one enters the Blue or Black Road that is the world of the grandfathers and grandmothers. In spirit, one will continue to learn by counseling those remaining on the Good Red Road. The Blue Road of the spirit runs East to West. The medicine wheel is life, afterlife, rebirth, and the honoring of each step along the way.

The medicine shield is an expression of the unique gifts that its maker wishes to impart about his or her current life journey. This can be a new level of personal growth or illustrate the next mountain a person wishes to climb. Every shield carries medicine through its art and self-expression. Each shield is the essence of a time and space that carries certain aspects of knowledge. All persons carry shields of the lessons they learned from the four directions on the medicine wheel. They are the healing tools we give ourselves to soothe the spirit and empower the will. The truth needs no explanation, just reflection. This allows intuition to guide the heart so that humanity may celebrate more than it mourns.

The medicine wheel is sacred, the native people believe, because the Great Spirit caused everything in nature to be round. The Sun, Sky, Earth and Moon are round. Thus, man should look upon the Medicine Wheel (circle of life) as sacred. It is the symbol of the circle that marks the edge of the world and therefore, the Four Winds that travel there. It is also the symbol of the year. The Sky, the Night, and the Moon go in a circle above the Sky, therefore, the Circle is a symbol of these divisions of time. It is the symbol of all times throughout creation.

The elements and majestic forces in nature, Lightning, Wind, Water, Fire, and Frost, were regarded with awe as spiritual powers, but always secondary and intermediate in character. Natives believe that the spirit pervades all creation and that every creature possesses a soul in some degree, though not necessarily a soul conscious of itself. The tree, the waterfall, the grizzly bear, each is an embodied Force, and as such an object of reverence.

B. Native American's Words of Wisdom

Love your life, perfect your life, beautify all things in your life. Seek to make your life long and of service to your people. Prepare a noble death song for the day when you go over the great divide. Always give a word or sign of salute when meeting or passing a stranger if in a lonely place. Show respect to all people, but grovel to none. When you arise in the morning, give thanks for the light, for your life and strength. Give thanks for your food and for the joy of living. If you see no reason for giving thanks, the fault lies in yourself. (Tecumseh, 1768–1813)

The first peace, which is the most important, is that which comes within the souls of people when they realize their relationship, their oneness with the universe and all its powers, and when they realize that at the center of the universe dwells the Great Spirit, and that this center is really everywhere, it is within each of us. (Black Elk, 1863–1950)

Black Elk Speaks is a 1932 book that relates the story of Black Elk, an Oglala Sioux medicine man, as told by John Neihardt (1932). Black Elk's son Ben Black Elk translated Black Elk's words from Lakota into English. In the summer of 1930, as part of his research into the Native American perspective on the Ghost Dance movement, Neihardt contacted an Oglala holy man named Black Elk, who was present as a young man at the 1876 Battle of the Little Big Horn and the 1890 Wounded Knee Massacre.

As Neihardt tells the story, Black Elk gave him the gift of his life's narrative, including the visions he had had and some of the Oglala rituals he had performed. The two men developed a close friendship. The book *Black Elk Speaks* grew from their conversations continuing in the spring of 1931. The current popularity of the book shows the growth of interest in the social and ethical analysis of Native American tribes.

The Ghost Dance was a religious movement that was incorporated into numerous Native American belief systems. The traditional ritual used in the Ghost Dance, the circle dance, has been used by many Native Americans since prehistoric times. Referred to as the "round dance," this ritual form characteristically includes a circular community dance held around an individual who leads the ceremony. It was used in many community rituals. Often accompanying the ritual are intermissions of trance, exhortations, and prophesying.

Native American myths include all the types found worldwide, such as stories of creation and of heroic journeys. They are particularly rich in trickster myths, however. Notable examples are Coyote and Iktome. The trickster is an ambiguous figure who demonstrates the qualities of early human development (both cultural and psychological) that make civilization possible and yet cause problems. He is an expression of the least developed stage of life, which is dominated by physical appetites. Spirituality is not religion to Native American. Religion is not a native concept, it is a nonnative word, with implications of things that often end badly, like holy wars in the name of individuals' gods, and so on. Native people do not ask what religion another native is because they already know the answer. To Native people, spirituality is the Creator.

> May the Warm Winds of Heaven
> Blow softly upon your house.
> May the Great Spirit
> Bless all who enter there.
> May your Moccasins
> Make happy tracks
> in many snows,

and may the Rainbow
Always touch your shoulder. (Ancient Cherokee Prayer Blessing)

C. Ancient Lakota Instructions for Living

Friend do it this way—that is,
whatever you do in life,
do the very best you can
with both your heart and mind.
And if you do it that way,
the Power of The Universe
will come to your assistance,
if your heart and mind are in Unity.

9. TAOISM'S WU WEI MEDITATION

Taoism originated in China long ago and is composed of a number of different disciplines that together help the individual live in harmony with nature and advance toward states of greater happiness and fulfillment. Taoist meditation is more like a sort of wisdom achieved by close observation of the things and phenomena in the world surrounding us. Such wisdom should help us go along with things and not against them and is surely related to the nondoing concept and practice. Chinese wu (not); wei (doing) is a term with various translations (e.g., inaction, nonaction, nothing doing) and interpretations designed to distinguish it from passivity. From a nondual perspective, it refers to activity that does not imply an "I." What is Nondoing (Wu Wei)?

Wu Wei, usually translated as nonaction, inaction, or nondoing, is one of the most important Taoist concepts. When linked to the Tao, the creator and sustainer of everything in the Universe, nondoing means the actionless of Heaven, like in the following abstract from Tao De Ching (Lao Tze):

> The Tao in its regular course does nothing (for the sake of doing it), and so there is nothing which it does not do. Linked with the human behavior, nondoing refers to not forcing the things on their way, on the action without effort. (Tao De Ching, Lao Tze)

Thus nondoing refers to a specific form of intelligence and, at the same time, to the urge of following the Tao (Way). These two are linked: one follows the Tao because it has (holds) the intelligence to do so, or because it has this intelligence he or she is able to follow the Tao.

A. The Way

The Way that can be experienced is not true;
The world that can be constructed is not true.
The Way manifests all that happens and may happen;
The world represents all that exists and may exist.
To experience without intention is to sense the world;
To experience with intention is to anticipate the world.
These two experiences are indistinguishable;
Their construction differs but their effect is the same.
Beyond the gate of experience flows the Way,
Which is ever greater and more subtle than the world. (Tao De Ching, Lao Tze)

Taoist meditation methods, have many points in common with Hindu and Buddhist systems, but the Taoist way is less abstract and far more down-to-earth than the contemplative traditions that evolved in India. The primary hallmark of Taoist meditation is the generation, transformation, and circulation of internal energy.

Once the meditator has "achieved energy" (deh-chee), it can be applied to promoting health and longevity, nurturing the spiritual embryo of immortality, martial arts, healing, painting and poetry, sensual self-indulgence, or whatever else the adept wishes to do with it. The two primary guidelines in Taoist meditation are jing (quiet, stillness, calm) and ding (concentration, focus). The purpose of stillness, both mental and physical, is to turn attention inward and cut off external sensory input, thereby muzzling the "Five Thieves." Within that silent stillness, one concentrates the mind and focuses attention, usually on the breath, in order to develop what is called one-pointed awareness, a totally undistracted, undisturbed, undifferentiated state of mind which permits intuitive insights to arise spontaneously.

Without Action
Not praising the worthy prevents contention,
Not esteeming the valuable prevents theft,
Not displaying the beautiful prevents desire.
In this manner the sage governs people:
Emptying their minds,
Filling their bellies,
Weakening their ambitions,
And strengthening their bones.
If people lack knowledge and desire
Then they can not act;
If no action is taken
Harmony remains. (Tao De Ching, Lao Tze)

Harmony
Embracing the Way, you become embraced;
Breathing gently, you become newborn;
Clearing your mind, you become clear;
Nurturing your children, you become impartial;
Opening your heart, you become accepted;
Accepting the world, you embrace the Way.
Bearing and nurturing,
Creating but not owning,
Giving without demanding,
This is harmony. (Tao De Ching, Lao Tze)

Taoist masters suggest that when you first begin to practice meditation, you will find that your mind is very uncooperative. That is your ego, or emotional mind, fighting against its own extinction by the higher forces of spiritual awareness.

Self
Both praise and blame cause concern,
For they bring people hope and fear.
The object of hope and fear is the self
For, without self, to whom may fortune and disaster occur?
Therefore,
Who distinguishes himself from the world may be given the world,
But who regards himself as the world may accept the world.
(Tao De Ching, Lao Tze)

The last thing your ego and emotions want is to be harnessed: they revel in the day-to-day circus of sensory entertainment and emotional turmoil, even though this game depletes your energy, degenerates your body, and exhausts your spirit. When you catch your mind drifting into fantasy or drawing attention away from internal alchemy to external phenomena, there are six ways you can use to "catch the monkey," clarify the mind, and reestablish the internal focus:

1. Shift attention back to the inflow and outflow of air streaming through the nostrils or energy streaming in and out of a vital point such as between the brows.
2. Focus attention on the rising and falling of the navel, the expansion and contraction of the abdomen, as you breathe.
3. With eyes half-closed, focus vision on a candle flame or a mandala (geometric meditation picture). Focus on the center of the flame or picture but also take in the edges with peripheral vision. The concentra-

tion required to do this usually clears all other distractions from the mind.

4. Practice a few minutes of mantra, the "sacred syllables" that harmonize energy and focus the mind. Although mantras are usually associated with Hindu and Tibetan Buddhist practices, Taoists have also employed them for many millennia. The three most effective syllables are "Om," which stabilizes the body; "ah," which harmonizes energy; and "hum," which concentrates the spirit. Om vibrates between the brows, ah in the throat, and hum in the heart, and their associated colors are white, red, and blue, respectively. Chant the syllables in a deep, low-pitched tone and use long, complete exhalations for each one. Other mantras are equally effective.

5. Beat the "Heavenly Drum" as a cool-down energy-collection technique. The vibrations tend to clear discursive thoughts and sensory distractions from the mind.

6. Visualize a deity or a sacred symbol of personal significance to you shining above the crown of your head or suspended in space before you. When your mind is once again still, stable, and undistracted, let the vision fade away and refocus your mind on whatever meditative technique you were practicing.

B. The Three Treasures or San Bao: Essence (Body), Energy (Breath), Spirit (Mind)

The Three Treasures or Three Jewels are basic virtues in Taoism. The *Tao Te Ching* originally used san bao to mean compassion, frugality, and humility. San bao first occurs in *Tao Te Ching*, Chapter 67, which Lin Yutang (1948; 292) says contains Lao-tzu's "most beautiful teachings":

> Every one under heaven says that our Way is greatly like folly. But it is just because it is great, that it seems like folly. As for things that do not seem like folly, well, there can be no question about their smallness!
> Here are my three treasures. Guard and keep them! The first is pity; the second, frugality; the third, refusal to be "foremost of all things under heaven."
> For only he that pities is truly able to be brave;
> Only he that is frugal is able to be profuse.
> Only he that refuses to be foremost of all things
> Is truly able to become chief of all Ministers.
> At present your bravery is not based on pity, nor your profusion on frugality, nor your vanguard on your rear; and this is death. But pity cannot fight without conquering or guard without saving. Heaven arms with pity those whom it would not see destroyed. (Waley, 1958)

In the millenary Taoist tradition, the concept of San Bao refers to three mysterious subtle structures of the human being, known as the three tan tien, structures that are particularly important. They are regarded by the Taoist sages to be some real treasures inside every human being, and their knowledge through direct experience is extremely valuable in spiritual practice. They correspond to a potential of a primordial natural innate force, on which the very life of the human being depends.

In short, we could define the tan tien as a subtle cavity, a kind of a reservoir, where the elixir of immortality obtained through alchemy is stored. The Taoist tradition states that in every human being's microcosm the subtle energy travels through a complex network of subtle energy channels, but alongside them there are certain mysterious places of concentration of energy that constitute genuine focal points. Out of these, the three tan tien are the most important structures.

These real "inner treasures," the three tan tien, are associated with the three basic energies of the human being, which in the Taoist tradition are associated with the vital energy, the pranic energy and the energy of the soul. These are known as Jing (essence), Chi (energy), and Shen (the soul).

Like all genuine spiritual traditions of our planet, Taoism has a complex and global vision of humans and their existential condition. Thus, the desire of inner evolution and spiritual transformation that allows the achievement of the state of godhood is founded by a coherent and consistent philosophical vision that describes the process of the universal creation, and how the creation (and by implication humans) can return to its divine unique Source.

Taoist meditation works on all three levels of the Three Treasures: essence (body), energy (breath), and spirit (mind).

1. The first step is to adopt a comfortable posture for the body; balance your weight evenly, straighten the spine, and pay attention to physical sensations such as heat, cold, tingling, trembling, or whatever else arises.
2. When your body is comfortable and balanced, shift attention to the second level, which is breath and energy. You may focus on the breath itself as it flows in and out of the lungs through the nostrils or on energy streaming in and out of a particular point in tune with the breath.
3. The third level is spirit. When the breath is regulated and energy is flowing smoothly through the channels, focus attention on thoughts and feelings forming and dissolving in your mind, awareness expanding and contracting with each breath, insights and inspirations arising spontaneously, visions and images appearing and disappearing. Eventually you may even be rewarded with intuitive flashes of insight re-

garding the ultimate nature of the mind: open and empty as space; clear and luminous as a cloudless sky at sunrise; infinite and unimpeded.

Just as all the rules of Qigong (chee gung) practice can be boiled down to the three Ss: slow, soft, smooth, so the main points of meditation practice may be summed up in the three Cs: calm, cool, clear. As for proper postures for practice, the two positions most frequently used in Taoist meditation are:

- Sitting cross-legged on the floor in half-lotus position, with the buttocks elevated on a cushion or pad. The advantages of this method are that this position is more stable and encourages energy to flow upwards toward the brain.
- Sitting erect on a low stool or chair, feet parallel and shoulder width apart, knees bent at a 90-degree angle, spine erect. The advantages of sitting on a stool are that the legs do not cramp, the soles of the feet are in direct contact with the energy of the earth, and internal energy tends to flow more freely throughout the lower as well as the upper torso.

Most meditators who follow Taoist meditation use both methods, depending on conditions. When sitting cross-legged, those whose legs tend to cramp easily, are advised to sit on thick firm cushions, perhaps with a phone book or two underneath, in order to elevate the pelvis and take pressure off the legs and knees. This also helps keep the spine straight without straining the lower back. The way the hands are placed is also important. The most natural and comfortable position is to rest the palms lightly on the thighs, just above the knees. Some meditators, however, find it more effective to use one of the traditional mudras, or hand gestures. Experiment with different combinations of posture and mudra until you find the style that suits you best. Taoist meditation masters teach three basic ways to control the Fire mind of emotion with the Water mind of intent, so that the adept's goals in meditation may be realized.

C. Taoist Meditations

1. The first method is called *stop and observe.* This involves paying close attention to how thoughts arise and fade in the mind, learning to let them pass like a freight train in the night, without clinging to any particular one. This develops awareness of the basic emptiness of all

thought, as well as nonattachment to the rise and fall of emotional impulses. Gradually one learns simply to ignore the intrusion of discursive thoughts, at which point they cease arising for sheer lack of attention.

2. The second technique is called *observe and imagine,* which refers to visualization. The adept employs intent to visualize an image, such as Buddha, Jesus, a sacred symbol, the moon, or a star, in order to shift mental focus away from thoughts and emotions and stabilize the mind in one-pointed awareness. You may also visualize a particular energy center in your body, or listen to the real or imagined sound of a bell, gong, or cymbal ringing in your ears. The point of focus is not important; what counts is shifting the focus of your attention away from idle thoughts, conflicting emotions, fantasies, and other distracting antics of the monkey mind and concentrating attention instead on a stable point of focus established by the mind of intent, or 'wisdom mind'.

3. The third step in cultivating control over your own mind is called *using the mind of intent to guide energy.* When the emotional mind is calm and the breath is regulated, focus attention on the internal energy. Learn how to guide it through the meridian network in order to energize vital organs, raise energy from the sacrum to the head to nourish the spirit and brain, and exchange stale energy for fresh energy from the external sources of heaven (sky) and earth (ground). Begin by focusing attention on the Lower Elixir Field below the abdomen, then moving energy from there down to the perineum, up through the coccyx, and up along the spinal centers into the head, after which attention shifts to the Upper Elixir Field between the brows. Although this sounds rather vague and esoteric to the uninitiated, a few months of practice, especially in conjunction with Qigong and proper dietary habits, usually suffices to unveil the swirling world of energy and awareness hidden within our bodies and minds. All you have to do is sit still and be quiet long enough for your mind to become aware of it.

It is always a good idea to warm up your body and open your energy channels with some Qigong exercises before you sit down to meditate. This facilitates internal energy circulation and enables you to sit for longer periods without getting stiff or numb. After sitting, you should avoid bathing for at least 20 minutes in order to prevent loss of energy through open pores and energy points.

If you live in the northern hemisphere, it is best to sit facing south or east, in the general direction of the sun. In the southern hemisphere, sit facing north or east. Still, what is Tao's Movement and what does it mean to empty your mind of the wishes not fitted with it? The answer is simple, but our minds are very complicated, so we are not able to enjoy it. Chuang-tzu (Master Chuang), who followed the teachings of Lao-tzu, describes the empty mind in his monumental work that bears his name by stating,

> The still mind of the sage is the mirror of heaven and earth, the glass of all things. Vacancy, stillness, placidity, tastelessness, quietude, silence, and non-action–this is the Level of heaven and earth, and the perfection of the Tao and its characteristics. (Lao-tzu)

The still mind is a mind that is not moving, or put another way, it is the mirror of the universe. This is the pure mind of ancient Taoist masters. When we speak about emptiness, we think of the verses Lao-tzu himself dedicated to it. In his *Tao Te Ching,* emptiness is related to the Tao, the Great Principle, the Creator and Sustainer of everything in the universe (the 10,000 things). Emptiness is also the state of mind of the Taoist disciple who follows the Tao. In this respect, to be empty means to have your mind empty of all wishes and ideas not fitted with the Tao's Movement (direction).

D. The Enlightenment in Taoist Meditation

Enlightenment
The enlightened possess understanding
So profound they can not be understood.
Because they cannot be understood
I can only describe their appearance:
Cautious as one crossing thin ice,
Undecided as one surrounded by danger,
Modest as one who is a guest,
Unbounded as melting ice,
Genuine as unshaped wood,
Broad as a valley,
Seamless as muddy water.
Who stills the water that the mud may settle,
Who seeks to stop that he may travel on,
Who desires less than may transpire,
Decays, but will not renew. (Tao De Ching, Lao Tze)

REFERENCES

Green, E. E. (1972). Biofeedback for mind/body self-regulation, healing and creativity. In *The varieties of healing experience: Exploring psychic phenomena in healing.*

Transcript of the Interdisciplinary Symposium, Los Altos, California, October 30, 1971. Academy of Parapsychology and Medicine.

Lao Tzu. (1958). *Tao Te Ching* (Wordsworth Classics of World Literature) (A. Waley, Trans.). Ware, UK: Wordsworth Editions.

Lin Yutang. (1948). *Tao Te Ching.*

Neihardt, J. (1932). *Black Elk speaks.* Albany, NY: State University of New York.

Nhat Hanh, T. (1999) *The heart of the Buddha's teaching.* New York: Broadway Books.

Rama, S. (1982). *Mandukya Upanishad: Enlightenment without God.* Honesdale, PA: Himalayan Institute Press.

Saraswati, P. S. (1974). *Tantra-Yoga Panorama.* Mangrove Creek, Australia: International Yoga Fellowship Movement.

SUGGESTED READINGS

Alcock, J. E. (1979). Psychology and near-death experiences. *Skeptical Inquirer, 3*(3), 25–41.

Allen, R. S. (2009). *Tecumseh* [Online]. Available at http://www.thecanadianencyclo pedia.com/index.cfm?PgNm=TCE&Params=A1ARTA0007898

Arieti, S. (1979). *Creatività la sintesi magica.* Italy: Il Pensiero Scientifico.

Armstrong, K. (2001). *Buddha.* London: Penguin Books.

Austin, J. H. (1999). *Zen and the brain: Toward an understanding of meditation and consciousness.* Cambridge, MA: First MIT Press paperback edition.

Barendregt, H. P. (1988). Buddhist phenomenology. In *Atti del Congresso Temi e prospettive della logica e della filosofia della scienza contemporanea.* (Cesena 1987. Vol. 11, pp. 37–55). CLUEB, Bologna.

Basham, A. L. (1959). *The wonder that was India.* New York: Grove Press.

Bechert, H., & Gombrich, R. (Eds.). (1984). *The world of Buddhism.* London: Thames & Hudson.

Bechert, H. (Ed.). (1996). *When did the Buddha live? The controversy on the dating of the historical Buddha.* Delhi: Sri Satguru.

Bertoletti, P. (1986). *Mito e Simbolo.* Dedalo.

Bettelheim, B. (1977). *Il mondo incantato.* Feltrinelli.

Bhikkhu, T. (2001). *Refuge: An introduction to the Buddha, Dhamma, & Sangha.* Valley Center, CA: Metta Forest Monastery.

Blackmore, S. (2003). *Consciousness: An introduction.* London: Hodder & Stoughton.

Bower, B. (2007, September 15). Consciousness in the raw: The brain stem may orchestrate the basics of awareness [Online]. *Science News.*

Brugnoli, A. (2004). *Stato di coscienza totalizzante, alla ricerca del profondo Se.* Verona, Italy: La Grafica Editrice.

Brugnoli, A. (2005). *Stati di coscienza modificati neurofisiologici.* Verona, Italy: La Grafica Editrice.

Brugnoli, M. P. (2001). Neurofisiologia di realtà percepita e realtà rappresentata: quale relazione tra working memory e visualizzazione mentale in ipnosi. *Acta*

Hypnologica, 3, 21–22.

Brugnoli, M. P. (2004). Tecniche di rilassamento e ipnosi nel controllo della sofferenza del paziente terminale. *Acta Hypnologica, 7*(1–2), 3–14.

Brugnoli, M. P. (2009). Tecniche di rilassamento e ipnosi clinica in terapia del dolore e cure palliative [Clinical hypnosis, spirituality and palliation: The way of inner peace]. Verona, Italy: Del Miglio Editore.

Brugnoli, M. P., & Shivchandra Parolini, M. (2009). *La via della pace interiore: tecniche di rilassamento e di meditazione per il benessere dell'anima.* Verona, Italy: Del Miglio Editore.

Buswell, R. E. (Ed.). (2003). *Encyclopedia of Buddhism.* New York: Macmillan Reference Books.

Capra, F. (1996). *The web of life: A new scientific understanding of living systems.* New York: Random House.

Carrithers, M. (1986). The Buddha. In *Founders of faith* (pp. 13–14), Oxford, UK: Oxford University Press.

Charon, J. E. (2004). *The spirit: That stranger inside us.* Califormula Publishing.

Coogan, M. D. (Ed.). (2003). *The illustrated guide to world religions.* New York: Oxford University Press.

Coomaraswamy, A. (1975). *Buddha and the gospel of Buddhism.* Boston: University Books.

Cousins, L. S. (1996). The Dating of the Historical Buddha: A Review Article. *Journal of the Royal Asiatic Society Series, 3*(6.1), 57–63.

Crosley, R. O. (2004). *Alternative medicine and miracles: A grand unified theory.* Lanham, MD: University Press of America.

Dandekar, P. H., Harrison, J. B., Raghavan, V., Weiler, R., & Yarrow, A. (1988). *Sources of Indian tradition: From the beginning to 1800.* (Vol. 1, 2nd ed.). New York: Columbia University Press.

Davidson, R. J., Kabat-Zinn, J., Schumacher, J., Rosenkranz, M., Muller, D., Santorelli, S. F., ... Sheridan, J. F. (2003). Alterations in brain and immune function produced by mindfulness meditation. *Psychosomatic Medicine, 65*(4), 564–570.

Davidson, R. M. (2003). *Indian esoteric Buddhism: A social history of the tantric movement.* New York: Columbia University Press.

De Give, B. (2006). *Les rapports de l'Inde et de l'Occident des origines au règne d'Asoka.* Paris: Les Indes Savants.

Dhamma, R. (2001). *The Buddha and his disciples.* Birmingham, UK: Dhamma-Talaka Publications.

Donath, D. C. (1971). *Buddhism for the West: Theravāda, Mahāyāna and Vajrayāna: A comprehensive review of Buddhist history, philosophy, and teachings from the time of the Buddha to the present day.* New York: Julian Press.

Dossey, L. (2001). *Il potere curativo della mente.* Red, Italy.

Eliot (1935). *Japanese Buddhism.* London: Edward Arnold.

Ellis, H. (1897). A note on hypnagogic paramnesia. *Mind, New Series, 6*(22), 283–287.

Ferrari, M., & Sternberg, R. J. (Eds.). (1998). *Self-Awareness: Its nature and development.* New York: Guilford Press.

Frost, S. E. (1989). *Basic teachings of the great philosophers.* New York: Anchor Books.

Fuller, R. C. (1996). Holistic health practices. In P. H. Van Ness (Ed.), *Spirituality and the secular quest* (pp. 230–234). New York: Crossroad Publishing Company.

Gethin, R. (1998). *Foundations of Buddhism.* New York: Oxford University Press.

Goldstein, J. (1983). *The experience of insight.* Boston: Shambhala.

Gombrich, R. F. (1988). *Theravāda Buddhism: A social history from ancient Benares to modern Colombo.* London: Routledge.

Gunaratana, B. H. (2002). *Mindfulness in plain English.* Somerville, MA: Wisdom Publications.

Harvey, P. (1990). *An introduction to Buddhism: Teachings, history and practices.* Cambridge, UK: Cambridge University Press.

Hefner, A. G. (2008). The MYSTICA™. Copyright © 1997. Alan G. Hefner. http://www.law.cornell.edu/uscode/17/107.shtml.

Hinnels, J. R. (1998). *The new penguin handbook of living religions.* London: Penguin Books.

Hofstadter, D. E. (1979). *Gödel Escher Bach [An eternal golden braid].* Hassocks, Sussex: Harvester Press.

James, W. (1902). *Lectures 16 & 17: Mysticism. In The varieties of religious experience: A study in nature* (pp. 206–234). Huntington, MA: Seven Treasures Publications.

James, W. (1890). *The principles of psychology* (Vol. 1). New York: Henry Holt.

Juergensmeyer, M. (Ed.). (2006). *The Oxford handbook of global religions.* Oxford: Oxford University Press.

Kabat-Zinn, J., Lipworth, L., & Burney, R. (1985). The clinical use of mindfulness meditation for the self-regulation of chronic pain. *Journal of Behavioral Medicine, 8*(2), 163–190.

Kasulis, T. P. (2006). Zen as a social ethics of responsiveness. *Journal of Buddhist Ethics, 13.*

Kehoe, B. A. (1989). *The ghost dance: Ethnohistory and revitalization.* Washington, DC: Thompson Publishing.

Kennet, W. M. (1953). *The religion of the Hindus.* New York: The Ronald Press Co.

Keown, D., & Prebish, C. S. (Eds.). (2004). *Encyclopedia of Buddhism.* London: Routledge.

Klein, A. C. (1995). *Meeting the great bliss queen: Buddhists, feminists, and the art of the self.* Boston, Beacon Press.

Knudsen, E. I. (2007). Fundamental components of attention. *Annual Review of Neuroscience, 30*(1), 57–78.

Lamotte, É. (1976). *Teaching of Vimalakirti* (Sara Boin, Trans.). London: Pali Text Society.

Lao Tzu. (1963). *Tao Te Ching.* London: Penguin Books.

Law, B. C. (2012). *A history of Pali literature* (Vol. I). Ulan Press.

Lazar, S. W., Bush, G., Gollub, R. L., Fricchione, G. L., Khalsa, G., & Benson, H. (2000). Functional brain mapping of the relaxation response and meditation. *NeuroReport, 11*(7), 1581–1585.

Leaning, F. E. (1925). An introductory study of hypnagogic phenomena. *Proceedings of the Society for Psychical Research.*

Lindtner, C. (1997). *Master of wisdom.* Berkeley, CA: Dharma Publishing.

Longhi Paripurna, M. (2001). *Bhagavad-Gita.* Verona, Italy: Demetra.

Lopez, D. S. (1995). *Buddhism in practice.* Princeton, NJ: Princeton University Press.

Lopez, D. S. (2001). *Story of Buddhism.* New York: HarperCollins.

Lowenstein, T. (1996). *The vision of the Buddha.* London: Duncan Baird Publishers.

Lu K'uan Yu. (1978). *The Surangama Sutra.* Bombay: B.I. Publications.

Miller, G. A., Galanter, E., & Pribram, K. H. (1960). *Plans and the structure of behavior.* New York: Holt, Rinehart & Winston.

Mizuno, K. (1972). *Essentials of Buddhism: Basic terminology and concepts of Buddhist philosophy and practice.* Tokyo: Kosei Publishing Co.

Morgan, K. W. (1956). *The path of the Buddha: Buddhism interpreted by Buddhists.* New York: Ronald Press; reprinted in 1997 by Motilal Banarsidass (Delhi).

Morin, A. (2004). Possible links between self-awareness and inner speech: Theoretical background, underlying mechanisms, and empirical evidence. Unpublished journal.

Muller, A. C. (1999). *The sutra of perfect enlightenment.* Albany, NY: State University Press of New York.

Namkai, N. (1983). *Il libro tibetano dei morti.* Newton Compton Editori.

Nattier, J. (2003). *A few good men: The Bodhisattva path according to the inquiry of Ugra* (Ugrapariprccha). Honolulu, HA: University of Hawaii Press.

Ospina, M. B., Bond, K., Karkhaneh, M., Tjosvold, L., Vandermeer, B., Liang, Y., ..., & Klassen, T. P. (2007). Meditation practices for health: State of the research. *Evidence Report/Technology Assessment (Full Report), June* (155), 1–263.

Page, T. (2000). *The Mahayana Mahaparinirvana Sutra* (Kosho Yamamoto, Trans.). Nepal: Nirvana Publications.

Perez-De-Albeniz, A., & Holmes, J. (2000). Meditation: Concepts, effects and uses in therapy. *International Journal of Psychotherapy, 5*(1), 49–59.

Petersen, R. (1997). *Out of body experiences.* Charlottesville, VA: Hampton Roads Publishing Company, Inc.

Radhakrishnan, S. (1977). *The Bhagavadgita.* New Delhi, India: Blackie and Son.

Rahula, W. (1974). *What the Buddha taught* (Rev. ed.). New York: Grove Press.

Rammurti, S. M. (1973). *Yoga sutras.* Garden City, NY: Doubleday.

Rinpoche, S. (1994). *The Tibetan book of living and dying.* London: Rider.

Robinson, R. H., Johnson, W. L., & Bhikkhu, T. (2004). *The Buddhist religion: A historical introduction* (5th ed.). Belmont, CA: Wadsworth Publishing.

Samraj, A. D. (2005). *What is required to realize the non-dual truth?: The controversy between the "talking" school and the "practicing" school of advaitism* (The Basket of Tolerance Booklet Series, Number 9). Self-published.

Schuhmacher, S., & Woerner, G. (1991). *Shambhala dictionary of Buddhism and zen.* (Michael H. Kohn, Trans.). Boston: Shambhala Publishing.

Sinha, H. P. (1993). *Bhāratīya Darshan kī rūprekhā* [*Features of Indian philosophy*]. Delhi: Motilal Banarasidas Publishers.

Skilton, A. (1997). *A concise history of Buddhism.* Cambridge, UK: Windhorse Publications.

Smith, H., & Novak, P. (2003). *Buddhism: A concise introduction.* San Francisco: Harper.

Staal, F. (1975). *Exploring mysticism.* London: Penguin.

Thera, D. (1992). *Jewels of the doctrine.* (Ranjini Obeyesekere, Trans.). New Delhi: Sri Satguru Publications.

Thera, P. (1999). *Dhammacakkappavattana Sutta [The book of protection].* Kandy, Sri Lanka: Buddhist Publication Society.

Thompson, M. (1997/2003). *Philosophy of religion.* Columbus, OH: McGraw-Hill Companies.

Thurman, R. A. F. (Trans.). (1976). *Holy reaching of Vimalakirti: Mahayana scripture.* State College, PA: Pennsylvania State University Press.

Tibetan Buddhism. (n.d.). *American heritage dictionary of the English language.* Bellmawr, NJ: Houghton Mifflin Company.

Tolle, E. (1999). *The power of now: A guide to spiritual enlightenment.* Vancouver, BC, Canada: Namaste Publishing.

Upanishad. (2001). *La via della liberazione.* Verona, Italy: Demetra.

Utley, R. (1964). *The last days of the Sioux nation.* New Haven, CT: Yale University Press.

Vaitl, D., Birbaumer, N., Gruzelier, J., Jamieson, G. A., Kotchoubey, B., Kübler, A., ... & Weiss, T. (2005, January). Psychobiology of altered states of consciousness. *Psychological Bulletin, 131*(1), 98–127.

Veith, I. (1976). Huang Ti Nei Ching Su Wen, *Canone di Medicina Interna dell'Imperatore Giallo.* Edizioni Mediterranee Roma.

Venerable Yin Shun. (1998). *The way to Buddhahood: Instructions from a modern Chinese master* (Wing H. Yeung, Trans.). Somerville, MA: Wisdom Publications.

Visuddhimagga. (Nyanamoli, Trans.) *The path of purification, appeared originally in the fifth century AD.* London: Shambhala.

Warder, A. K. (1963). *Introduction to Pali.* Bristol: PaliText Society.

Webb, R. (Ed.). (1975). *Analysis of the Pali Canon.* Somerville, MA: Wisdom Publications

Welch, H. (1967). *The practice of Chinese Buddhism.* Cambridge, MA: Harvard University Press.

White, K. (2005). *The role of Bodhicitta in Buddhist enlightenment including a translation into English of Bodhicitta-sastra, Benkemmitsu-nikyoron, and Sammaya-kaijo.* The Edwin Mellen Press.

Williams, P. (1989). *Mahayana Buddhism: The doctrinal foundations.* London: Routledge.

Williams, P. (Ed.). (2005). *Buddhism: Critical concepts in religious studies.* London: Routledge.

Williams, P., & Tribe, A. (2000). *Buddhist thought.* London: Routledge.

Chapter VI

CLINICAL HYPNOSIS, MINDFULNESS, AND MUSIC THERAPY

1. NEUROPHYSIOLOGY OF MUSIC

Neurophysiology of music may be regarded as a branch of either psychology or musicology. It aims to explain and understand musical behavior and melodious experience. The modern international field of music psychology is gradually exploring a multitude of neurophysiological issues that surround this central question. Music neurophysiology may be regarded as scientific research about human culture. Music affects the brain at different levels. The results of many researchers have, and will continue to have, direct implications for matters of general concern: compassionate values, human identity, human neurophysiology and nature, and quality of life.

Music consists of sound sequences and experiences that require a neuronal integration over time. As we become familiar with music, the associations among notes, melodies, and entire symphonic movements become stronger and more complex. These associations can become so tight that, for example, hearing the end of one album track can elicit a robust image of the upcoming track while anticipating it in total silence.

Leaver and associates (2009) studied this predictive "anticipatory imagery" at various stages, throughout learning and investigate activity changes, in corresponding neural structures, using functional magnetic resonance imaging. The anticipatory imagery (in silence) for highly familiar naturalistic music was accompanied by pronounced activity in rostral prefrontal cortex and premotor areas. Examining changes in the neural bases of anticipatory imagery during two stages of learning conditional associations between simple melodies, however, demonstrates the importance of frontostriatal connections consistent with a role of the basal ganglia in "training" the frontal cortex (Pasupathy & Miller, 2005).

People have used music and song to comfort one another since time immemorial. Aristotle and Plato wrote about their beliefs in the healing power of music. Pythagoras of Samos conducted perhaps the world's first physics experiment. By playing strings of different lengths, Pythagoras discovered that sound vibrations naturally occur in a sequence of whole tones or notes that repeat in a pattern of seven: like the seven naturally occurring colors of the rainbow, the octave of seven tones. His experience affirms Pythagoras's assertion in the fifth century BC that "There is geometry in the humming of the strings. There is music in the spacings of the spheres."

Since the time of the ancient Romans, music has been a basic art, largely used in the recovering process. This is very well-represented by the Greek and Roman god Apollo, who was a master of both music and medicine.

During medieval times, the tradition of monastic chants developed. The Benedictine Order, which embraced communal living, supported their ill or dying community members through formal musical rituals.

Today in the Western world, most doctors and people consider chants, music, and medicine to be different methods belonging to completely separated fields. We never hear things like "you are in your awareness, what you are listening to" or "let the music be your medicine."

In the 1800s, the era of romanticism in music, some composers and music critics, argued that music should and could express ideas, images, emotions, or even a whole literary plot. In 1832, composer Robert Schumann stated that his piano work "Papillon" was "intended as a musical representation" of the final scene of *Flegeljahre,* a novel by Jean Paul. A group of modernist writers in the early twentieth century, including Walter Pater and Ezra Pound, believed that music was essentially pure, because it did not represent anything or refer to anything beyond itself. Bucknell (2002) disagreed with this view and argued against the alleged purity of music in the classic work on Bach, stimulating our emotions and imagery.

At McGill University (Montreal, Canada), two fMRI experiments, explored the neural substrates of a musical imagery task that required manipulation of the imagined sounds: temporal reversal of a melody. Musicians were presented with the first few notes of a familiar tune (Experiment 1) or its title (Experiment 2), followed by a string of notes that was either an exact or an inexact reversal. The task was to judge whether the second string was correct or not by mentally reversing all its notes, thus requiring both maintenance and manipulation of the represented string. Both experiments showed considerable activation of the superior parietal lobe (intraparietal sulcus) during the reversal process. Ventrolateral and dorsolateral frontal cortices were also activated, consistent with the memory load required during the task. They also found weaker evidence for some activation of the right auditory cortex in both studies, congruent with results from previous simpler music imagery tasks. They interpreted these results in the context of other cerebral transformation tasks, such as mental rotation in the visual domain, which are known to recruit the intraparietal sulcus region, and they proposed that this region, subserves general computations that require transformations of a sensory input.

Mental imagery tasks may thus have both task or modality-specific components as well as components that supersede any specific codes and instead represent an amodal mental manipulation (Zatorre, Halpern & Bouffard, 2010).

Sound has, therefore, been with us throughout the evolutionary process, and it is an integral part of all our activities. Music is a product of sound and is, therefore, a natural outcome of this evolutionary process.

Each single element in the universe is in a state of constant physical vibration that becomes apparent to us as light, sound, or music. The human senses can be aware of only a fraction of the infinite scale of vibrations.

In Western science, sounds, music, voice, and silence are seen as air vibrations that can vary in specific frequencies measured in Hertz, which includes the entire range of audible or inaudible sounds.

Let us consider the electron, the molecule, or any bigger form of matter. We know that each form of matter constantly emits some kind of energy. Each form has its own characteristic resonance or "radiation" in time and space. The electron's (or the molecule's) typical radiations are well-known and have already been the subject of several studies. We can suppose that this pulse or "sound" is characteristic of the same frequency band initially emitted when the universe was created and that kept resounding.

The human senses can be aware of just a fraction of the infinite scale of vibrations. In fact, our ears can perceive only few frequencies that we can also use to produce various genres of music. What we feel as music is a mental content generated by the ears and the brain, responding to external vibration stimuli. These stimuli cause the musical perception but are substantially different than is. Because each person is unique, cerebrally and psychologically, each has his or her own particular way to respond to the external stimuli, having thus a more or less distinctive experience from listening to the same piece of music.

It is impossible to express objective and absolute judgments about a tune in the absence of a reference version of it; in a certain sense, there are as many versions as there are listeners. We may say that what we call music, and its beauty (or feeling), exists only in the subjectivity (the minds) of the listeners.

Music is generated by the brain from external stimuli, and because they are aesthetic sensations, they are based on our mental musical content. Certainly sometimes the environment (at visual andv social levels and emotions) in which the listening takes place has a certain influence on the listening. The biological and psychological structure of the listener may also enter into play; it creates the mental representations of the environment and feelings.

Thus, generalizing, it is very improbable that two or more persons can have identical listening experiences of a sound. The next frontier in the research on awareness could be represented by the discover of the effects of music and rhythm on the brain functions. Recently, the interest has been mainly focused on

- Music to increase the learning process
- Music therapy
- Emotional reactions to music
- The connection between tonality and physics
- The beneficial and pathological effects of certain sounds and/or rhythms
- Music has been a help or supplement to meditation practices and to different state of consciousness.

Steven Halpern, musician and director of the Palo Alto Spectrum Research Institute (California), believes that "dissonance can literally knock out the body's tuning." Halpern argues that "noises, even the ones under the threshold of consciousness, could provoke a permanent tension which irritates both mind and body in a substantial way." His label produces a specific genre of music aimed to counter this effect.

Music involves the right hemisphere of the brain. This could explain its effectiveness in therapy. Harmonic sounds are a logarithmic sequence, acoustically perceptible and traceable in each single sound (as the sound of wind, the murmuring of a stream, a musical instrument, the human voice). In each of these sounds, there is an ascending and infinite harmonic sequence as the prime numbers. This harmonic sequence is not clearly perceptible by the average human ear, for the most part, subjugated by a mind that is not very aware (Silva, 1999).

2. NEUROPSYCHOLOGY OF MUSIC

What is music? What is silence?
Silence transcends thoughts, concepts, images, and reasoning. It is a state

of consciousness, in which there are no words or images. In silence, any words or images should merge from inside and not from outside. Silence recharges our body and mind.

In psychology, we can look for silence in two ways: inner silence and outer silence. Outer silence helps us to find inner silence. Inner silence is more precious, however. There are two kinds of inner silence: passive and active. In passive inner silence, the heart and mind are at rest at the unconscious level, whereas in active inner silence, the heart and mind are at rest at the conscious level.

Modern life, with all its distractions and features, seems particularly unsuited to silence. Even if we have actual outer silence, our mind is rarely silent. If we analyze our thoughts, there seems to be a never-ending stream of worries, anxieties, and regrets. In clinical hypnosis and in mindfulness, we try to do a very difficult thing, silence our thoughts completely. It is difficult only because we are so unused to this idea. The mind is so used to thinking that it is easy to think and our existence is defined by our thoughts, and this must be our only existence.

Descartes said, "I think, therefore, I am." Clinical hypnosis and mindfulness, however, teach us, that what we are is unencumbered by thoughts. The real "I" is ourselves, which is beyond thought. There is some inner self that can decide whether to pursue thoughts or not. It is when we are able to stop thoughts entering our mind that we will start to experience real silence.

In musical theory, silence is not always referred to as the point where musical sounds actually cease to exist. Moments of silence are experienced during sustained fermatas and extreme pianissimos or when a complex harmony dissipates into a sparing use of the tone material.

Cage says there is no such thing as silence. If so, what is what we thought was silence? Is silence sound? Music? Emotions? Mindfulness? Silence is not just the canvas on which music is painted. Music and silence move humans to a deeply interiority. Music and silence calm the mind and produce a great sense of well-being and energy. Music and silence have the ability to affect our emotions, intellect, and psychology; lyrics can assuage our loneliness or incite our passions. Some kinds of music and silence could be used to help patients in relief of pain and suffering.

Emotion, in its most general definition, is an intense mental state that arises autonomically in the nervous system, rather than through conscious effort, and evokes either a positive or negative psychological response. An emotion is often differentiated from a feeling.

According to Plutchik (1980), feeling can be viewed as the subjective experience of an emotion that arises physiologically in the brain. As such, music is a powerful art of feelings, whose aesthetic appeal is highly dependent on the culture in which it is practiced. Many psychologists adopt the ABC model, which defines emotions in terms of three fundamental attributes:

A. physiological arousal;
B. behavioral expression (e.g., facial expressions);
C. conscious experience, the subjective feeling of an emotion.

All three attributes are necessary for a full-fledged emotional event, although the intensity of each may vary greatly.

Some scientists make the following distinctions among affect, feeling, and emotion:

- *affect* is an innately structured, noncognitive appraising sensation that may or may not register in consciousness
- *feeling* is affect made conscious, possessing an evaluative capacity that is not only physiologically based but also often psychologically (and sometimes relationally) oriented
- *emotion* is a psychosocially constructed, dramatized feeling

Some of the aesthetic elements expressed in music include feelings, emotions, lyricism, harmony, hypnotism, resonance, playfulness, and colors. Music and science may seem to inhabit different universes, one of beauty and emotion, the other of logic and reason. Now, however, neuroscientists are placing them in the same solar system.

Norman M. Weinberger, professor of neurobiology and behavior at the University of California at Irvine has explained that new researches are beginning to reveal the role of music in brain function and in our lives. He explained that a particular chunk of brain is musical. It is complex because music has many elements: rhythm, melody, and so on. For example, certain cells in the right hemisphere respond more to melody than to language. Neurons learn to prioritize some sounds. This finding revolutionized thinking about brain organization by showing that learning is not a "higher" brain function but rather one that occurs in the sensory systems themselves.

Music exercises the brain. Playing an instrument, for instance, involves vision, hearing, touch, motor planning, emotion, and symbol interpretation, all of which activate different brain systems. This may be why some Alzheimer's patients can perform music long after they have forgotten other things (Ruytjens, Willemsen, Van Dijk, Wit & Albers, 2006).

Music psychologists investigate all aspects of melodic behavior by applying methods and knowledge from all aspects of psychology. Because music reaches a deep, nonrational part of the human spirit, it is ideally suited as an adjunct service that can affect feelings such as grief, fear, anxiety, sadness, and anger that stand in the way of a clear passage. Music can release blocked or painful feelings and can stimulate positive ones, such as hope, love, and gratitude. Sharing music together, can lead to sharing of the emotions that the music brings up.

A. The Main Psychophysiological Elements of Music in Assagioli's Studies

A scientific music therapy should be founded on the exact knowledge of each single musical element and on the effect that each of these elements produces, both on the physiological functions and on the psychological conditions. Concerning this last regard Assagioli's studies about music therapy are extremely interesting.

Roberto Assagioli (1888-1974) was the first Western psychologist to incorporate psychology, feelings, and spirituality into an overall view of the human psyche. He began psychosynthesis in 1910. He wanted to expand beyond Freud's analysis and "talking cure." He added synthesis and a broader use of our human abilities, such as will, imagination, and intuition. He included even our spiritual side, our higher aspirations, and our center, which he called the self. People use psychosynthesis as a way of life and in a wide variety of fields, such as education, psychology, business, and spirituality.

Psychosynthesis offers delightful tools for many purposes: embracing opposed parts of our inner worlds, enriching each other with our differences, making groups and organizations function with greater purpose, and enjoying a respectful interchange with the world that envelops us. The main goal of the broad-ranging theory and methods of psychosynthesis is to enhance the full range of human experience and support our movement toward self-realization (Assagioli, 1977).

According to Assagioli, the main psychophysiological elements (that we can find in music) are (1) rhythm, (2) tone, (3) melody or tune, (4) harmony, and (5) timbre.

1. *Rhythm.* The primordial and fundamental element of music, rhythm influences the human being more intensely and immediately. This great influence is basically due to direct action on body and emotions. Organic life is based on the different kind of rhythms: the rhythm of breathing and heart. Therefore, it should not come as a surprise that the musical rhythms exert a powerful influence on those organic and psychological rhythms, at times stimulating them and sometimes calming them, creating either harmony or inconsonance.

2. *Tone.* Each note, while it is physically produced by a specific vibratory frequency, generates particular psychological and physical effects.

3. *Melody.* The combination of rhythms, tones, and accents produces those musical "units" called melodies. Melodies, being a synthesis of various musical elements, are very suitable means to express emotions.

4. *Harmony.* Whereas melody is produced by a succession of sounds, harmony is created by the superimposition of various notes and different vibratory frequencies.

5. *Timbre.* Various musical instruments, including the human voice, are very different in nature and structure. This gives a peculiar quality to the sound, which, therefore, generates very specific emotional reactions.

We can use all these elements in clinical hypnosis and in mindfulness, with the association of music, silence and our voice. Through the rhythm and the sweet sound of music, silence, and voice, in clinical hypnosis and mindfulness, and through the rhythm and emotions of our verbal suggestions of calm . . . tranquility . . . comfort . . . more and more intense . . . more and more profound . . . (and pauses of silence . . .) holding us in a warm embrace . . . we can create an indirect hypnosis, in the patient. We can help a patient stir up a positive thought about pleasant emotions, so to diminish the perception of pain and suffering.

Rhythm and sound in music can acquire different values when they come in contact. In general, with the word rhythm we indicate a regular succession (in a certain period of time) of sounds, cadences, and movements. In harmony terms, this concept can be further specified: with the term rhythm we indicate the succession of the accents and their position in the musical phrase or simply the structure of the musical beat. Cyclicity indicates the modalities of the recurring repetition of the rhythmic phenomenon. The cyclic irregularities can have a strong expressive meaning, especially when they modify an otherwise regular rhythm.

Music provides tools that patients can learn to use to decrease their experience of pain and suffering at the end of life. In almost all cases, this should occur within the context of a setting that includes medical and psychological support and education.

Alteration in the experience of pain can include changes in affect, as well. Willmarth (1998) demonstrated that hypnotic modification of mood also resulted in changes in the perception of pain. As we said, music can also be used as a powerful curative or healing element.

As Assagioli underlines, "There are several ways in which it (i.e., music) can exert a beneficial influence on the body and on the soul. First of all, the effect of music can be relaxing and comforting" (Assagioli, 1977). It is not necessary to emphasize how this can be valuable in these days of physical exhaustion, nervous strain, and mental and emotional excitation. A period of rest is the generic and obvious prescription in order to eliminate such conditions. Chronic pain often requires more effort, but music, hypnosis, and mindfulness provide many individuals with a way to experience focused, narrow attention that redirects attention to thoughts or memories more pleasant than the pain. We can use music with or without hypnosis and mindfulness in pain therapy.

We can measure the physiological parameters causing or maintaining pain. These parameters may include excessive muscle tension or improper breathing, among others (Sherman, 2004).

The studies on the mechanism of suggestions and on the importance of the subconscious in the psychic life have demonstrated that unconsciously received impressions can have broad positive (or negative) repercussions, not only on the psyche, but also on the body (Assagioli, 1977).

Music is a real "spiritual alchemy," able to transform the most resistant and dark pain to some sort of "sweeter" pain, and then into acceptance, and lately even into joy, self-expansion, and even an expansion of personal awareness.

Therese Schroeder-Sheker developed a field, specifically of music in palliative care, called "music thanatology." The term thanatology is derived from "Thanatos," the Greek god of death. Music thanatology sometimes is used in a strict sense to refer to a specific way of using live harp music at the bedside of acutely dying patients. Music thanatologists view their work as a compassionate, spiritual, and contemplative practice. Music thanatology does not presume that the listener has a reserve of energy that can respond actively to the music. A person who is actively dying may be very weak, with limited communication capacity. In some cases, the person may be comatose or in an altered state of consciousness on the threshold of death.

Music in pain therapy and palliative care recognizes the need to care for the whole person, including mind, body, and spirit. The principles that should govern care at the end of life are well-accepted. They include responsiveness to the patients' wishes—truthful, sensitive, empathic communication and meticulous attention to the physical, spiritual, and psychosocial needs of patients and family (American Society of Clinical Oncology, 1998). Music applied to the experience of pain and suffering at the end of life permits a clinician to address the source of felt pain and the perception of pain itself.

With the use of hypnosis, we have studied that "pain is real if you feel it."

"Why suffering? Does my doctor think this pain is all in my head and in my mind?" These are not uncommon questions from patients who have been referred for behavioral medicine services connected to a pain management program.

Before one can begin using hypnosis, music, and mindfulness for pain management, the properties of the pain itself must be considered. In his excellent book *Pain Assessment and Intervention from a Psychophysiological Perspective,* Rich Sherman (2004) points out that the simplest classification, considers pain as either inflammatory or neuropathic. This system focuses primarily on identifying the underlying cause of the pain. No one can argue that identifying the source of pain is not a wonderful achievement. Unfortunately, in the real world of pain management, two obstacles appear.

First, in spite of numerous new diagnostic imaging and assessment tools, we still often fail to identify the cause of pain.

Second, often, when we do identify the problem generating the pain, there is nothing that can be done to directly "fix" the problem.

It is the perception of pain and the individual's physical and emotional reaction to the pain perception that give us the opportunity to create treatment approaches that can provide relief. The underlying principle of music in pain therapy and in palliative care focuses on improving the patient's physical, psychological, and spiritual comfort and quality of life.

In whatever setting it is administered, palliative care is generally provided by an interdisciplinary team, which may include physicians, nurses, social workers, home-health aides, pharmacists, chaplains, physical and occupational therapists, musicians, and trained volunteers (Last Acts®, 2001).

To better describe and provide care with music during the current chronic trajectory that many cancer patients experience, it will be necessary to integrate palliative and supportive efforts long before patients are within days to hours of dying. For example, advance care planning with music may be beneficial after diagnosis and after treatment has begun, when the patient feels less anxious.

Improving the quality of end-of-life care for patients will require the improved awareness, knowledge, and skills of the health professionals who provide their care. Patients would benefit greatly from end-of-life resources, with music made available in a wide variety of settings.

B. Music as Help and Supplement to Clinical Hypnosis and Mindfulness in Pain Therapy and Palliative Care

The music is offered uniquely for the needs of that patient. If family or friends are present in the room, naturally they will also react to the music. The entire group present may be affected, but the process of creating the music is primarily guided by the state of the patient.

People who use music in health care are convinced that music can have somatic benefits when used as one component of holistic multidisciplinary palliative care. Creating a supportive musical field, may be helpful to the patients who are anxious to calm down or become more at peace. Many scientific studies have demonstrated that music with or without therapeutic suggestions (as clinical hypnosis) may have some beneficial effects on pain.

At Linköping University, Sweden, Nilsson, Rawal, Enquist, and Unosson (2004) demonstrated that music with or without therapeutic suggestions in the early postoperative period has a beneficial effect on patients' experience of analgesia. They have also observed that intraoperative music and music in combination with therapeutic suggestions may have some beneficial effects on postoperative recovery (Frid, Berezkin, Evtiukhin, Beliaev & Aleksandrin, 1981; Nilsson, Rawal, Uneståhl, Zetterberg & Unosson, 2001).

In recent years, Tsao and Zeltzer at David Geffen School of Medicine at UCLA, studied the use of complementary and alternative medicine (CAM) in pediatric populations. The efficacy of the CAM interventions was evaluated according to the framework developed by the American Psychological Association (APA) Division 12 Task Force on Promotion and Dissemination of Psychological Procedures. According to these criteria, only one CAM approach reviewed herein (self-hypnosis/guided imagery/relaxation for recurrent pediatric headache) qualified as an empirically supported therapy, although many may be considered possibly efficacious or promising treatments for pediatric pain. Several methodological limitations of the existing literature on CAM interventions for pain problems in children are highlighted and future avenues for research are outlined (Tsao, 2005).

Distraction with music therapy may facilitate habituation to painful stimuli (Arntz, Dreessen & Merckelbach, 1991), perhaps because engaging in an alternative, attentionally demanding task limits the capacity to process pain, thereby reducing pain sensitivity (Farthing, Venturino & Brown, 1984). In an early study, Fowler-Kerry and Lander (1987) compared the following four conditions on injection pain in 200 children (age 4.5–6.5 years): (1) music distraction (music played over headphones before and during injection), (2) suggestion (verbal instructions that the experimenter would help the child during the injection), (3) distraction plus suggestion, and (4) two control groups (i.e., no intervention; headphones without music). Music distraction was superior to a suggestion in reducing pain. More recently, another study (Megel, Houser & Gleaves, 1999) in ninety-nine children (age 3–6 years) found that those who listened to lullabies during immunization showed fewer behavioral distress than no intervention controls, although the groups did not differ on physiological responses or reported pain.

Another study examined the effects of live music therapy for pain related to intravenous starts, venipunctures, injections, and heel sticks in twenty pediatric patients age 0–7 years and twenty children matched for age and type of needle insertion who did not receive the intervention (Malone, 1996). The results indicated that the music group showed less behavioral distress than the control group during pre-needle and postneedle stages.

Music may be considered a promising intervention for procedural pain (American Society of Clinical Oncology, 1998).

Before the music performance, it is necessary for the patients to be informed about the piece and its effects so that they can contribute to the influence of the music on their consciousness. It is advisable to have the patients relax, before and during the performance, in order "to open the doors to the unconscious."

According to Assagioli (1977), there is a specific psychosynthesis process feasible even through music, constituted of three stages:

Spiritual psychosynthesis produces the inclusion and the integration of superior psychospiritual elements (higher self or higher consciousness) in the conscious personality. Good examples of this kind of music are the Gregorian chant; Palestrina's compositions; and the music of some great composers, such as Bach, Handel, Wagner, César Franck, and Scriabin.

Interindividual psycho-synthesis takes place between individuals and other people belonging to a group to which they belong (interaction therapist-patient or self-help groups). In this situation, the consciousness of the single individual embraces in a harmonic relationship, all humanity.

We may mention Beethoven's Ninth Symphony, which reaches its apex with Schiller's words "Seid umschlungen, Millionen" (Be embraced, millions).

Cosmic psychosynthesis consists of increasing the individual's acknowledgment and acceptance of the laws governing the relationship and rhythms of the life of the universe itself: spirituality and the relationship between life and death.

3. MUSIC AND THE HIGHER CONSCIOUSNESS

This is where all our higher feelings and thoughts enter consciousness, such as artistic or scientific intuition and inspiration. All our noble ethical feelings, such as altruistic love or self-sacrifice, are derived from this higher consciousness. It is also the place of genius and higher spiritual forms, such as ecstasy and the power of enlightenment. Here, the hidden psychic energies are enormous.

The music choice requires a great care for the different effects it can produce in the unconscious. Each person can react differently to the same piece, according to his or her experiences, emotions, and background. The analogies traceable in physics, biology, astronomy, and acoustics are of great interest for us.

History tells us that Pythagoras introduced his disciples to mathematical and astronomical theories using the monochord, and it is well-known that Kepler used this instrument for his studies and his "harmonic model" of the universe. This is coherent with the most recent discoveries. The latest theories of important physicists, such as Bohm and Sheldrake, describe a universe in which the smallest particles are not to be considered as matter but instead as pure energy. This takes us back to considering the acoustic phenomenon as the sound and silence, pure energy.

The allusion of various mystical traditions, unanimous in affirming that at the origin of the creation there was the "Logos," or the Word or that the creation is nothing else than a mantra, does not seem to be accidental.

A Tibetan tradition says that elements are the essence of the universe, the essence of the elements is color, the essence of color is light, that the essence of light is sound. We could agree here with Bohm, who says that the origin of matter is not matter itself but vibration or pure energy.

Great music moves humans and gods alike, deeply. Music calms the mind and produces an extreme sense of well-being and euphoria. One also gets a similar experience during deep meditation and samadhi.

In the beginning was the Word. Almost all the great religions of the world talk about it. In Patanjali's Yoga Darshan, Ishwara is defined as a special Being who is expressed by the original word Pranav.

> Life should be happiness and if you're not happy, you're wasting your existence and the time remaining you to live your life. Happiness is the final goal of creation and evolution and his expansion. Therefore, have you to consider it if you decide to undertake any action. If it derives no happiness from an action, this action fails its very own goal, and his accomplishment cannot be justified. (Bhagavad-Gita)

What that original word was nobody is sure although in major yoga commentaries, it is called "om." Recently, however, scientists have discovered that very soon after the Big Bang, and before anything else appeared in the universe, primordial sound waves were produced. This could have formed the basis of Brahma Nad, mentioned in the Upanishads. Sound has, for that reason, been with us throughout the evolutionary process and is an integral part of all our activities. Music is a product of sound and is, therefore, a natural outcome of this evolutionary process.

Music affects the brain at different levels. Our moods change with distinct types of music. At a deeper level, however, its effect is similar to that of meditation. This is probably why all great religions have stressed the need for music as a means for praying and meditation. Hindu classical music, one of the oldest musical systems of the world, has spiritual roots and traces its origins to Vedic hymns. Similarly, in other religions, harmonious chants, hymns, and other forms of music have been used since ancient times to express the glory of God or to help focus the mind on the transcendent thoughts.

Recent PET studies conducted by scientists have shown that certain types of music activate neural pathways similar to those associated with euphoria and reward. Although fMRI is replacing PET in many neuroimaging studies, PET still holds unique advantages and can give us valuable knowledge about the auditory cortex and auditory perception (Ruytjens et al., 2006). These same pathways are activated in response to other pleasurable activities that give emotional happiness. Similarly, in deep meditation, the mind focuses on a single thought for a long time. Thus, when contemplation, reflection, and samadhi (together called sanyam according to *Patanjali's Yoga Darshan*) are done on a single thought, it produces the sense of well-being and happiness.

In this process, a major portion of the 100 billion neurons of the brain are being used in a laser-like fashion for a single thought. This deep meditation process helps stimulate or "tickle" the pituitary gland, which gives the feeling of well-being. The exact mechanism, however, is still not understood.

When we hear soul-stirring music, we feel good, very like what we feel during deep meditation. This is the principle of equivalence. The brain, therefore, appreciates and absorbs the music by creating the same complex thought pattern as that during meditation. Similar effects are also seen in different types of music, which stimulate feelings of anger, sadness, and other emotions.

Music

- It reaches the deepest levels of sensations and consciousness
- It obtains greater clarity and insight
- It enters higher states of awareness
- It reduces stress and anxiety
- It deepens your spiritual connection

A. Music and the Self-Hypnosis Technique

Music, in a modified state of consciousness and in hypnosis, provides all the benefits of profound meditation without endless hours of discipline. Within minutes, you feel yourself lifted from physical tension and mental anxieties. As stress dissolves, you feel a higher, more refined energy moving through your body. A powerful combination of brain wave frequencies guides you into the extraordinary self-hypnosis state known as body asleep-mind awake. While your mind vibrates in resonance with the music, it becomes balanced, energized, and open. You feel refreshed, revitalized, and nourished at the deepest levels.

Self-hypnosis techniques with music are not new. They have been around for thousands of years. Anyone can do self-hypnosis, regardless of religious or cultural background. Consider these suggestions to get you started:

- Select a hypnosis technique that fits your lifestyle and belief system and a music you like. Many people build self-hypnosis into their daily routine.
- Set aside some time. Start with 5-minute relaxation sessions once or twice a day and work up to 20 minutes each time.
- Keep trying. Be kind to yourself as you get started. If you are relaxing and your attention wanders, slowly return to the object, sensation, or movement you are focusing on.
- Make relaxation and self-hypnosis part of your life.

Many people prefer to start and end their day with a period of relaxation. Others prefer to take relaxation breaks during the day. Experiment and find out what works best for you.

We live in a universe of infinite complexity, and many forces operate on us. Yes, it is true that we are not in control of everything that happens because we are not in control of most of those infinite other parts of the universe. In fact, the only thing you have total and complete control over is your own mind.

Listening to music increases your ability to be consciously aware. As you continue with the program, doing this becomes easier and more automatic. That "watcher" part of you becomes stronger and stronger until it is watching over everything, and with that degree of conscious awareness, it is pretty difficult to create anything that is not beneficial for you.

Some of the motives for which we can use music and self-hypnosis are

1. To relax the body and mind and to rejuvenate one's flow of energy in order to more effectively face the responsibilities of one's demanding and active life.
2. To heal illnesses (especially psychosomatic ones).
3. To overcome emotional problems.
4. To develop a more relaxed and positive view towards life.
5. To develop a peaceful and more clearly functioning mind.
6. For greater ability to penetrate into the core of problems and find

inspirational solutions. This has been found especially useful by scientists and businessmen.

7. To increase relief of pain and suffering.
8. As a method of self-observation and self-discovery.
9. To develop the latent powers of the mind.
10. Locus of Self. The experiencing of one's self borrows from several dimensions, some physical, some psychological, others spiritual.
11. Complete word silence in the context of profound peacefulness.
12. Perceptible lapses in the experience of the continuity of time.
13. Sensation of the irrelevance of time passing, in the context of feeling enlightened by this new perception.
14. Nonduality.
15. Higher Consciousness.

With music, you learn that you are your mind, body, spirit, and emotions and that you are not separate from everything else. Once you begin to experience the fact that everything is connected in an infinitely complex matrix and an infinitely complex dance of creation and that you are that dance, something shifts.

The pioneering studies of Dr. Marcel Vogel and Irzhak Bentov revealed that, in a state of deep relaxation or meditation, the electromagnetic field surrounding our head literally attunes to the basic electromagnetic field of the earth itself. The earth's harmonic resonance has been measured at approximately eight cycles per second, or 8 Hz. The frequency range of the electrical activity of the brain that we access in states of deep relaxation is also centered around 8 Hz. Is this correspondence just a coincidence? Perhaps that is why we feel so rejuvenated when surrounded by nature in a forest, in the mountains, or by the ocean. Perhaps this is also a key to understanding how our inner and outer environments can be orchestrated to a higher level of harmony. At this point, the search for what to be or do, where to go, what to avoid or get, or what to change in order to be happy and peaceful ceases.

Exploring the inner space of the human spirit has to equal the exploration of outer space. Music, silence, mindfulness, hypnosis, and self-hypnosis all have the capacity to reach special states of the mind, which center upon an universal consciousness.

Indeed, hypnosis may be called the most potent nonpharmacological relaxant known to science. They may seem like separate entities. On closer look and in their long-term practice, however, they are found to share common principles. Most importantly, they all can bring to light the knowledge of higher self: comprehension, relaxed self-control, relief of pain and suffering, existential centeredness, and spiritual blossoming in dying patients.

4. MUSIC AND MINDFULNESS

Each single element in the universe is in a state of constant vibration that becomes apparent to us either as light, or sound, or music. At the beginning, there were aeons of silence. From the Big Bang to the whole universe, everything could be interpreted as music.

In many gnostic systems, the various emanations of God, who is also known by such names as the One, the Monad, Aion teleos (The Broadest Aeon), Bythos ("depth or profundity"), Proarkhe ("before the beginning"), the Arkhe ("the beginning"), are called aeons. This first being is also an æon and has an inner being within itself, known as Ennoea ("thought, intent"), Charis ("grace"), or Sige ("silence"). Along with the male Caen comes the female æon Akhana ("love").

What is silence? Aeons? Love? Music? It is to retreat in wordless inner self, gazing out the window of our heart and going for slow meandering walks through a garden. Silence transcends thoughts, concepts, images, and reasoning. It is a higher state of consciousness in which there are no words or images. There is a time for silence. There is a time to let go and allow people to hurl themselves into their own destiny. There is a time to prepare to pick up the pieces when it is all over.

According to the philosopher Plato, there are five mathematical sciences:

1. Arithmetic
2. Plane geometry, or the study of numerical proportions
3. Three-dimensional geometry, including the "Platonic Solids"
4. Astronomy
5. Music, which illustrates the harmonious composition of the universe

Near the end of Kant's book on the structure of the cosmos, he declared, "In the universal silence of nature and in the calm of the senses, the immortal spirit's hidden faculty of knowledge, speaks an ineffable language and gives (us) undeveloped concepts, which are indeed felt, but do not let themselves be described."

Mindfulness is an open, kind, nonjudging attention to what is happening in the present moment as it is happening. It shapes a wise and compassionate relationship with and response to experience as it unfolds moment by moment. This is a moment-to-moment intimate spiritual experience. When we are in silence, all that becomes moot. In silence, nothing more is needed.

Spiritual teaching should always be received with caution and ambivalence, by teachers and students alike. When we attempt to convey spiritual truth, we are tending towards transcendent meaning. Transcendence, by definition, is above or beyond the separative, cognitive world of words and concepts. Mental cognition imposes structure and form, which clarify most areas of knowledge. Spirituality and transcendence, however, are always compromised by description and definition. We might try to convey the ecstatic qualities of great music, but words, at best, will lead only to a pale imitation of what they attempt to describe. As Krishnamurti pointed out, "The description is never the described." You have to experience and be affected by art and nature to truly commune with them.

At the beginning, there were aeons of silence. In the beginning was the Word. What that original word was nobody is sure, although in major yoga commentaries, it is called "om."

Recently, however, scientists have discovered that very soon after the Big Bang and before anything else appeared in the universe, primordial sound waves were produced. This could have formed the basis of "Brahma Nad," mentioned in the Upanishads.

The Om (or Aum) sign and sound are the main symbols of Hinduism. Most religions indicate that creation began with sound. For the Hindus and Buddhists, Om is the primordial sound, the first breath of creation, the vibration that ensures existence. Om sign and sound signify God, Creation, and the Oneness of all creations. This mystical and sacred Hindu word Om is the highest mantra (chant), symbolizing the vibration of the Supreme and of divine energy (Shakti). It is believed that the whole universe, in its fundamental form, is made up of vibrating, pulsating energy and Om is considered the humming sound of this cosmic energy. It means oneness and a merging of our physical body with our spiritual being. The great Hindu sage Patanjali once said, "He who knows Om, knows God." Using Om or Aum is a way of deepening the concentration of the mind.

Sound has, therefore, been with us throughout the evolutionary process and is an integral part of all our activities. Music is a product of sound and is, therefore, a natural outcome of this evolutionary process. This is probably why all great religions have stressed music as a means for praying, mantra, and meditation.

A mantra is a spiritual word, poem, or prayer repeated during meditation. Traditionally, mantras are used by Hindus and Buddhists as a means to focus the mind and attain a form of spiritual enlightenment or realization. The repetition of a mantra that has either a spiritual significance linked to a sacred text or a personal significance allows the individual to consistently explore and reflect upon spirituality on a subconscious level. At the same time, deep focus on a single phrase helps to clear the mind, restoring it to a state that is free from the physical and time-bound concerns of our everyday life.

Om begins many Hindu mantras and is also used by Buddhists. The Buddhist mantra "Om Mani Padme Hum" is one example of a mantra for which Om is the root.

Indian classical music, one of the oldest musical systems of the world, has spiritual roots and traces its origins to Vedic hymns. In other religions, musical chants, hymns, and other forms of music have also been used since ancient times to express the glory of God or to help focus the mind on spiritual thoughts.

Om is the most often chanted sound among all the sacred sounds on earth. This sound is considered as the sound of the existence. It is believed that the whole universe, in its fundamental form, is made up of vibrating, pulsating energy. Om is considered as the humming sound of this cosmic energy. Om is said to be the original primordial creative sound from which the entire universe has been manifested. It is the primal sound of the universe that contains all sounds in itself. It is the sound of the supreme consciousness. Om is said to be the essence of all mantras, the highest of all mantras or divine word (shabda), Brahman (ultimate reality) itself. Om is said to be the essence of the Vedas. By sound and form, Om (the sound is Aum) symbolizes the infinite Brahman (ultimate reality) and the entire universe. A stands for creation, U stands for preservation, M stands for destruction or dissolution. Repetition of Om or Aum dissolves the mind it its divine source.

A. Mindfulness and the Chanting of Om

Sit in a comfortable undisturbed place . . .
Take some deep breaths . . .
Now chant Om in succession at least seven times . . .
Make each breath last as long as possible . . .
Take deep breath and chant
Oooooo . . . hhhhhhhh . . . Mmmmmmm . . .
Then again, repeat this chanting of Om . . .
Do this for seven times . . .
After this, stop chanting and sit for a moment of silence . . .
You will be amazed by the inner peace you will get in such a small chanting of Om . . .
Listen to the sound of universe . . .
Let us listen to the sound of Om . . .
You are requested to listen carefully . . .
This sound of Om produces instant positive vibrations and takes the listener to a state of mental stillness . . .

Thus when silence, contemplation, reflection, and samadhi (together called Sanyam according to *Patanjali's Yoga Darshan*) are done on a single feeling, then it produces the sense of well-being and happiness. In this process, a major portion of the 100 billion neurons of the brain are being used in a laser-like fashion for a single thought.

In the Vedas, Om is the sound of the Sun, the sound of Light. Om is the sound of nonduality. Silence is the sound of nonduality.

To understand how delusion arises, practice watching your mind.

Begin by simply letting it relax. Without thinking of the past or the future, without feeling hope or fear about this thing or that, let it rest comfortably, open and natural. In this space of the mind, there is no problem, no suffering. (Chagdud Rinpoche's)

The Soul of Thoughts
The soul is dyed the colour of its thoughts.
Think only on those things that are in line with your principles
and can bear the full light of the day.
The content of your character is your choice.
Day by day, what you choose, what you think, and what you do is what you become.
Your integrity is your destiny . . . it is the light that guides your way. (Heraclitus)

The separate self dissolves in the sea of pure consciousness, infinite and immortal. Separateness arises from identifying the Self with the body, which is made up of the elements; when this physical identification dissolves, there can be no more separate self. This is what I want to tell you, beloved. (Brihadaranyaka Upanishad, Chapter 2, 4:12)

As the rivers flowing east and west
merge in the sea and become one with it,
Forgetting they were ever separate rivers,
So do all creatures lose their separateness.
When they merge at last into pure Being. (Chandogya Upanishad, 10:1-2)

The Self who is free from sin, free from old age, from death and from grief, from hunger and thirst, which desires nothing but what it ought to desire, and imagines nothing but what it ought to imagine, that it is which we must search out, that it is which we must try to understand. He who has searched out that Self and understands it, obtains all worlds and all desires. (Chandogya Upanishad, 8.7.1)

According to the teaching of the Indian philosophy of Chandogya Upanishad (Vedic text), there is no separate self, all is One. It is only illusion,

Maya, that clouds our vision. If we accept this premise, then we can say that the absolute self, the one, or whatever name you give to the absolute principle, "creates" bodies and looks at its "creations" through the body's eyes. This causes the illusion of many selves. The absolute is one, homogenous whole, but through illusion, delusion, ignorance, and wrong thinking, there is a belief in separation of multitudes of units.

Music, silence, hypnosis, self-hypnosis and mindfulness all have the capacity to reach special states of the mind that center on relaxation. Indeed, mindfulness may be called the most potent nonpharmacological relaxant known to science. They may seem like separate entities. On closer look and in their long-term practice, however, they are found to share common principles. Most importantly, they all can bring to light the knowledge of higher self: comprehension, relaxed self-control, relief of pain and suffering, existential centeredness, and higher consciousness.

Look inside yourself and try to examine and be conscious of the feeling or sensation you have of yourself. I mean just the feeling that you are alive and existing. Concentrate on what you sense to be your essence.

This feeling of universal consciousness is actually always with you, no matter what you are doing or where you are. It is an invariable and continuous factor, but it is clouded by the five senses and by thoughts. It is not something theoretical, metaphorical, or mystical. It is a fact. It is knowledge.

Inner silence is a peculiar state of being in which thoughts are canceled out and one can function from a level other than that of daily awareness. Inner silence means the suspension of the internal dialogue, the perennial companion of thought, and is therefore, a state of profound quietude.

B. The Technique of Inner Silence

> I become aware of the sounds around me . . .
> where I am now . . .
> Both near and distant sounds . . .
> nothing bothers me any more . . .
> my heart contemplates this peace . . .
> Then, I imagine I am sitting on my favorite river bank . . .
> and watching the whirlpools forming and dissolving in the water . . .
> flowing before me . . .
> I have no desire to interfere with or disturb the water or the whorls . . .
> I am just witnessing the unfolding patterns as they arise and move on in the river of mind . . .
> Now I bring my awareness back to the sounds around me . . .
> where I am now . . .
> and I move on in the river of mind . . .

and I move on in the river of mind . . .
I listen to the sound of my breathing . . .
I develop a dispassionate witness . . .
that doesn't get involved in the experience . . .
that leaves it alone to unfold and surrenders to its effect in the body . . .
without limitation or judgment . . .
and move on in the river of mind . . .
and move on in the river of mind . . .
and listen to the sound of the breathing . . .
and silence . . .

Inner silence is the avenue that leads to a true suspension of judgment, to a moment when sensory data emanating from the universe at large ceases to be interpreted by the senses; a moment when cognition ceases. At the beginning, there were aeons of silence. It is in the vessel of silence, that inner transformation can appear.

REFERENCES

American Society of Clinical Oncology. (1998). *Policy on Cancer Care During the Last Phase of Life.* Available at http://www.asco.org/ac/1,1003,12-002174-00_18-0010346-00_19 0010351-00-20-001,00.asp

Arntz. A., Dreessen, L., & Merckelbach, H. (1991). Attention, not anxiety, influences pain. *Behaviour Research and Therapy, 29,* 41–50.

Assagioli, R. (1977). *Psicosintesi terapeutica.* Rome, Italy: Casa Editrice Astrolabio.

Bucknell, B. (2002). *Literary modernism and musical aesthetics.* Cambridge, UK: Cambridge University Press.

Farthing, G. W., Venturino, M., & Brown, S. W. (1984). Suggestion and distraction in the control of pain: Test of two hypotheses. *Journal of Abnormal Psychology, 93,* 266–276.

Fowler-Kerry, S., & Lander, J. R. (1987). Management of injection pain in children. *Pain, 30,* 169–175.

Frid, I.A., Berezkin, D. P., Evtiukhin, A. I., Beliaev, D. G., & Aleksandrin, G. P. (1981). Hypnosis and music analgesia in the postoperative period. *Anesteziologiia i Reanimatologiia, September-October* (5), 30–32.

Last Acts®. (2001). *Care Beyond Cure-Palliative Care and Hospice.* Fact Sheet. Accessed February 24, 2003 at http://www.lastacts.org/scripts/la_res01.exe FNC= FactSheets__Ala_res_NewHome_html)

Leaver, A. M., Van Lare, J., Zielinski, B., Halpern, A. R., & Rauschecker, J. P. (2009). Brain activation during anticipation of sound sequences. *Journal of Neuroscience, 29*(8), 2477–2485.

Malone, A. B. (1996). The effects of live music on the distress of pediatric patients receiving intravenous starts, venipunctures, injections, and heel sticks. *Journal of Music Therapy, 33,* 19–33.

Megel, M. E., Houser, C. W., & Gleaves, L. S. (1999). Children's responses to immunizations: Lullabies as a distraction. *Issues in Comprehensive Pediatric Nursing, 21,* 129–145.

Nilsson, U., Rawal, N., Enqvist, B., & Unosson, M. (2003). Analgesia following music and therapeutic suggestions in the PACU in ambulatory surgery: A randomized controlled trial. *Acta Anaesthesiologica Scandinavica, 47*(3), 278–283.

Nilsson, U., Rawal, N., Unestȧhl, L.E., Zetterberg, C., & Unosson, M. (2001). Improved recovery after music and therapeutic suggestions during general anaesthesia: A double-blind randomised controlled trial. *Acta Anaesthesiologica Scandinavica, 45*(7), 812–817.

Plutchik, R. (1980). A general psychoevolutionary theory of emotion. In R. Plutchik & H. Kellerman (Eds.), *Emotion: Theory, research, and experience* (Vol. 1. Theories of Emotion, pp. 3–33). New York: Academic Press.

Ruytjens, L., Willemsen, A. T., Van Dijk, P., Wit, H. P., & Albers, F. W. (2006). Functional imaging of the central auditory system using PET [Review]. *Acta Otolaryngology, 126*(12), 1236–1244.

Sherman, R. A. (2004). *Pain assessment and intervention from a psychophysiological perspective.* Wheat Ridge, CO.: Association of Applied Psychophysiology and Biofeedback.

Silva, M. (1999). *Music for peace.* Firenze, Italy

Tsao, J. C. I. (2005). *Pediatric pain program.* Oxford University Press.

Zatorre, R. J., Halpern, A. R., & Bouffard, M. (2010). Mental reversal of imagined melodies: A role for the posterior parietal cortex. *Journal of Cognitive Neuroscience, 22*(4), 775–789.

SUGGESTED READINGS

Aitken, J. C., Wilson, S., Coury, D., & Moursi, A. M. (2002). The effect of music distraction on pain, anxiety and behavior in pediatric dental patients. *Pediatric Dentistry, 24,* 114–118.

Andrasik, F., & Blanchard, E. B. (1987). Biofeedback treatment of muscle contraction headache. In J. P. Hatch, J. G. Fisher & J. D. Rugh (Eds.), *Biofeedback: Studies in clinical efficacy* (pp. 281–315). New York: Plenum Press.

Arena, J. G., & Blanchard, E. B. (1996). Biofeedback and relaxation therapy for chronic pain disorders. In R. J. Gatchel & D. C. Turk (Eds.), *Psychological approaches to pain management* (pp. 179–230). New York: The Guilford Press.

Arts, S. E., Abu-Saad, H. H., Champion, G. D., Crawford, M. R., Fisher, R. J., Juniper, K. H., & Ziegler, J. B. (1994). Age-related response to lidocaine-prilocaine (EMLA) emulsion and effect of music distraction on the pain of intravenous cannulation. *Pediatrics, 93,* 797–801.

Barrera, M. E., Rykov, M. H., & Doyle, S. L. (2002).The effects of interactive music therapy on hospitalized children with cancer: A pilot study. *Psychooncology, 11,* 379–388.

Blanchard, E. B. (1992). Psychological treatment of benign headache disorders. *Journal of Consulting and Clinical Psychology, 60,* 537–551.

Bloom, P. (2004). *Advances in neuroscience relevant to the clinical practice of hypnosis: A clinician's perspective.* Keynote address to the 16th International Congress of Hypnosis and Hypnotherapy, Singapore.

Chambless, D. L., & Hollon, S. D. (1998). Defining empirically supported therapies. *Journal of Consulting and Clinical Psychology, 66,* 7–18.

Ewin, D. (1986). The effect of hypnosis and mind set on burns. *Psychiatric Annals, 16,* 115–118.

Faymonville, M. E., Laureys, S., Degueldre, C., Del Fiore, G., Luxen, A., Franck, G., ..., & Maquet, P. (2000). Neural mechanisms of antinociceptive effects of hypnosis. *Anesthesiology, 92,* 1257–1267.

Field, M. J., & Cassel, C. K. (1997). *Approaching death: Improving care at the end of life.* Washington, DC: National Academy Press.

Hilgard, E. R., & Hilgard, J. R. (1994). *Hypnosis in the relief of pain.* New York: Brunner/Mazel.

Hipple, W. J. Jr. (1957). *The beautiful, the sublime and the picturesque in eighteenth-century British aesthetic theory* (Chapter 4, William Hogarth, pp. 54–66), Carbondale, IL: The Southern Illinois University Press.

Kant, I. (1929). *Critique of pure reason* (Norman Kemp Smith, Trans.). London: The Macmillan Press Ltd.

Kant, I. (1981). *Universal natural history and theory of the heavens* (Stanley L. Jaki, Trans.). Edinburgh, Scotland: Scottish Academic Press.

Lo, B. (1995). Improving care near the end of life: Why is it so hard? *JAMA, 274,* 1634–1636.

Mach, E. (1897/1959). *The analysis of sensations and the relation of the physical to the psychical* (C. M. Williams & Sydney Waterlow, Trans.). Mineola, NY: Dover Editions.

Maryland Health Care Commission, Health Resources Division. Issue Policy Brief (2002, May). *Hospice Services.*

Merskey, H., & Bogduk, N. (1994). *Classification of chronic pain. Descriptions of chronic pain syndromes and definitions of pain terms* (2nd ed.). Seattle, WA: IASP Press.

Patterson, D. R., & Jensen, M. P. (2003). Hypnosis and clinical pain. *Psychological Bulletin, 129,* 495–521.

Rosenberg, H. M., Ventura, S. J., Maurer, J. D., Heuser, R. L., & Freedman, M. A. (1996). *Births and deaths: United States, 1995. Monthly Vital Statistics Report* (Vol. 45, Issue 3, Suppl. 2). Hyattsville, MD: National Center for Health Statistics.

Schwartz, M. S. (Ed.). (1995). *Biofeedback: A practitioner's guide.* New York: The Guilford Press.

Silva, M. (2004). *Beyond music.* Firenze, Italy.

Sundaram, R. (1995). Art therapy with a hospitalized child. *American Journal of Art Therapy, 34,* 2–8.

Task Force on Promotion and Dissemination of Psychological Procedures. (1995). Training in and dissemination of empirically validated psychological treatments: Report and recommendations. *Clinical Psychology, 48,* 3–23.

Wenrich, M. D., Curtis, J. R., Shannon, S. E., Carline, J. D., Ambrozy, D. M., & Ramsey, P. G. (2001). Communicating with dying patients within the spectrum of medical care from terminal diagnosis to death. *Archives of Internal Medicine, 161,* 2623–2624.

Willmarth, E. K., & Willmarth, K. J. (2005, Spring). Biofeedback and hypnosis in pain management. *Biofeedback, 33*(1), 20–24.

Wittgenstein, L. (1961). *Tractatus logico-philosophicus* (D. F. Pears & B. F. McGuinness, Trans.). London: Routledge.

Chapter VII

CLINICAL HYPNOSIS, MINDFULNESS, AND THE LANGUAGE OF METAPHORS

1. ALLEGORIES AND METAPHORS IN POETRY AND SPIRITUAL VERSES

Every time we read poetry or a meditative spiritual verse we are engaged in a miracle that we do not even recognize: the wind; a blue sky; white clouds; green leaves; the black; curious eyes of a child; the unnatural atmospheres; and feelings. Feelings, love and death—Eros and Thanatos, are the themes of the play. Communication in clinical hypnosis is speech, feelings, and emotions: the language plays a basic role in emotions.

> Your soul is as a moonlit landscape fair,
> Peopled with maskers delicate and dim,
> That play on lutes and dance and have an air
> Of being sad in their fantastic trim. (. . .)
> The melancholy moonlight, sweet and lone,
> That makes to dream the birds upon the tree,
> And in their polished basins of white stone
> The fountains tall to sob with ecstasy. ("Clair de Lune," Paul Verlaine)

Don't run after your thoughts . . . find joy and peace in this very moment . . .

Mindfulness is not a discursive reflection on philosophy; it is a penetration of mind into mind itself. Images flow in a quick succession and often swiftly change their field of reference: from science to theology, from astronomy to philosophy and to the soul.

Everything in poetry and metaphor could become a meaning and even the meaning of meaning. Hypnosis, metaphors, and mindfulness can be the power of emotions and the door to higher consciousness in relief of suffering.

269

A. Is Poetry Mindfulness?

Poetry is mindfulness, and we are told to set our minds on the higher consciousness. Mindfulness or meditation is a spiritual practice that forms part of the believer's prayer life. It creates awareness and aligns our being to the will and purposes of inner awareness. Spiritual verses in many different religions involve more than just talking and asking God for things. It involves listening and being filled with the streams of living water.

Through the practice of spiritual verses you can experience many benefits:

- Quiet your racing thoughts
- Increase your ability to concentrate
- Increase creativity
- Increase wisdom
- Decrease generalized anxiety
- Reduce panic attack
- Promote a sense of well-being
- Keep you centered and rooted in love and truth
- Help you to understand life
- Give you peace of mind
- Help you make contact with yourself and discover who you really are.

As long as the Self is in bondage to the false personal self of evil, so long is there not even a possibility of freedom, for these two are contraries. However, when free from the grasp of selfish personality, he reaches his real nature; Bliss and Being shine forth by their own light, like the full moon, free from blackness. But he who in the body thinks "this is I," a delusion built up by the mind through darkness; when this delusion is destroyed for him without remainder, there arises for him the realization of Self as the Eternal, free from all bondage. (Vedanta, Verses 299–378).

Commit to the Lord whatever you do, and your plans will succeed.
(Proverbs, 16:3 NIV)

Delight yourself in the Lord and he will give you the desires of your heart.
(Psalms, 37:11 NIV)

The imagery in hypnosis, mindfulness, and spiritual care is a network that has a great semantic and psychological relevance in verses, and it should be not considered a mere decorative pattern superimposed on a given theme. Hypnosis, mindfulness and spiritual care, are usually associated with suggestions and allegories. In all the world, people know the inner strength of Psalm 23:

> The Lord is my shepherd, I lack nothing.
> He makes me lie down in green pastures,
> he leads me beside quiet waters,
> he refreshes my soul.
> He guides me along the right paths
> for his name's sake.
> Even though I walk
> through the darkest valley,
> I will fear no evil,
> for you are with me;
> your rod and your staff,
> they comfort me.
> You prepare a table before me
> in the presence of my enemies.
> You anoint my head with oil;
> my cup overflows.
> Surely your goodness and love will follow me
> all the days of my life,
> and I will dwell in the house of the Lord forever. (Psalm 23, A Psalm of David)

There are two therapeutic "hypnotic" allegories in this psalm that are admirably well-adapted to the purpose for which they are produced and supported to induce both a state of mindfulness and inner strength. The first is that of a shepherd; the second is that of a great feast. They have the most excellent pasture; as guests, they have the most nutritive and abundant fare. God condescends to call himself the Shepherd of his people, and his followers are considered as a flock under his guidance and direction; He who called them from darkness into his marvelous light.

1. He leads them out and in, so that they find pasture and safety.
2. He knows where to feed them, and through his grace and providence, leads them in the way in which they should go.
3. He watches over them and keeps them from being destroyed by ravenous beasts.
4. If any have strayed, he brings them back.
5. He brings them to the shade in times of scorching heat; in times of persecution and affliction, he finds an asylum for them.
6. He takes care that they shall lack no manner of thing that is good.

"The Lord is my shepherd." In these words and allegory, the believer is taught to express his or her satisfaction in the care of the great Pastor of the Universe, the Redeemer and Preserver of men in a universal love. Are we blessed with the green pastures of the ordinances? Let us not think it enough to pass through them, but let us abide in them. The consolations of the Holy Spirit are the still waters by which the saints are led and the streams that flow from the fountain of living waters. In these paths, we cannot walk unless God leads us into them and leads us on in them.

B. Hypnosis and Allegory

Allegory is a device in which characters or events represent or symbolize ideas and concepts. Allegory has been used widely throughout the history of philosophy and spirituality in different religions. A reason for this is that allegory has an immense power of illustrating complex ideas and concepts in a digestible, concrete way. In allegory, a message is communicated by means of symbolic figures, actions, or symbolic representation.

As a literary device, an allegory in its most general sense is an extended metaphor. One of the best known examples is Plato's allegory of the cave. In this allegory, there are a group of people who have lived chained to the wall of a cave, facing a blank wall all of their lives. The people watch shadows projected on the wall by things passing in front of a fire behind them and begin to ascribe forms to these shadows. According to the allegory, the shadows are as close as the prisoners get to viewing reality.

The history of imaginative hypnosis is very ancient. We can consider as imaginative hypnosis the symbolic contents in ancient philosophy, verses, and prayers.

As Jung studied, the archetypes have been inside ourselves since a long time before us and come back in our dreams, memories, and images through metaphors. The metaphors get filled with symbolic contents that stay alive and are activated during the hypnotic sessions.

Metaphors and poetry in hypnosis and spiritual care are a trance state characterized by a very relaxed, drowsy, and lethargic appearance. During this trance state, the person who has been hypnotized loses initiative to carry out his or her own plans, redirects attention away from the activity in which he or she was engaged toward the instructions of the hypnotist, has heightened ability to produce fantasies, and has an increased susceptibility to suggestions.

In pain therapy, we have begun to discover the various therapeutic benefits of these practices. The state of relaxation and the altered state of consciousness in hypnosis are especially effective in chronic pain and in the therapy for suffering. Relaxation, mindfulness, and hypnosis are intensely personal and spiritual experiences. The desired purpose of each technique is to channel our consciousness into a more positive direction, by totally transforming one's state of mind. A modified state of consciousness is to turn inward and concentrate on the inner self.

It is quite difficult to understand the internal functioning and management of information of the brain. Pavlov coined the word conditioning. Watson adopted it and invented "behaviorism" and later Skinner came up with "reinforcement." The school of epiphenomenologists considered the mind as the product of the brain's "hardware" and "wiring" complexity, however, all of them failed to address only one key linked to the brain.

A number of cognitive scientists, including George Lakoff, Mark Turner, and their colleagues, have recently argued that metaphor should not be seen as a linguistic device but rather as a form of thought that is pervasive, systematic, and fundamental (Hopkins, 2004). Spanos and Barber (1974) indicated that "hypnosis is, in part, a process of involvement in suggestion-related imaginings." By using metaphors, a language full of analogies, the hypnotist can activate phenomena that have been defined as "transderivational" (Casula, 2001; Casula, Preti & Portaluri, 2005; Gulotta, 1980).

According to Haley (1963), "one way of confronting the problem of a subject who is resistant to the directives of the therapist, is to communicate in analogical or metaphorical manner. If the subject shows resistance to A, the therapist can speak of B, and when A and B are on metaphorical terms, the subject will make this connection spontaneously and will respond adequately. In the complex situation of hypnotic induction, the metaphor can be communicate both at a verbal and non verbal level."

In the past, I have engaged in research examining the relationship between various forms of hypnosis. I believe that the form of consciousness with poetry and metaphors is a bridge to modified states of consciousness and inner self. When the main road is blocked, as Milton Erickson often said, then we must find other roads, perhaps more winding, that will ultimately take us to our destination (Casula, 2001; Casula, Preti & Portaluri, 2005).

Humanity is increasingly turning toward various mindfulness and meditation techniques in order to cope with the increasing stress of modern-day lifestyles and to attain peace of mind.

C. Hypnosis and Poetry

The metaphorical, rhetorical, and linguistic aspects are very important in the study of the door to consciousness and to enter into the inner self of the patient. Poetry text can become a good catalyzer within a hypnotic treatment. In poetry and metaphors, images and the rhythm of the voice and sound are what make the deep communication. We can experiment with the hypnotically power of the rhythm and suggestions in one of Shakespeare's sonnets.

> Shall I compare thee to a summer's day?
> Thou art more lovely and more temperate:
> Rough winds do shake the darling buds of May,
> And summer's lease hath all too short a date;
> Sometime too hot the eye of heaven shines,
> And often is his gold complexion dimm'd;
> And every fair from fair sometime declines,
> By chance or nature's changing course untrimm'd;
> But thy eternal summer shall not fade,
> Nor lose possession of that fair thou ow'st;
> Nor shall Death brag thou wandrest in his shade,
> When in eternal lines to time thou grow'st:
> So long as men can breathe or eyes can see,
> So long lives this, and this gives life to thee. (Sonnet 18, Shakespeare)

Sound and rhythm, are very important in the relationship with the patient. Rhythm in hypnosis is a musical quality produced by the repetition of stressed and unstressed syllables (Casula, 2001; Casula, Preti & Portaluri, 2005; Preminger & Brogan, 1993). The sonnet consists of three quatrains followed by a couplet and has the characteristic rhyme scheme: *abab cdcd efef gg.*

The durations of time ("day" in line one, "May" in line three, "summer" in line four) lead toward the "eternal" in lines nine and twelve. Whereas the first two quatrains are characterized by constant change, the second half of the sonnet is increasingly focused on the eternal (González, 2006).

In the first interpretation, the poem reads that beautiful things naturally lose their fanciness over time. In the second, it reads that nature is a ship with sails not adjusted to wind changes in order to correct course. This, in combination with "nature's changing course," creates an oxymoron: the unchanging change of nature or the fact that the only thing that does not change is change. This line in the poem creates a shift from the mutability of the first eight lines, into the eternity of the last six. Both change and eternity are then acknowledged and challenged by the metaphor in the final line (Jungman, 2003).

Rhythm occurs in all forms of language, both written and spoken, but is particularly important in clinical hypnosis. The original form of a sonnet's rhythm was the ancient Italian sonnet, developed by the fourteenth-century poet Petrarch. It consisted of an octet (eight line) (also known as the "Italian octave") and a sestet (six lines) (also known as the "Sicilian sestet"). Each section of an Italian sestet has a specific rhyme scheme and a specific purpose. The rhyme scheme for the octet is ABBA ABBA, and the purpose of the octet is to present a situation or a problem. The rhyme scheme for the sestet can be either CDECDE or CDCDCD, and the purpose of the sestet is to comment on or resolve the situation or problem posed in the octet.

The poem carries the meaning of an Italian or Petrarchan sonnet, which typically discussed love (Jungman, 2003).

The most obvious king of rhythm, is the regular repetition of stressed and unstressed syllables found in some poetry. The rhyme scheme of the English sonnet is aab cdcd efef gg. As noted, Shakespeare has eliminated the close linking, via rhymes, of the individual quatrains, presumably to allow more flexibility in English, which does not provide as many rhyming possibilities as Italian does.

Rhythm is the distinguishing founding element in a metaphor, or in a poetic or spiritual text, rhythm is unique and privileged in communication with the patient (Casula, 2001; Casula, Preti & Portaluri, 2005).

D. The Movement of the Verses and Rhythm in Hypnosis Suggestions

Whitman's use of metaphors and hypnotic rhythms is notable. A line of his verse, if scanned in the routine way, seems like a prose sentence, or an advancing wave of prose rhythm. The line is the unit of sense in Whitman. Whitman experimented with meter, rhythm, and form because he thought that experimentation was the law of the changing times and that innovation was the gospel of the modern world.

Imagery means a figurative use of language in hypnosis. Whitman's use of imagery shows his imaginative power, the depth of his sensory perceptions, and his capacity to capture reality instantaneously. He expresses his impressions of the world in language that mirrors the present. He makes the past come alive in his images and makes the future seem immediate. Whitman's imagery has some logical order on the conscious level, but it also delves into the subconscious, into the world of memories, producing a stream of consciousness of images. These images seem like parts of a dream, pictures of fragments of a world.

> This is thy hour O Soul, thy free flight into the wordless,
> Away from books, away from art, the day erased, the lesson done,
> Thee fully forth emerging, silent, gazing, pondering the themes thou lovest best.
> Night, sleep, death, and the stars. ("A Clear Midnight," Walt Whitman)

From this point of view, poems, thanks to their symbolic, metaphorical, and visual content, are quite up to carrying the therapeutic messages used by clinical hypnotic treatments. If the first rule within the therapeutic rapport is to synchronize your breath according to the rhythm of your patient and then lead it, little by little, varying yours, then, in a parallel way, as soon as the meter of the poetic lines varies, the nonverbal underlying deep message varies too.

Metaphors, poetry, spiritual verses, and hypnosis have much in common. They interpret the universe through sensory perceptions. The symbols are highly personal; in poetry the use of the symbol is governed by the objects observed: the sea, the wind, nature, the universe.

Next to the rhythm, another important nonverbal element is the "sound" of vowels, consonants, and syllable groups that all help build it. This is achieved by making the rhythm slower, faster, softer, harsher, soothing, and sweet or by means of devices you can easily recognize, rhymes, assonances, different shades of sounds, suggesting different shades of inner meaning and emotions.

Descriptive words in poetry and rhythm make their sound like a feeling; mindfulness of feeling is the mind experiencing awareness of the thoughts.

> Sweet love, renew thy force; be it not said
> Thy edge should blunter be than appetite,
> Which but to-day by feeding is allay'd,
> To-morrow sharp'ned in his former might.
> So, love, be thou; although to-day thou fill
> Thy hungry eyes even till they wink with fullness,
> To-morrow see again, and do not kill
> The spirit of love with a perpetual dullness.
> Let this sad int'rim like the ocean be
> Which parts the shore, where two contracted new
> Come daily to the banks, that, when they see
> Return of love, more blest may be the view;
> [Or] call it winter, which being full of care,
> Makes summer's welcome, thrice more wish'd, more rare.
> (Sonnet 56, Shakespeare)

Sweet love is an adjuration initially to the beloved, but the syntax soon changes the direction of the appeal to the love that the poet himself feels, which he fears is in danger of atrophying. On the other hand, an ocean is such a wide expanse that one could hardly expect to catch a glimpse of the beloved on the other side. The expectation is therefore perhaps of a ship coming in to view, the *"return of love"* which carries the loved one.

Can you see that ocean? Can you feel the slow rhythm of the waves? Can you sense the essence of feelings? Once you really understand that it is not the words, but the event of the poem or message that lies beyond the words, you will be able to make sense of the metaphor in general and open up your world in a significant way.

The most recent psychologist to have an impact in the field of hypnosis was the father of modern hypnosis, Milton Erickson. His nonverbal and verbal pacing techniques with metaphors are still used today.

The term metaphor comes from the Greek word metapherein, meaning "to carry over, or transfer." Rhythm (or "measure") in writing and metaphors, is like the beat in music.

In poetry, metaphors, and hypnosis, rhythm implies that certain words are produced more forcefully than others and may be held for longer duration. The repetition of a pattern of such emphasis, is what produces a rhythmic effect.

The biology of cognition attributes a practical and connotative role to language but also gives importance to emotions, which together with language form the consensual domain of conversations. In hypnosis, we use rhythm with consciously creating recognizable patterns.

In poetry, hypnosis, and metaphors, language becomes the medium for producing aesthetic events that grasp the domain of emotions of hypnotist and patient. When applied to deeper levels of experience, what is carried over by a metaphor are relationships and placement of attention, feelings, beliefs, and thoughts. A language more and more spontaneously and hypnotically indirect, implicit, and symbolic can activates new mental associations (Casula, 2004; Casula & Clerici, 1995).

2. METAPHORS, SPIRITUAL VERSES, POETRY, HYPNOSIS, AND FIGURES OF SPEECH

Figures of speech are a mode of expression in which words are used out of their literal meaning, or out of their ordinary use, in order to add beauty or emotional intensity or to transfer the poet's sense impressions by comparing or identifying one thing with another that has a meaning familiar to the reader. Some important figures of speech in poetry, spiritual verses, and hypnosis are simile, metaphor, personification, hyperbole, and symbol.

According to Padgett (2000), we can consider these figure of speech:

SIMILE: An explicit comparison is made between two essentially unlike things, usually using like, as, or than, as in Burns' "O my Love's like a red, red rose. . . ."

METAPHOR: A word or phrase literally denoting that one object or idea is applied to another, thereby suggesting a likeness or analogy between them.

PERSONIFICATION: Distinctive human characteristics, for example, honesty, emotion, volition, and so on, are attributed to an object or idea. Personification is commonly used in allegory.

SYMBOL: An image transferred by something that stands for or represents something else, like flag for country or autumn for maturity. Symbols can transfer the ideas embodied in the image without stating them.

HYPERBOLE: A bold, deliberate overstatement not intended to be taken literally; it is used as a means of emphasizing the truth of a statement.

LITOTES: A type of meiosis (understatement) in which an affirmative is expressed by the negative of the contrary, as in "not unhappy" or "a poet of no small stature."

IMAGERY, IMAGE: The elements in a literary work used to evoke mental images, not only of the visual sense, but also of sensation and emotion. Although most commonly used in reference to figurative language, imagery is a variable term that can apply to any and all components of a poem that evoke sensory experience, whether figurative or literal, and also to the concrete things so imaged.

FIGURE OF SOUND: Sometimes called sound devices, these include onomatopoeia, alliteration, assonance, consonance, euphony, resonance, and others. Not all of these are considered figures of speech, exactly, but they are included here because they are part of what you will find if you look closely at the language and word choice of a poem. They work hand in hand with rhythm and all types of rhyme.

ALLITERATION: Also called head rhyme or initial rhyme, the repetition of the initial sounds (usually consonants) of stressed syllables in neighboring words or at short intervals within a line or passage. Alliteration has a gratifying effect on the sound, gives a reinforcement to stresses, and can also serve as a subtle connection or emphasis of key words in the line. Alliterated words, however, should not "call attention" to themselves by strained usage.

ASSONANCE: The relatively close juxtaposition of the same or similar vowel sounds but with different end consonants in a line or passage, thus a vowel rhyme, as in the words date and fade.

ONOMATOPOEIA: Strictly speaking, the formation or use of words that imitate sounds, like whispering, clang, and sizzle, but the term is generally expanded to refer to any word whose sound is suggestive of its meaning. Because sound is an important part of poetry, the use of onomatopoeia is another subtle weapon in the poet's arsenal for the transfer of sense impressions through imagery.

CACOPHONY: Discordant sounds in the jarring juxtaposition of harsh letters or syllables, sometimes inadvertent but often deliberately used in poetry for effect, as in the lines from Whitman's "The Dalliance of the Eagles":

... The clinching interlocking claws, a living, fierce, gyrating wheel,
Four beating wings, two beaks, a swirling mass tight grappling,
In tumbling turning clustering loops, straight downward falling. ...

Sound devices are important to poetic and hypnotic effects to create sounds appropriate to the content. The use of words with the consonants b, k, and p, for example, produce harsher sounds than do the soft f and v or the liquid l, m, and n.

CAESURA: A rhythmic break or pause in the flow of sound that is commonly introduced in about the middle of a line of verse but may be varied for different effects. Usually placed between syllables rhythmically connected in order to aid the recital as well as to convey the meaning more clearly, it is a pause dictated by the sense of the content or by natural speech patterns, rather than by metrics. It may coincide with conventional punctuation marks, but not necessarily.

We can use the different figures of speech, metaphors, verses, and poems as indirect suggestion in hypnosis and during therapeutic modified states of consciousness.

The departure point of metaphor is indicated in the problem presented by the subject requesting therapeutic intervention. The hypnotist must first accurately note the content of the problem because to be able to use metaphor, he or she must create a structure analogous to this content. The arrival point to be reached through metaphor is indicated by the request of the subject. The request may take many forms: for help, for change, to stop suffering, to stop pain, and so on. The motivations can be used by the hypnotist to reach the therapeutic goal more easily. To arrive at the destination by means of the metaphor, we must proceed along a new path that allows us to avoid obstacles blocking the main route.

Through poetry, spiritual verses, and metaphors, we can have a real possibility that we should misconstrue a representation of the physical space inside our consciousness in this way (Hopkins, 2004).

Hypnosis can be a kind of relationship made up of unrepeatable moments when it is experienced in an integrated way, using the indirect Ericksonian communication through the poetry, the metaphors, the hypnotic trance. Hypnosis becomes than a creative experience when the choice of a certain tool or a different one from the therapist's knowledge stock can even be extemporary or unconscious. Its power, if activated in a relationship, open to the future and to changes, allows a person to feel and experience unrepeatable moments of synchronicity, such as to reveal new opportunities and interventions (Piazza & Carletti, 2006).

How can I use poetry, metaphor and rhythm in mindfulness and clinical hypnosis?

According to Battino (2002),

1. listen to the problem as offered
2. be guided by the areas of desired outcomes
3. list dramatic themes that are part of the current and desired situation
4. choose a poem, or a metaphor or a mindfulness technique that parallels those themes
5. design appropriate general outcomes
6. arrange the outcome to create suspense or mystery

With poetry, spiritual verses, and metaphor, any creative space is opened, followed, listened to, but then encircled and defined within one's way of individuation.

Repetition of a sound, rhythm, syllable, word, phrase, line, stanza, or metrical pattern is a basic unifying device in hypnosis. Repetition of sounds is the basis for rhyme and alliteration. Repetition of patterns of accents is the basis for rhythm. Repetition of key words, phrases, and sentence patterns is often important in hypnosis. The repetition of similar endings of words, or even of identical syllables (rime riche), constitutes rhyme, used generally to set up relationships within the same line (internal rhyme). Sometimes, repetition reinforces, or even substitutes for, meter (the beat), the other chief controlling factor of poetry and metaphors. Ancient spiritual chants from all cultures, show repetition. Repetition is found extensively in free verse, which does not have a traditional, recognizable metrical pattern. Repetition in free verse includes parallelism (repetition of a grammar pattern) and the repetition of important words and phrases, and is always used in clinical hypnosis.

3. CLINICAL HYPNOSIS, MINDFULNESS AND THE LANGUAGE OF METAPHORS: THE TECHNIQUES

The procedures for inducing relaxation and hypnosis are many and varied, but certain steps are common also with metaphor induction. The first such step usually involves having you sit or lie comfortably so you do not have to exert any effort to maintain your bodily position and telling you not to move and to relax your body as much as possible. This step has a variety of effects. For one thing, if you are somewhat anxious about what is going to happen, your anxiety, which intimately related to bodily tension, is at least partially relieved if you relax. You limit your ability to feel anxiety. This makes it easier for you to alter your state of consciousness.

Second, the hypnotist commonly tells you to listen only to his or her voice and ignore other thoughts or sensations that come into your mind, or the therapist simply tells you the metaphor. Ordinarily, you constantly scan the environment to see if important stimuli are present. This constant scanning keeps up a continuous, varied pattern of information and energy exchanges among subsystems, which tends to keep subsystems active in the waking state pattern.

The metaphor can be a kind of relationship made of unrepeatable moments when it is experienced in an integrated way, between the indirect Ericksonian communication through the metaphor and the hypnotic trance. The psychotherapeutic journey with the patient becomes then a creative experience. Good poets have a repertoire of stories that they can pull out on any occasion. The following will be provided for each theme:

- A title
- The intended audience, in other words, the purpose of this particular metaphor
- Opening: setting the stage by giving basic elements such as time, setting ambience, conditions, background
- Development: components of the narrative in step-by-step sequence
- Closing: morals, punch lines, special reorientation. (Battino, 2002).

There are many approaches to teaching the patient for the simple use of metaphors and poetry in self-relaxation. The following exercise is very easy:

- Following your breath while reading a poem
- Read a poem
- Breathe long, light, and even breaths
- Follow your breath and be master of it while remaining aware of the feelings and sentiments of the poetry
- Continue as with the poetry
- This can be practiced in any time and place
- Breathe quietly and more deeply than usual

During hypnosis, metaphors, poetry, spiritual verses, and suggestions may be proffer creativity, fluidity of associations, spontaneity, primary process thinking, and comfort. As they are focused on a single concept, they give a single aligned image in return; if we want to talk about combinations of concepts, question, and answers or explore a topic further and wider, we get combinations of metaphors, or sequences of metaphors leading from one into another.

Do you like poems? Do you think of scenarios and play them in your mind, dreaming and living dreams in an altered state of consciousness? In hypnosis with poetry, spiritual verses, and metaphors, some factors are absolutely important:

- You must use "all five senses" in your descriptions. If you see waves on the ocean, for example, do not just describe how it looks. Describe its light, its smell, and the sound of the wind howling across the waves.
- Phrase all your descriptions in the present tense.
- Close your eyes and describe out loud anything you can "see."
- Later on in the image streaming process, you can use it for problem solving and a great many other metaphors besides.

Metaphors and poetry need emotion, but we need to create positive emotion with words and this creation is called imagery. A metaphor is the comparison of two unlike things by saying one is the other. Remember the nursery rhyme (author unknown): "Twinkle, twinkle little star, How I wonder what you are. Up above the world so high, Like a diamond in the sky. . . ." Comparing the star to a diamond is a simile that creates imagery.

Psychologists identify seven kinds of mental images: those of sight, sound, taste, smell, touch, bodily awareness, and muscular tension. All are available to poets and are used by poets. Metaphor, simile, allegory, personification, metonymy (attribute for whole) and synecdoche (part) all involve imagery. The following list of hypnosuggestions with metaphors should be considered as a frame of work:

- Simply relax and feel happy
- Have a fantasy accompanied by feelings of relaxation and well-being
- Go in fantasy to a favorite place
- Have a fantasy about himself or herself
- Fantasize about a specific problem (and its resolution)
- Imagine the future when the problem will be resolved
- Imagine possible solutions and their consequences
- Enact, in fantasy, an interpersonal problem or conflict that involves interaction or confrontation with an antagonist (Lynn, Neufeld & Matyi, 1987)

A. Metaphors and Healing

That metaphor is the omnipresent principle of language can be shown by mere observation. We cannot get through three sentences of ordinary fluid discourse without it (Richards, 1936). Therapeutic metaphor is one of the most important tools available for assisting people in the process of personal transformation, well-being and healing.

> As darkness, which is distinct (from sunshine), vanishes in the sun's radiance, so the whole objective universe dissolves in Brahman. (Vivekachudamani, Verses 564–6)

The major purpose of therapeutic metaphor is to pace and lead an individual's experience through the telling of a story that helps that individual access resources necessary for change. In a therapeutic context metaphors are used as tools for transformation, facilitating new patterns of thoughts, feelings and behavior. Consider using imagery to:

- Externalize thought
- Create mood and atmosphere
- Give continuity by recurring leitmotifs
- Develop plot or increase dramatic effect by abrupt changes in imagery
- Exploit the etymology of words to subtly revive their original meanings

The first object using metaphors is the knowledge of our own mind. Every object of the mind is itself mind. In Buddhism and mindfulness, we call the object of mind the dharmas. Dharmas are usually grouped into five categories:

1. bodily and physical forms
2. feelings
3. perceptions
4. mental functionings
5. consciousness

These five categories are called the five aggregates. The fifth category, consciousness, however, contains all the other categories and is the basis of their existence (Nhat Hanh, 2007).

Through hypnosis with metaphors, we are conscious of the presence of bodily form, feelings, perception, mental functioning, and consciousness. With the use of poetry, mindfulness, and metaphors–the language, more and more spontaneously and hypnotically indirect, implicit, symbolic, and imaginative—can activate new mental associations and knowledge.

When this phenomenon is expressed in a state in which the conscience level is modified, the cathartic and metaphoric effect may be slower and more intense. The employment of a hypnotic methodology can be inserted magically into some eye-opening moments of the therapy, according to the experienced life, the resistances, and the metaphorical spontaneous content of the emotions. The metaphor is perhaps one of man's most fruitful potentialities. Its efficacy verges on magic, and it seems a tool for creation that God forgot inside one of His creatures when he made him (Ortega y Gasset, 1925).

> The milky sky, the hazy, slender trees,
> Seem smiling on the light costumes we wear,
> Our gauzy floating veils that have an air
> Of wings, our satins fluttering in the breeze.
> And in the marble bowl the ripples gleam,
> And through the lindens of the avenue
> The sifted golden sun comes to us blue. (A La Promenade, Paul Verlaine)

> At night, when the sea cradles me
> And the pale star gleam
> Lies down on its broad waves,
> Then I free myself wholly
> From all activity and all the love
> And stand silent and breathe purely,
> Alone, alone cradled by the sea
> That lies there, cold and silent, with a thousand lights.
> (Hermann Hesse, At Night On The High Seas)

The compulsion of Hermann Hesse to make explicit in language what was implicit in his deepest experience typifies our own present day problem of the cognitive exploration of our inner self. The words go from personal to cosmic level. Can you feel that sea? Can you feel the slow rhythm of the waves? Can you sense the essence of tranquility? Do you understand the concept of tranquility better now? Do you feel more tranquil in having touched this?

The intensity of therapeutic suggestion in poetry derives from the extremely thick verbal interplay in the poem, whose rhetorical structure and visual imagery establish an extraordinary semantic concentration in each stanza. Several of Hesse's novels depict the protagonist's journey into the inner self. A spiritual guide assists the hero, in his quest for self-knowledge and shows the way beyond the world "deluded by money, number and time." The poem carries all the emotional power of direct and indirect speech.

"Indirect" suggestion is conceptualized in two distinct ways in the literature. From an Ericksonian perspective, indirect suggestions are theoretically approached as suggestions that can circumvent the censorship of consciousness, to reach the unconscious, where they can activate dormant potentials. In contrast, from a research perspective, indirect suggestion is operationally defined as a technique. Based on Ericksonian theory, it was claimed that "indirect" suggestion was more effective than traditional, direct suggestion (Fourie, 1997).

A symbol is the smallest unit of metaphor, consisting of a single object, image, or word representing the essence of the quality or an attribute it stands for.

The following is a Jung's definition of a symbol: "A word or an image is symbolic when it implies something more than its obvious and immediate meaning. It has a wider 'unconscious' aspect that is never precisely defined or fully explained. Nor can one hope to define or explain it. As the mind explores the symbol, it is led to ideas that lie beyond the grasp of reason." The underlying assumption, is that in order to be effective a metaphor needs to be processed outside of conscious awareness (Matthews & Langdell, 1989). The value of metaphor is that it can bypass conscious resistances and serve to stimulate creativity, and lateral thinking, in relation to a problem.

Neuroscientists believe the brain exists in real, objective space and is as devoid of consciousness as is the physical space conceived of by physicists. Neither the external space of the physical senses nor the internal space of the mind exists in the brain. Within the context of the experienced world, the demarcation between external and internal space is one of convention, not absolute reality. We may experience mental images, for example, not only in our "mind's eye," with our eyes closed, and our attention withdrawn from the physical world (Wallace, 2006).

The philosophy of consciousness was pronounced by many studies of the human being, long before we knew about the source of self-knowledge and its pros and cons. The experience of the suffering-pleasure dimension has been historically accepted as an intrinsic part of life from various religious traditions and by various anthropologists, doctors, philosophers, and literary authors (Hayes, Stroshal, & Wilson, 1999; Luciano, 2001; Wilson & Luciano, 2002).

Therapeutic metaphors encourage people to focus on the deeper structure relationships between their reality and that of the story. The therapeutic value of the metaphor lies in the similarity of its deep structure to the deep structure of the problem (formal properties), even though the surface level characters and details (the content) are very different. Metaphors, spiritual verses, and poetry, in a hypnosis therapeutic context, may be useful

- To have good relaxation of body and mind
- To have good relief of pain
- To have good relief of suffering
- As distraction, to have good relief of pain
- To provide a key mechanism for improving a sense of greater connectedness with others
- To open up possibilities and strategies
- To facilitate new patterns of thoughts, feelings, and consciousness
- To stimulate lateral thinking and creativity
- To reframe or redefine a problem or situation
- To introduce doubt into a position that holds that there is only one way
- To bypass normal ego defences
- To allow the client to process directly at a subconscious level (indirect suggestions)
- To suggest solutions and new options
- To provide a gateway between the conscious and the unconscious
- To understand the subconscious mind
- To increase communication
- To facilitate retrieval of resource experiences
- To lighten up the "spiritual" dimension
- To involve a higher mode of consciousness in which the ordinary mental-egoic self is transcended
- To improve mind-body relationship
- To accept near-death experiences, death, and dying
- To improve psychology of self and self-realization
- To understand the higher self
- To understand the evolution of consciousness
- To understand the Integral approaches to knowledge

A land whose suns' moist rays,
Through the skies' misty haze,
Hold quite the same charms for my spirit
As do your scheming eyes
There all is only order:
Comfort and beauty, calm and bliss.
See how the ships, asleep
They who would ply the deep!
Line the canals: to satisfy
Your merest whim they come

From far-flung heathendom
And skim the seven seas.
On high, the sunset's rays enfold
In hyacinth and gold,
Field and canal; and, with the night,
As shadows gently fall,
Life sleeps, and all
Lies bathed in warmth and evening light.
There all is only order:
Comfort and beauty, calm and bliss.
("Invitation to the Voyage," Charles Baudelaire)

Central to Baudelaire's poetry is the platonic division between the body and the soul and its rebuttal by the philosophers of the Enlightenment Movement. According to Plato, what belongs to the body is temporary, open to error and corruption, and can never achieve perfection. What belongs to the soul, however, is infinite and may attain true knowledge and perfection through acquaintance with the ultimate forms of truth and beauty. Thus, when philosophers such as Locke, Hume, Voltaire, Rousseau, and even Descartes proffered philosophies based on reason, and knowledge based on the bodily senses rather than through the soul, this represented an immense challenge, even an attack, on the status quo. Baudelaire frequently emphasizes the temporary nature of moments of pleasure. These are fleeting moments that make life more bearable, but the pleasure he takes from them is double-edged. He is left with the feeling that physical experience is lacking in some way. He is happy to indulge in his freedom but regrets the lack of spirituality and the depth that would lend the experience, and a sense of control over these events.

Very often, imagery experiences are understood by their subjects as echoes, copies, or reconstructions of actual perceptual experiences from their past. At other times, they may seem to anticipate possible, often desired or feared, future experiences. Thus imagery has often been believed to play a very large, even pivotal, role in both memory (Paivio, 1986; Yates, 1966) and motivation. It is also commonly believed to be centrally involved in visuo-spatial reasoning and inventive or creative thought.

Recent experiments have shown that the saccadic eye movements that a subject spontaneously and unconsciously makes when experiencing a visual mental image do indeed tend to reenact the stimulus-specific pattern of saccades made when actually looking at the equivalent visual stimulus (Richardson, 1999). Thomas (1999) argues that enactive theory depicts both imagery and creative thinking as manifestations of the more basic imaginative capacity of intentionalistic perception or "seeing as."

This solitary hill has always been dear to me
And this hedge, which prevents me from seeing most of
The endless horizon.
But when I sit and gaze, I imagine, in my thoughts
Endless spaces beyond the hedge,
An all encompassing silence and a deeply profound quiet,
To the point that my heart is almost overwhelmed.
And when I hear the wind rustling through the trees
I compare its voice to the infinite silence.
And eternity occurs to me, and all the ages past,
And the present time, and its sound.
Amidst this immensity my thought drowns:
And to flounder in this sea is sweet to me. ("The Infinite," Giacomo Leopardi)

This Italian poem concentrates in a few lines the theme of philosophical and psychological progression from circumstance to inner consciousness and awareness. The solidarity of man and creation stated in the final line links the man to divinity, and it is such a revelation that it will replace all previous questioning. In this poem the world is as a vast divine system of metaphors, and the mind is at its fullest stretch when observing them.

The ever-recurring microcosm-macrocosm conceit in this poetry appeals greatly to an original relation to the universe, a relation in which every man could express his peculiar self. The metaphoric success of this determination is linked to each man's ability to transcend the limitation of experience by submitting external events to his mind. Leopardi's keen sensitivity to the larger aspects of nature, his mastery and daring with the visual image, and his appreciation of the connotative value of single words place him among the most original and provocative poets in the language of inner self.

Metaphor and poetry, being a powerful distillate of human emotional experience, can translate the theorical proposals into effective procedures that are words written in a communicative emotional code, speaking directly to the unconscious mind. Everybody's personal imaginative journey developed and got enriched more and more, stimulated by feelings.

Whitman brought vitality and picturesque metaphors to his descriptions of the physical world. He was particularly sensitive to sounds and described them with acute awareness. His view of the world was dominated by its change and fluidity in imagery. "Spirit That Form'd This Scene" was written in Platte Canyon, Colorado.

Spirit that form'd this scene,
These tumbled rock-piles grim and red,
These reckless heaven-ambitious peaks,

These gorges, turbulent-clear streams, this naked freshness,
These formless wild arrays, for reasons of their own,
I know thee, savage spirit—we have communed together,
Mine too such wild arrays, for reasons of their own;
Wast charged against my chants they had forgotten art?
To fuse within themselves its rules precise and delicatesse?
The lyrist's measur'd beat, the wrought-out temple's grace—column
and polish'd arch forgot?
But thou that revelest here—spirit that form'd this scene,
They have remember'd thee. ("Spirit That Form'd This Scene," Walt Whitman)

Metaphor presents some undeniable advantages in the relationship with
patient:

- reduction of the patient's attention field
- suggestions toward conditions of well-being
- consolidation of the state of well-being as a personal affective and emotional experience
- possibility of talking about the trouble in acceptable emotional conditions
- the development of symbolic processes and their interpretation in an alert state
- posthypnotic suggestions

The method allows the patient to reach an objective as a result of direct personal action, in as much as he realizes he has a new instrument: the knowledge of the state of well-being. The spoken, verbal message achieves the maximum effectiveness when verbal and nonverbal are synchronized so that they flow together and harmoniously. It is this great opportunity, given by the poetic text, for an emotional communication that suggests its therapeutic potentiality.

After having defined for the patient the field of therapeutic intervention, metaphor and poetry are used with the specific intention of letting the patient perceive feelings and, consequently, sense a condition of well-being that gives the patient an inner motivation to recover.

Your consciousness is simultaneously experiencing many realities in the slinky loops of time. The base, linear time, is part of the illusion of third dimension or physical reality to enable souls to experience emotions. The third dimension is the slowest moving level of consciousness, the base of the slinky. Once there, you forget the other realities, dots on the slinky above, and the experience you are having can give you the peace of mind.

Poetry and spiritual verses are primarily about capturing and recording a fleeting image of emotion. Feelings frequently rise and fall without any examination, putting them into words, recording them for feelings. Poetry and spiritual verses are ways to examine our inner thoughts and recognize the fleeting and impermanent nature of emotion. Poetry and spiritual verses hold magical emollient for each of us—if we enthusiastically embrace them. In doing so, we will extemporize our ardent devotion where indoctrination and intellect abound, where inspiration is sublime, and where the mind is captive but surrenders into a radiance of zeal and harmony.

> If beyond earthly wont, the flame of love
> Illume me, so that I o'ercome thy power
> Of vision, marvel not: but learn the cause
> In that perfection of the sight, which soon
> As apprehending, hasteneth on to reach
> The good it apprehends. I well discern,
> How in thine intellect already shines
> The light eternal, which to view alone
> Ne'er fails to kindle love; and if aught else
> Your love seduces, 't is but that it shows
> Some ill-mark'd vestige of that primal beam.
> This would'st thou know, if failure of the vow
> By other service may be so supplied,
> As from self-question to assure the soul.
> (The Divine Comedy. Paradise: Canto V, Dante Alighieri.
> Translated by The Rev. H. F. Cary, Trans.)

. . . and the original Italian version with the rhythm and musical sound:

> S'io ti fiammeggio nel caldo d'amore
> di là dal modo che 'n terra si vede,
> sì che del viso tuo vinco il valore,
> non ti maravigliar; ché ciò procede
> da perfetto veder, che, come apprende,
> così nel bene appreso move il piede.
> Io veggio ben sì come già resplende
> ne l'intelletto tuo l'etterna luce,
> che, vista, sola e sempre amore accende;
> e s'altra cosa vostro amor seduce,
> non è se non di quella alcun vestigio,
> mal conosciuto, che quivi traluce.
> Tu vuo' saper se con altro servigio,
> per manco voto, si può render tanto
> che l'anima sicuri di letigio.

In Dante's Christian universe, every motion, from the petty choices of humans to the cosmic revolutions of the stars, is motivated by love. Thus love for God gives the entire universe its proper order, for everything moves in accord with God's will. Appropriately then, God's love is represented as light, which grows ever brighter the closer to heaven one gets. Death is something that all must face at some time or another or in one way or another. Dante sees something reflected in Beatrice's eyes as in a mirror and turns to see a single intense point of light *un punto,* around which nine concentric circles wheel (the different levels of the modified states of consciousness?), turning faster and brighter, the nearer they are to the inner point, through their closeness to the ultimate truth (higher consciousness, God).

As in Aristotle (Metaphysics), heaven and all nature hang from this point, the prime mover, which is without magnitude, but without parts and indivisible: the nonduality. In spiritual verses, images and the rhythm of the voice and sound, are what makes the deep communication with higher consciousness.

> True nature is always elusive,
> Only the heart of no-heart
> can grasp-it.
> Up in the mountain,
> the burning jade stays brilliant.
> And in the roaring furnace,
> lotus blossoms keep their fragrance.
> (Ngo An, Korea, Zen (Chan) Buddhism, 1090)

Dualistic conceptions in the Atman, the Infinite Knowledge, the Absolute, are like imagining castles in the air. Therefore, always identifying thyself with the Bliss Absolute, the One without a second, and thereby attaining Supreme Peace, remain quiet. (Vivekachudamani, verses 524–526)

REFERENCES

Alighieri, D. (1990). La Divina Commedia. a cura di S. Jacomuzzi, A. Dughera, G. Ioli, V. Jacomuzzi, S. E. I., *Torino.*

Alighieri, D. (2007). *Paradise* (H. F. Cary, Trans.). eBooks@Adelaide.

Battino, R. (2002). *Metaphoria.* New York: Crown House Publishing Co.

Baudelaire, C. (1972). *Tutte le poesie; Petit poemes en prose. Per Club del libro Fratelli Melita.* Rome, Italy: Newton Compton Editori.

Casula, C. (2001). *La forza della vulnerabilità. Utilizzare la resilienza per superare le avversità.* Milan, Italy: Franco Angeli Editore.

Casula, C. (2004). *Giardinieri, principesse, porcospini. Metafore per l'evoluzione personale e professionale.* Editore Franco Angeli, Italy.

Casula, C., & Clerici, A. M. (1995). *Parole terapeutiche: uso del linguaggio e approcci terapeutici.* Cattolica, Italy: Editore ISU Università.

Casula, C., Preti, M., & Portaluri, S. (2005). *7 meditazioni guidate. Per risvegliare l'energia dei chakra.* Con CD Audio. Italy: Red Edizioni.

Fourie, D. P. (1997). Indirect suggestion in hypnosis: Theoretical and experimental issues. *Psychological Report, 80*(3 Pt. 2), 1255–1266.

González, F. (2006). *Spanish studies in Shakespeare and his contemporaries.* Newark, DE: University of Delaware Press.

Gulotta, G. (1980). *Ipnosi. Aspetti psicologici, clinici, legali e criminologici.* Milan, Italy: Giuffrè.

Haley, J. (1963). *Strategies of psychotherapy.* New York: Grune and Stratton.

Hopkins, J. (2004). *Mind as metaphor: A physicalistic approach to the problem of consciousness.*

Jungman, R. E. (2003). Trimming Shakespeare's Sonnet 18. *ANQ, 16*(1), 18–19.

Lynn, S. J., Neufeld, V., & Matyi, C. L. (1987). Inductions versus suggestions: Effects of direct and indirect wording on hypnotic responding and experience. *Journal of Abnormal Psychology, 96*(1), 76–79.

Matthews, W. J., & Langdell, S. (1989). What do clients think about the metaphors they receive? An initial inquiry. *American Journal of Clinical Hypnosis, 31*(4), 242–251.

Nhat Hanh, T. (1999) *The heart of the Buddha's teaching.* New York: Broadway Books.

Ortega y Gasset, J. (1925) *The dehumanization of art.*

Padgett, R. (Ed.). (2000). *The teachers and writers handbook of poetic forms.* New York: Teachers & Writers Collaborative.

Paivio, A. (1986). *Mental representations: A dual coding approach.* New York: Oxford University Press.

Piazza, C., & Carletti, C. (2006). Hypnosis and poetry. A use of rhythm and metaphor in a group training experiences. *Acta Hypnologica, 10*(2), 19–24.

Preminger, A., & Brogan, T. (1993). *The new Princeton encyclopedia of poetry and poetics* (p. 894). Princeton: Princeton University Press.

Richardson, J. (1999). *Mental imagery.* Hove, UK: Psychology Press.

Spanos, N. P., & Barber, T. X. (1974). Toward a convergence in hypnosis research. *American Psychologist, 29,* 500–511.

Thomas, N. J. T. (1999). Are theories of imagery theories of imagination? An Active Perception approach to conscious mental content. *Cognitive Science, 23,* 207–245.

Wallace, B. A. (2006). Vacuum states of consciousness: A Tibetan Buddhist view. In D. K. Nauriyal (Ed.), *Buddhist thought and applied psychology: Transcending the boundaries.* London: Routledge Curzon.

Wilson, K. G., & Luciano, M. C. (2002). *Terapia de aceptación y compromiso. Un tratamiento conductual orientado a los valores* [*Acceptance and commitment therapy. A behavioral treatment oriented towards values*]. Madrid: Pirámide.

Yates, F. A. (1966). *The art of memory.* London: Routledge & Kegan Paul.

SUGGESTED READINGS

Bandura, A. (1977). Self-efficacy: Toward a unifying theory of behavioral change. *Psychological Review, 84*(2), 191–215.

Barnes-Holmes, Y., Barnes-Holmes, D., McHugh, L., & Hayes, S. C. (2004). Relational frame theory: Some implications for understanding and treating human psychopathology. *International Journal of Psychology and Psychological Therapy, 4*(2), 355–375.

Battino, R., & South, T. L. (2005). *Ericksonian approaches.* New York: Crown House Publishing Co.

Berman, M., & Brown, D. (2000). *The power of metaphor.* New York: Crown House Publishing Co.

Damasio, A. (1999). *The feeling of what happens: Body, emotion and the making of consciousness.* London: Heinemann.

Erickson, M. H., & Rossi, E. L. (1976, January). Two level communication and the microdynamics of trance and suggestion. *American Journal of Clinical Hypnosis, 18*(3), 153–171.

Erickson, M. H., & Rossi, E. L. (1980). *The nature of hypnosis and suggestion* (Vol. b1). New York: Irvington Publishers.

Erickson, M. H., Rossi, E. L., & Rossi, S. I. (1976). *Hypnotic realities: The induction of clinical hypnosis and forms of indirect suggestion.* New York: Irvington Publishers.

Gheorghiu, V. A. (1972). On suggestion and suggestibility. *Scientia, 107.*

Hayes, S. C., Barnes-Holmes, D., & Roche, B. (Eds.). (2001). *Relational frame theory: A post-Skinnerian account of human language and cognition* (pp. 211–238). New York: Kluwer Academic/Plenum Publishers.

Heal J. (2004). *Minds, brains and indexical draft.* Manuscript in preparation.

Honderich, T. (1995). Consciousness, neural functionalism, real subjectivity. *American Philosophical Quarterly, 32,* 369–381.

Kosslyn, S. M. (1980). *Image and mind.* Cambridge, MA: Harvard University Press.

Locatelli, C. (1981). *Texts and contexts. Storia della letteratura inglese ed americana.* Milan, Italy: Signorelli Editore.

Luciano, M. C. (1999). La psicoterapia analítico funcional (FAP) y la terapia de aceptación y compromiso (ACT) [Analytic functional psychotherapy (AFP) and acceptance and commitment therapy (ACT)]. *Análisis y Modificación de Conducta, 25,* 497–584.

Luciano, M. C., & Hayes, S. C. (2001). Trastorno de evitación experiencial [Experiential avoidance disorder]. *Revista Internacional de Psicología Clínica y de la Salud, 1,* 109–157.

Luciano, M. C., Rodríguez, M., & Gutiérrez, O. (2004). A proposal for synthesizing verbal contexts in experiential avoidance disorder and acceptance and commitment therapy. *International Journal of Psychology and Psychological Therapy, 4,* 377–394.

Luciano, M. C., & Törneke, N. (2006). *Experimental basis of ACT clinical methods from an RFT perspective.* Presented at Workshop II International Institute of RFT-ACT, London.

Ray, R. H. (1994). Shakespeare's sonnet 18. *The Explicator, 53*(1), 10–11.

Richardson, A. (1969). *Mental imagery.* London: Routledge & Kegan Paul.

Simpson, P. (2004). *Stylistics.* New York: Routledge.

Shepard, R. N., & Cooper, L. (1982). *Mental images and their transformations.* Cambridge, MA: The MIT Press.

Shor, R. E. (1979). The fundamental problem in hypnosis research as viewed from historic perspectives. In E. Fromm & R. E. Shor (Eds), *Hypnosis: Developments in research and new perspectives.* New York: Aldine Publ. Co.

Wilson, K. G., Hayes, S.C., Gregg, J., & Zettle, R. (2001). Psychopathology and psychotherapy. In S. C. Hayes, D. Barnes-Holmes, & B. Roche (Eds.), *Relational frame theory: A post-Skinnerian account of human language and cognition.* New York: Kluwer Academic/Plenum Publishers.

Chapter VIII

RELAXATION AND HYPNOSIS IN PEDIATRIC PATIENTS: TECHNIQUES FOR PAIN RELIEF AND PALLIATIVE CARE

1. PAIN THERAPY AND PALLIATIVE CARE IN INFANTS AND CHILDREN

Pediatric suffering in chronic diseases is a significant and psychophysiologically complex problem, involving the fundamental interaction of a neurophysiological response with age, cognitive set, personality, ethnic culture, and emotive state (Legrain et al., 2009).

Acute and chronic pain management in children is increasingly characterized by either a multimodal or a preventive analgesia approach. Smaller doses of opioid and nonopioid analgesics, such as nonsteroidal anti-inflammatory drugs, and local anaesthetics, are commonly used alone or in combination with nonpharmacological therapies to maximize pain control and minimize drug-induced adverse side effects. A multimodal approach uses nonpharmacological complementary and alternative medicine therapies. These include distraction, guided imagery, clinical hypnosis and relaxation techniques.

Using the neurophysiology of pain as a pattern, multimodal pain and suffering management, is described in this chapter.

The effects of tumor and its therapy, and the mechanisms and experience of pain in the child with cancer, have a serious impact on neurocognitive functioning and psychosocial issues of the children and family. At a time of enlarging interest in palliative care children's pediatric oncology programs may be failing to deliver adequate help to children with cancer. Not all cancer patients suffer pain from their disease, although most have pain related to treatments or procedures or to psychological suffering. The combination of pharmacological and non pharmacological approaches may be optimal for acute and chronic pain in children. The evaluation of pain and suffering in the newborn and children is difficult because pain is mainly a subjective phenomenon.

Until a few years ago, several myths persisted. First, the myth that children, especially infants, do not feel pain the way adults do, and therefore there are no untoward consequences for them. The second myth is the lack of assessment and reassessment for the presence of pain. The third myth is the misunderstanding of how to conceptualize and quantify a subjective experience (Loizzo, Loizzo & Capasso, 2009).

Pediatric oncologists and those charged with developing pediatric palliative care programs must deal with the different physiological and developmental stages encountered while caring for infants, children, and adolescents. When discussing palliative care in children with cancer, where few die but many suffer, a paradigm shift must occur that does not equate palliative care with end-of-life care (Harris, 2004).

> Palliative care for children represents a special, albeit closely related field to adult palliative care. Palliative care for children is the active total care of the child's body, mind and spirit, and also involves giving support to the family. It begins when illness is diagnosed, and continues regardless of whether or not a child receives treatment directed at the disease.

> Health providers must evaluate and alleviate a child's physical, psychological, and social distress. Effective palliative care requires a broad multidisciplinary approach that includes the family and makes use of available community resources; it can be successfully implemented, even if resources are limited. It can be provided in tertiary care facilities, in community health centers and even in children's homes. Palliative care improves the quality of life of patients and families who face life-threatening illness, by providing pain and symptom relief, spiritual and psychosocial support to from diagnosis to the end of life and bereavement. (WHO)

According to the WHO, palliative care in children

- provides relief from pain and other distressing symptoms
- affirms life and regards dying as a normal process
- intends neither to hasten nor postpone death
- integrates the psychological and spiritual aspects of patient care
- offers a support system to help patients live as actively as possible until death
- offers a support system to help the family cope during the patients' illness and in their own bereavement

- uses a team approach to address the needs of patients and their families, including bereavement counseling, if indicated
- will enhance quality of life and may also positively influence the course of illness
- is applicable early throughout the illness, in conjunction with other therapies that are intended to prolong life, such as chemotherapy or radiation therapy, and includes those investigations needed to better understand and manage distressing clinical complications

The care of disabled children or those at the end of life may be particularly complex.

A. Neurophysiology and Neuropsychology of Pain in Infants and Children

"Pain is an unpleasant sensory and emotional experience associated with actual or potential tissue damage, or described in terms of such damage. The inability to communicate verbally does not negate the possibility that an individual is experiencing pain and is in need of appropriate pain-relieving treatment. Pain is always subjective. Everyone learns the application of the word through experiences related to injury in early life" (IASP).

For most children with cancer, the primary goal of cure is to achieve the alleviation of pain. "Many people report pain in the absence of tissue damage or any likely pathophysiological cause; generally, this happens for psychological reasons. There is usually no way to distinguish their experience from that due to tissue damage if we take the subjective report. . . . If they regard their experience as pain, and if they report it in the same ways as pain caused by tissue damage, it should be accepted as pain" (IASP). Considerations of the toxicity of cancer therapy, the quality of life, and growth and development are usually secondary to this goal. As a result, it may be difficult for physicians to change their focus even when there is little hope of a cure (Anton, 2009). Children who die of cancer receive aggressive treatments and procedures at the end of life. Many have substantial suffering in the last month of life and attempts to control their symptoms are often unsuccessful. Greater attention must be paid to pain and suffering therapy for these children.

"As with the pain threshold, the pain tolerance level is the subjective experience of the individual. The stimuli which are normally measured in relation to its production are the pain tolerance level stimuli and not the level itself. Thus, the same argument applies to pain tolerance level as to the pain threshold, and it is not defined in terms of the external stimulation as such" (IASP).

Unrelieved pain and suffering in infants and children, can permanently change their nervous system and may give "prime" them, for having chronic pain. Barriers to good pain management are numerous and reflect biological, psychological, and social factors (Hester, Foster & Kristensen, 1990). The biological barriers to pediatric pain management are as follows (Andrews & Fitzgerald, 1997):

- Complete myelination of nerve pathways not required for pain transmission.
- C-fibers are unmyelinated and A-delta fibers are thinly myelinated.
- Incomplete myelination results in slower conduction velocity but offset by shorter distances.
- Complete myelination of pain pathways to brainstem and thalamus by 30-week gestation; thalamus to the cortex by 37 weeks.
- Nociceptive nerve endings in cutaneous and mucous surfaces by 20 weeks of gestation.
- Threshold for responding to cutaneous stimulation is lowest in the youngest neonates.
- Inhibitory pathways do not develop until after birth.

We must remember that children and adolescents do not tolerate pain and suffering better than adults:

- Infants feel pain (Loizzo, Loizzo & Capasso, 2009).
- The youngest premature infant has the anatomical and physiological components to perceive pain or "nociception" and demonstrates a severe stress response to painful stimuli (Silva, Gomez, Máximo & Silva, 2007).
- Children beyond childhood can accurately point to the body area or mark the painful site on a drawing; children can use pain scales.
- Inadequate analgesia for initial procedures (bone marrow aspiration, lumbar puncture, or both) in young children may diminish the effect of adequate analgesia in subsequent procedures (Weisman, Bernstein & Schechter, 1998).
- Pain is a common experience during childhood. All children encounter "everyday" pain associated with minor bumps and bruises, and many endure pain resulting from serious injuries, diseases, and other health conditions requiring medical care. Regardless of its prevalence, pain in infants, children, and adolescents, is often underestimated and undertreated.

- Survivors of cancer during adolescence show an elevated risk of demonstrating symptoms of posttraumatic stress, anxiety and/or depression during adulthood, which is also reflected in a greater number of *DSM-IV* diagnoses when in comparison to controls. Extensive follow-up assessments should include the examination of possible late psychological effects of a cancer diagnosis in adolescence in order to identify survivors needing psychosocial interventions even years after the conclusion of successful medical treatment (Seitz et al., 2010).

Recent advances in neonatal intensive care include, and are partly attributable to, growing attention for comfort and pain control for the term and preterm infant requiring intensive care or procedure in chronic illnesses. Limitation of painful procedures is certainly possible, but most critically ill infants require unavoidable painful or stressful procedures such as intubation, mechanical ventilation, or catheterization. Many analgesics (opioids and nonsteroidal anti-inflammatory drugs) and sedatives (benzodiazepines and other anesthetic agents) are available, but their use varies considerably among units (Durrmeyer, Vutskits, Anand & Rimensberger, 2010).

A child's pain is what finally gets his or her attention, and this pain is the result of a condition that has triggered a series of physical, psychological and neurological events. Since the 1980s, the problem of pain experienced by newborns has met with increasing interest both in research work and in clinical practice. It is worth noting that significant progress in the neurophysiological basis of pain and in diagnostic and therapeutic methods has occurred during that time.

The low tactile threshold of preterm infants when they are in the neonatal intensive care unit (NICU), while their physiological systems are unstable and immature, potentially renders them more vulnerable to the effects of repeated invasive procedures. There is a small but growing literature on pain and tactile responsive following procedural pain in the NICU.

Acute pain follows injury to the body and generally disappears when the bodily injury heals. It is often, but not always, associated with objective physical signs of autonomic nervous system activity. Chronic pain, in contrast to acute pain, rarely is accompanied by signs of sympathetic nervous system arousal. The lack of objective signs may prompt the inexperienced clinician to say the patient does not "look" like he or she is in pain (American Pain Society, 1999).

Chronic pain in children is the result of a dynamic integration of biological processes, psychological factors, and sociocultural context considered within a developmental trajectory. This category of pain includes persistent (ongoing) and recurrent (episodic) pain with possible fluctuations in severity, quality, regularity, and predictability. Chronic pain can occur in single or multiple body regions and can involve single or multiple organ systems. Ongoing nociception can result in a sensitization of the peripheral and central nervous systems to produce neuroanatomical, neurochemical, and neurophysiological changes. It is important that assessment and treatment strategies be based on this definition and related dimensions (American Pain Society).

Understanding the central modulation of pain perception was greatly advanced by the finding that electrical or pharmacological stimulation of certain regions of the midbrain produces relief of pain. This analgesic effect arises from activation of descending pain-modulating pathways that project, via the medulla, to neurons in the dorsal horn, particularly in Rexed's lamina II, that control the ascending information in the nociceptive system. The major brainstem regions that produce this effect are located in poorly defined nuclei in the periaqueductal gray matter and the rostral medulla (Latremoliere & Woolf, 2009). In acute and chronic pain central sensitization is a generator of pain hypersensitivity by central neural plasticity.

Central sensitization represents an enhancement in the function of neurons and circuits in nociceptive pathways caused by increases in membrane excitability and synaptic efficacy as well as to reduced inhibition and is a manifestation of the remarkable plasticity of the somatosensory nervous system in response to activity, inflammation, and neural injury. The net effect of central sensitization is to recruit previously subthreshold synaptic inputs to nociceptive neurons, generating an increased or augmented action potential output: a state of facilitation, potentiation, augmentation, or amplification. Central sensitization is responsible for many of the temporal, spatial, and threshold changes in pain sensibility in acute and chronic clinical pain settings and exemplifies the fundamental contribution of the central nervous system to the generation of pain hypersensitivity (Latremoliere & Woolf, 2009).

The sympathetic nervous system and pain interact on many levels of the neuraxis. The sympathetic nervous system is part of the autonomic nervous system (involuntary) and prepares the body for the "fight or flight" reaction. Its activity is normally balanced in pain by that of the parasympathetic nervous system, which tends to return the body to its normal state after a "Fight or flight" episode. In the sympathetic nervous system, the preganglionic nerves leave the central nervous system between T1 and L2 to join the sympathetic ganglia (junction box). The ganglia form a chain that runs down the front of the spinal vertebral bodies. Postganglionic nerves leave the ganglia to supply their target organ.

Of note is the fact that every part of the peripheral nervous system, from dorsal root ganglion all the way to the pain receptors in the periphery, has a postganglionic sympathetic supply that increases both sensory receptor sensitivity and nerve conduction speeds. In the peripheral nervous system, the preganglionic nerves leave the central nervous system via the tenth cranial nerve (vagus) and also via the sacral parasympathetic nerves (craniosacral outflow). They join ganglia just before their target organ. Postganglionic nerves then leave the ganglia to supply their target organ.

In light of recent advances in understanding of the neurophysiological basis of pain, mechanisms-based clinical reasoning strategies for pain were identified. These are (1) nociceptive, (2) peripheral neurogenic, (3) central, and (4) autonomic/sympathetic. There was some evidence to suggest that reasoning within these categories variously influenced therapists' prognostic decision making as well as the planning of physical assessments and treatment (Smart & Doody, 2007). Even subtle changes in pathophysiology can dramatically change the effect of sympathetic nervous system on pain, and vice versa. In the periphery, inflammation or nociceptive activation is enhanced, spinal descending inhibition is reversed to spinal facilitation, and finally the awareness of all these changes will induce anxiety, which furthermore amplifies pain perception, affects pain behavior, and depresses mood (Wright, 1999; Schlereth & Birklein, 2008).

Stress responses to acute pain in neonate provides physiological and biochemical changes include (Stallard et al., 2002)

- stress hormones
- corticosterone
- adrenaline, noradrenaline
- glucagon
- aldosterone
- metabolites
- glucose
- lactate
- pyruvate

Several studies have exhibited the psychological processes that are implied in the stress response and have shown, according to Selye's research, the participation of the hypothalamic-pituitary-adrenal (HPA) axis and the major role of cortisol. The activation of the HPA axis represents one of the several important responses to stressful events and pain in critical illnesses. The stress response takes a biological aspect: increased cortisol plasma levels is observed (Boudarene, Legros & Timsit-Berthier, 2002).

The metabolic effects of stress are known to have significant effects in children. Most of these effects are mediated by the major stress hormonal axis in the body, the HPA axis. Within the central nervous system, the hippocampus, the amygdala, and the prefrontal cortex, as part of the limbic system, are believed to play important roles in the regulation of the HPA axis. With the advent of structural and functional neuroimaging techniques, the role of different central nervous system structures, in the regulation of the HPA axis, can be investigated more directly in pain.

PET results demonstrated that stress causes the dopamine release if subjects reported low maternal care early in life. By employing fMRI, we can understand how exposure to stress and activation of the HPA axis is associated with decreased activity in major portions of the limbic system, a result that allows us to speculate on the effects of stress on cognitive and emotional regulation in the brain. Taken together, the use of neuroimaging techniques in psychoneuroendocrinology opens exciting new possibilities for the investigation of stress effects in the central nervous system (Pruessner et al., 2010).

B. Pain Assessment and Management in Children

To evaluate and treat chronic childhood pain efficiently and effectively, the mind-body dualism must be abandoned. It is meaningless to dichotomize chronic pain as organic versus nonorganic, because all pain is associated with, at a minimum, neurosensory changes. Maintaining this dichotomy is harmful because such faulty thinking leads to over-medicalization (inappropriate investigations, procedures, and interventions) or insufficient acknowledgment of the child's multidimensional experience and underlying neurophysiology (American Pain Society).

The measurements of pain are needed to identify patients who require intervention and to evaluate the effectiveness of intervention. The terms measurement and assessment are widely used in the pain literature and differentiated in the following manner. Measurement refers to the assignment of a number or value and is commonly associated with the dimension of pain intensity. Assessment describes a more complex process in which information about pain, its meaning, and its effect on the person is considered along with quantitative values (O'Rourke, 2004).

VAS have a number of convenient and favorable properties. A pain scale measures a patient's pain intensity or other features. Pain scales are based on self-report, observational (behavioral), or physiological data (Melzack & Katz, 2001). Self-report is considered primary and should be obtained if possible. Pain scales are available for neonates, infants, children, adolescents, adults, seniors, and disabled persons whose communication is impaired. Children ages eight and above can generally apply standard VAS successfully. Several self-report scales, have been developed for children ages three to eight; these have been primarily on scales that use pictures or drawings of faces (McGrath & Unruh, 1999; Johnston, 1998; Turk & Melzack, 2001; Pediatric Pain Sourcebook of Protocols, Policies and Pamphlets, 2007).

From Tears to Words: The Development of Language to Express Pain in Young Children

Behavioral observation is the primary assessment approach for preverbal and nonverbal children and is an adjunct to assessment for verbal children. Observations focus on vocalizations (e.g., crying, whining, or groaning), verbalizations, facial expressions, muscle tension and rigidity, ability to be consoled, guarding of body parts, temperament, activity, and general appearance.

For infants, very young children, and children with severe cognitive or communication impairments, it may be impossible to use self-report measures; therefore, behavioral measures are required. Behavioral measures include measures of crying, facial expression, body posture and movements, daily routines, or some combination of these items (Prkachin K. M., 2009). The Neonatal Facial Coding System and the Child Facial Coding System are behavioral measures of pain intensity (McGrath & Unruh, 1999; Johnston, 1998; Melzack & Kate, 2001).

A mother's responsiveness to her infant's signals and pain is important for developing their personal relationship and the child's social and cognitive competence. While interacting, both mother and infant emit signals to capture each other's attention and to indicate whether to join, sustain, or terminate their interaction. Maternal sensitivity to these signals is a central feature in the development of optimal or secure attachment (Leavitt, 1999).

Maternal love, which may be the core of maternal behavior, is essential for the mother-infant attachment relationship and is important for the infant's development and mental health. Little has been known about these neural mechanisms in human mothers, and the relationship between maternal love, pain and infant behavior, however.

When first-time mothers see their own infant's face, an extensive brain network seems to be activated wherein affective and cognitive information may be integrated and directed toward motor/behavioral outputs. Dopaminergic reward-related brain regions are activated specifically in response to happy, but not sad, infant faces.

304 Clinical Hypnosis in Pain Therapy and Palliative Care

Understanding how a mother responds uniquely to her own infant when she or he is smiling or crying, may be the first step in understanding the neural basis of mother-infant attachment and relief from pain and suffering (Strathearn, Li, Fonagy & Montague, 2008). The single cue of a screwed up or distressed-looking face is the strongest predictor, and on its own correctly classified 87 percent of pain and nonpain episodes (Stallard et al., 2002). Children rapidly develop an extensive vocabulary to describe pain between twelve and thirty months of age, with words for pain from injury emerging first and reflecting the development of normal speech acquisition.

The differences in verbal expressions in the context of illnesses and injuries suggest that children make a cognitive distinction between the origins and the sensory aspects of pain. These findings can help parents and childcare and healthcare professionals to appreciate the early communication capabilities of young children and to engage in more effective pain assessment and management for young children (Franck, Noble & Liossi, 2010).

Adequate reliability and validity documentation is lacking for behavioral observations; consequently, most such observations offer only a second-best approximation of the child's experience, even though clinicians often attribute greater importance to nonverbal expression than to self-report (Craig, 1992). Observations are problematic in that the stimulus for behaviors or changes is not always clear. For example, children cry in response to pain, as well as fear, loneliness, and overstimulation.

Infants and children with an intellectual disability are sometimes unable to verbalize and describe their painful experience; therefore, family members and health professionals can assess the intensity of the pain only from the behavior exhibited by the children.

Pain expression modalities are extremely different between children able to verbalize their pain and those unable to do so (Dubois, Capdevila, Bringuier & Pry, 2008). There is the necessity to take into account the particularities of each child in order to individualize the pain management and avoid misdiagnosis and the undertreating of pain in nonverbal children. The verbal indications of pain in children are are much less common than in adults. They may not understand a term, such as "pain." They speak globally, such as "I don't feel good," or deny pain for fear of being given an injection. They may cry, scream, groan, or moan or use a variety of words to describe pain, such as ow, boo-boo, ouch, hurt.

C. Pain Treatment in Children

Pain and suffering, are managed within a therapeutic alliance among the child, his or her parent(s), nurses, physicians, and other health-care professionals. The beliefs and preferences of the child and family should be elicited, respected, and carefully considered. At the same time, the primary obligation of the health-care professional is to ensure safe and competent care. The presence of divergent beliefs and goals among members of the team can interfere with effective pain and symptom management, but these can often be resolved through discussion and negotiation. Medical interventions include analgesics, adjuvant agents (e.g., corticosteroids, tricyclic antidepressants, stimulants), palliative chemotherapy, radiation therapy, regional analgesia-anesthesia, and neurosurgical approaches. In most cases, analgesics either alone or supplemented with chemotherapeutic agents, radiation therapy, and adjuvants provide adequate pain relief. Regional analgesia-anesthesia is occasionally helpful.

In children with chronic pain in palliative care we have to use the WHO's pain ladder. If pain occurs, there should be prompt oral administration of drugs in the following order (WHO):

1. nonopioids (aspirin and paracetamol)
2. then, as necessary, mild opioids (codeine)
3. then strong opioids such as morphine, until the patient is free of pain

To calm fears and anxiety, additional drugs, "adjuvants," should be used. To maintain freedom from pain, drugs should be given "by the clock." In other words, every three to six hours, rather than "on demand" (WHO). This three-step approach of administering the right drug, in the right dose, at the right time, is inexpensive and 80 to 90 percent effective. Local anesthesia and regional nerve block anesthesia or surgical intervention on appropriate nerves may provide further pain relief, if drugs are not wholly effective.

The physical examination should include an appropriately directed neurological and musculoskeletal evaluation. Appropriate diagnostic procedures may be conducted as part of a patient's evaluation, based on a patient's clinical presentation. The choice of an interventional diagnostic procedure (e.g., selective nerve root blocks, medial branch blocks) should be based on the patient's specific history and physical examination and anticipated course of treatment. Standard dosing of opioids adequately treats most cancer pain in children; however, a significant group requires more extensive management. These problems occur more commonly among patients with solid tumors metastatic to the spine and major nerves (Collins, Grier, Kinney & Berde, 1995).

Drugs for cancer and chronic pain include anticonvulsants, antidepressants, benzodiazepines, N-methyl-D-aspartate receptor antagonists, nonsteroidal anti-inflammatories, opioid therapy, skeletal muscle relaxants, and topical agents (American Society of Anesthesiologists, 2010).

The purpose of these guidelines for chronic pain management is to optimize pain control, enhance functional abilities and physical and psychological well-being, enhance quality of life, and minimize adverse outcomes. The psychosocial evaluation should include information about the presence of psychological symptoms (e.g., anxiety, depression, or anger), psychiatric disorders, personality traits or states, history of substance in adolescents or current medication use or misuse, and coping mechanisms.

D. Psychological and Behavioral Factors in Pain Treatment in Children and Adolescents

Children and adolescents with chronic illnesses or cancer present an exceptional stress. The emotional needs of adolescents with cancer are a serious factor in the recommendation for the establishment of adolescent cancer units, in major cancer centers, and parental anxiety scores, especially those of mothers, is much higher than reported norms (Allen, Newman & Souhami, 1997).

In a study conducted at the Royal Children's Hospital, Melbourne, parents of children who had died of cancer over the period from 1996 to 2004 were interviewed between February 2004 and August 2006. Parents also completed and returned self-report questionnaires. Eighty-four percent of parents reported that their child had suffered "a lot" or "a great deal" from at least one symptom in their last month of life, most commonly pain (46%), fatigue (43%), and poor appetite (30%). Of the children treated for specific symptoms, treatment was successful in 47 percent of those with pain, 18 percent of those with fatigue and 17 percent of those with poor appetite. Relatively high rates of death at home, and low rates of unsuccessful medical interventions suggest a realistic approach at the end of life for Australian children dying of cancer. Many suffer from unresolved symptoms, however, and greater attention should be paid to palliative care for these children (Heath et al., 2010).

What is needed is a systematic and comprehensive approach to all children with significant life-threatening diseases to ensure that their special needs are met. If timely palliative care is to be available to the terminally ill child, a shift in perspective is required as to how and when such support is introduced. Developing resources with the people who provide frontline care for these children and their families enables health professionals to assume this special aspect of care with more confidence and competence.

In children and adolescent, nonpharmacological methods demonstrated efficacy for procedures–lumbar punctures, bone marrow aspirations, biopsies and anesthesiology procedures–and include

1. clinical hypnosis used in the therapy of pain, suffering, and procedures in children (Brugnoli, 2009, Jensen & Patterson, 2006; Richardson, Smith, McCall & Pilkington, 2002; Ziltzer & LeBaron, 1982).
2. a multidimensional psychological intervention that includes disctraction, breathing exercises, relaxation, reinforcement, and imagery (Brugnoli, A., 2005; Brugnoli, M. P., 2009; Jay et al., 1985).

Clinical hypnosis appears effective in reducing pain and anxiety in children undergoing lumbar punctures (Accardi & Milling, 2009). Lumbar puncture, also known as spinal tap, involves the removal of cerebral spinal fluid from the spinal canal. This fluid contains glucose, proteins, white blood cells, and many other substances that are also found in blood. Doctors use lumbar punctures to diagnose and monitor many different severe neurological diseases, including cancers of the spinal cord and brain.

Hypnosis was shown to be more effective than nonhypnotic techniques were for reducing procedural distress in children and adolescents with cancer (Zeltzer & LeBaron, 1982). As defined by the American Cancer Society, hypnosis "is a state of restful alertness during which a person can be relatively unaware of, but not completely blind to, their surroundings."

A team of researchers in the psychology department at the University of Wales conducted a controlled clinical trial of eighty pediatric cancer patients between the ages of six and sixteen. Each group of children received one of four different types of treatment:

1. direct hypnosis with standard medical treatment
2. indirect hypnosis with standard medical treatment
3. attention control with standard medical treatment
4. standard medical treatment alone.

Standard medical treatment for all patients consisted of lumbar puncture. Patients who underwent hypnosis, direct or indirect, reported less anxiety and pain than did their unhypnotized counterparts. In addition, all the forms of hypnosis appeared equally effective. Hypnotized patients were also rated by the investigators as demonstrating less behavioral distress than the control groups did. An important factor associated with the efficacy of hypnosis was the ease with which a patient could become hypnotized. These British researchers concluded that hypnosis appears effective in preparing children with cancer for lumbar puncture and procedures (Liossi & Hatira, 2003). A comprehensive, methodologically informed review of studies of the effectiveness of hypnosis for reducing procedure-related pain in children and adolescents was provided. To be included in the review, studies were required to use a between-subjects or mixed model design in which hypnosis was compared with a control condition or an alternative intervention in reducing the procedure-related pain of patients younger than age nineteen. An exhaustive search identified thirteen studies satisfying these criteria. Hypnosis was consistently found to be more effective than control conditions were in alleviating the discomfort associated with bone marrow aspirations, lumbar punctures, voiding cystourethrogram, and post-surgical pain (Accardi & Milling, 2009).

2. PERCEPTION, CONSCIOUSNESS, AND HYPNOSIS IN PEDIATRIC AGE

We can understand the use of clinical hypnosis in children's pain if we know the different interpretative hypotheses (according to the different approach of various theoretical trends or schools of thought) concerning the cognitive and the consciousness development.

A. Perception and Mind in Children

How do perception and consciousness develop in children? What role does experience play? Are there distinct phases in development? Is there a general common sequence in such phases? Psychology is called to answer to such and many other questions. To exemplify, we could distinguish between two major schools, very far apart on the value to assign to experience.

The first school (Langer, 1973) recognizes–through theorization and empirical research–a key role for environmental influence. The individual development will be achieved modeling oneself to personal experience. Although a radically empiric interpretation of development finds less and less success nowadays, for many years, huge branches of developmental psychology were influenced by this model (Bandura, 1963; Skinner, 1959).

On the other hand, the second school–which includes Werner and Piaget among its most important scholars–assigns to the mind an active role in structuring the experience. According to this theory, the development takes place through a self-constructive activity that takes the child from a primitive stage, to more and more evolute ones.

As far as movement is concerned, we can say that a certain amount of physical exercise corresponds to a primary bodily need (Stevens, 1950).

Werner upholds the idea that the main principle of development has to be sought in the progressive differentiation of mental structures and distinctions and simultaneously in their advanced integration.

The mind is equipped with a self-regulation system aimed to balance the structure once an imbalance has occurred, either in one of its parts or in its whole. So the psychophysical balance becomes the fundamental element in the mental development because it does not simply "repair" the disturbance caused by experience but tends to restore the balance, considering both the disturbing elements and the mechanism activated by them. Therefore, the new balance will reach a higher level of organization. The latest generated mental action could then integrate and anticipate eventual future disturbances. This information is extremely relevant for the use of hypnosis in pain therapy. The cognition development in a child will have a spiral progression in which experience plays a key role in the coordination with the preexistent balance (Piaget, 1972; Travis, Arenander & Dubois, 2004).

In 1915, Groos already advanced the hypothesis that, in children, game represents a way to exert the same capabilities necessary at a more adult age to sustain anxiety itself, and even tensions generated by the relation with the world.

Cognitive abilities do not occur in isolation. Infants remember the items they have attended to and perceived, and their emotional state will influence their perception and representation of the events they encounter. Moreover, by examining the development of the whole cognitive system, or the whole child, we gain a deeper understanding of mechanisms developmental change (Oakes, 2009). Game has also to be seen as an organized expression of the primary needs of perception and manual ability (Benedetti, 1969). We should add that the role of the game in the hypnologic approach is really crucial, as will be explained later.

As far as the relationship psyche-soma is concerned, it is by now consolidated, so that the quantity of sensory information reaching the cortex can change with the variation of the state of consciousness. The sensory information reaches its apex in the states of selective attention, which do not necessarily correspond to the awake state and do not necessarily decrease in the absence of attention. The important research conducted on the subject by Hernandez Peon deserves a mention. He demonstrated that distraction induces a reduction in potentials in the visual cortex, evoked by flashing lights, until their complete disappearance for the modest intensity of the stimuli. Vice versa, the neurological reaction becomes iterative as a consequence of the increasing of the attention. The control of sensory information by central structures begins at a peripheral level, for example, retinal (Hernandez-Peon & Hagbarth, 1955) or cochlear, and then at reticular formation. Only a minimum part of the sensorial stimulation, as Moruzzi states, becomes probably part of our perceptive process.

Moruzzi could demonstrate this phenomenon through an electrophysiological study of sleep. He observed that the great activity of cortical neurons did not decrease compared to the awake state. The discharge of the labyrinthic receptors or of the retina, in a dark environment, are all examples of an independent nervous activity of consciousness. This research is extremely interesting for a better study of the psyche (Moruzzi, 1981; Wong et al., 2007; McKown & Strambler, 2009).

Perception of the dispositions of others, revealed by movements, is an essential ingredient of adaptive daily life social behavior. Brain's imaging points to several brain regions, involved in visual processing of social interaction, represented by the motion of geometric shapes.

Keeping in mind that successful visual social perception depends on intact communication throughout the brain, we focus here on analysis of the induced gamma neuromagnetic response to social interaction revealed by motion. A peak of induced gamma activity of 62 Hz was found at first from the stimulus onset over the right parietotemporal junction. Two further enhancements in gamma response of lower frequency of 44 Hz, occurred at 1.4 seconds over the medial prefrontal and posterior temporal cortices in the right hemisphere. Subsequent boosts of 44 Hz were found at 1.6 seconds over the left temporal and right posterior temporal cortices. For the first time, the findings identify the cortical network engaged in visual processing of social interaction, revealed by motion, and help to better understand proper functioning of the social brain circuitry (Pavlova, Guerreschi, Lutzenberger & Krägeloh-Mann, 2010). Neurophysiology also considers the possibility that the limits of unconscious could not be defined simply by the organic structure. The way in which the latter is used, especially in the human being (as Moruzzi noted), depends, for the most part, on the individual cultural formation, imagination, personality, and psyche (Eccles, 1966; Franck, Noble & Liossi, 2010).

Currently it is necessary to conceive in a dynamic way even the boundary between conscious and unconscious phenomena. The integration of all these data through a long learning process, constitutes the so-called "subjective integration" (Held, 1961). Consciousness poses the most enigmatic problems in the science of the mind. There is nothing that we know more familiarly than conscious knowledge, but there is nothing that is harder to explain. There is not just one problem of consciousness. Consciousness is an unclear term, referring to many different phenomena. Each of these phenomena needs to be explained, but some are easier to explain than others.

According with the philosopher David Chalmers, it is useful to divide the associated problems of consciousness into "hard" and "easy" problems. The easy problems of consciousness are those that seem directly susceptible to the standard methods of cognitive science, whereby a phenomenon is explained in terms of computational or neural mechanisms. The hard problems are those that seem to resist those methods (Chalmers, 1998). In line with Chalmers, the hard problems are related to these phenomena:

- The ability to discriminate, categorize, and react to environmental stimuli
- The integration of information by a cognitive system
- The different states of consciousness
- The ability of a system to access its own internal states
- The focus of attention
- The deliberate control of behavior
- The difference between awake state and sleep

The really hard problem of consciousness is the problem of experience. When we think and perceive, there are billions of pieces of information processing, but there is also a subjective aspect (Chalmers, 1998).

Damasio has suggested that the senses of vision, hearing, touch, taste and smell function by nerve activation patterns that correspond to the state of the external world. Emotions are nerve activation patterns that correspond to the state of the internal world. If we experience a state of fear, then our brains will record this body state in nerve cell activation patterns obtained from neural and hormonal feedback, and this information may then be used to adapt behavior appropriately. Emotions are based on internal body environment and act as input into the brain, just as visual or auditory information is an input to the brain from the external environment. Certainly in evolutionary terms, the brain is primarily an organ for homeostasis, a center that collects and collates feedback on body states and performs to maintain constancy of the internal environment. This concept vastly clarifies the role and nature of emotions and allows them to be studied using the full force of integrated modern neuroscience (Damasio, 1999).

We have already considered how, from a neurophysiological point of view, soma and psyche constitute a wholeness. Now it is important to analyze a new acquisition of modern neurophysiological thought: the involvement of emotions in perception.

The relevancy of the interaction between emotions and perceptions has already been demonstrated by several studies, and it has been shown in the congenital defects observed after a parietal damage. In this case we are in front of both a sensorial deficit and an emotional deficit for everything lying in such a space (Benedetti, 1969; Franck, Noble & Liossi, 2010).

Emotions exemplified well how an increasing of adaptability, in conjunction with the activation of an automatism suitable to predispose a prompt and appropriate body reaction, corresponds to the occurrence of unconscious process and mechanisms (Bandura, 2001). Emotions also clarify how the persistence of unconscious mechanisms could constitute an obstacle on the path of personal growth and of social progress.

Whereas in some cases, a good chunk of our intelligence and cultural realization is due to emotions, in other situations, we are able to preserve our well-being only by keeping them under control.

When we talk about relaxation and clinical hypnosis techniques in children, we earlier underlined how the soma-psyche interaction is important for the understanding of neuropsychomotricity. We have to remember also that knowledge about this interaction is in ongoing evolution and represents a vast sector of research. Psychomotricity plays a key role in individual development, and this premise makes it important to understand both the relation perception-soma-psyche and the hypnosis techniques.

It is useful to recall Milton H. Erickson's experiences in pediatric hypnosis since they could demonstrate themselves to be suitable for a wide range of situations.

As we said, a change in the state of consciousness could modify cortex perceptions, increasing their amount in a state of concentration and new abilities (Benedetti, 1969; Travis, Arenander & DuBois, 2004). This underlines the advantage in the formation of a balance in the psychosomatic development. Whereas psychomotricity develops only a deeper awareness of motion, relaxation techniques, including hypnosis, facilitate a deeper level of self-motion consciousness and a better perception of one's own body. Moreover, they help (through the data perceived and known during a situation of muscular relaxation and calmness) the self.

In pediatrics, according to Erickson, any kind of therapist-patient interaction has to be specifically adapted to the child, since he has his own needs. This requires an accurate physical and psychic assessment of the patient age. Therefore, any intervention must be based on the own child needs and never on an arbitrary classification. The psychologically oriented treatment, if used in an appropriated way, must refer to the child capability of expressing his feelings and of understanding the events.

The relaxation and hypnosis techniques used on children are the ones usually employed with adult patients. The only difference lies in the administration of the treatment. It is important to keep in mind that a child is indeed a "complete" person though a young and little one. His view of the world (and of the events) is not the adult's views. His experiences and his knowledge are limited and different. When we use the relaxation or hypnosis techniques with a child, the central aim is to make him understand in a more complete and in a better way, what is happening around him.

This "modus operandi" is not always necessary with adult patients and makes the use of specific techniques easier with a child, for in pediatric age, there is a pressing need of knowing and discovering.

Since relaxation, especially with hypnotic techniques, entails a deeper awareness, it could also offer a child a new and easy area of psychomotor exploration (Erickson, 1978). This work has to match with the child dignity, with his experiences, and with all he learned during his life. It would be a huge mistake to talk to the pediatric patient in a childish way or, even worse, to look down on him. It is therefore crucial that the therapist-patient interaction be first of all an interaction between "two persons."

The therapist must present to the patient a serious concept with sincerity in order to reach a common goal through a mutual understanding.

Independently of the age, the patient should never sense the presence of a threat. The adult physical or intellectual strength, his authority, and his status are so much superior to the child's that their undue use represent a threat to his adequacy as an individual. The effective verbalization of pain requires progressive cognitive development and acquisition of social communication skills.

Use of self-report in pediatric pain assessment assumes children have acquired a capacity to understand and use common words to describe pain (Stanford, Chambers & Craig, 2005). Because a child cannot rely on a solid ground of experiences, a therapist will necessarily work with the patient and not on the patient. It should be always kept in mind that for a child it is not easy to accept a passive participation in the treatment. It is fundamental to address a pediatric patient without altering the usual tone of voice and way of talking.

The best way to establish a relationship with a child is to use a familiar language and to support what is explained with images and ideas suitable for catching his attention. Talking to a child in a puerile way is usually perceived as some sort of insult because any average intelligent child knows that an adult can talk perfectly. It is also necessary to respect the child's ability without ever minimizing it, to grasp most concepts. It gives a better result to hope in a better understanding, rather than to hurt the patient by implying a lack of knowledge on his part.

Any child must be respected as a thinking being. He has his own feelings, he can formulate thoughts and ideas. He is also able to integrate his thoughts with his experience even if he has to do that according to his way of relating with the world (Erickson, 1978). No adult can do this for him, and this should always be taken into consideration in whatever therapeutic approach to a child.

The relaxation and hypnosis techniques to administer to children are often for them, the most intuitive ones. The treatment should resemble a game to which the child can respond actively and so personally participate in the development of a therapy. A child has an extraordinary power of imagination, and his curiosity, along with his quickness, enable him to have a competent and satisfying reaction to the most variegate techniques. The most adequate results have been achieved by giving a child the satisfaction of having learned something new.

Erickson reports an interesting example concerning the use of hypnotic relaxation technique in pediatrics. He describes the case of a very belligerent two-year-old girl. She did not want to deal with anyone, and she was ready to keep her position by all means. Erickson had noticed that the girl's favorite toy was a little rabbit. He therefore approached the girl in a challenging way by saying,

> I think your rabbit does not know how to sleep.
> "Oh no, my rabbit knows how to sleep," and the battle had so started.
> "Even if you show him how to sleep I think your rabbit is not able to lie down putting his head on the pillow."
> "The rabbit is able to do so. Look!"
> "And can he stretch his/its legs and arms as you do?"
> "Yes he can! Look!"
> "And can he also close his eyes, breath deeply and fall asleep?"
> "The rabbit sleeps."

The last declaration was made with some sort of satisfaction. The girl and her rabbit fell asleep and kept sleeping in a state of deep relaxation.

In this particular case, the adopted technique consisted of meeting the girl at her level, as an individual, and in second instance, in presenting ideas to which she could actively respond. So she was able to participate to the achievement of a common goal acceptable for both her and her therapist (Erickson, 1978).

The described technique of indirect suggestion can be useful to approach a child during procedures, in an emergency room, in a doctor's office, as well as in palliative care. It is in fact easy enough to make a toy by blowing up a latex glove and then painting eyes and a mouth on it. The reason for the success of this trick is simple: in pediatric psychology the main duty of a doctor or therapist is to meet the child's immediate needs. This is what the child can grasp, and once his needs have met it has also been created a better situation in which to treat him.

If it is necessary to treat a pediatric patient with any "traumatic therapy" or procedures (i.e., injections, stitches etc.), however, it is probably better to implement a different technique. In fact, Erickson describes another interesting way to deal with a pediatric patient suffering from a severe pain. The child, according to Erickson, wants not only sympathy but also the acknowledgement of his pain. This implies that there should not be a falsification of the real situation.

Another effective behavior could be helping the pediatric patients to develop their self-esteem with direct suggestions. This should be obtained by using affection rather than severity, by showing care for the children's needs (either physical or cognitive), and by the demonstration of knowing how to do interesting and beautiful games. To all of this should also be added the use of positive motivations.

One could therefore follow the interiorization of experiences with the subsequent reinforcement of the self, along with an ability to express opinions and of taking decisions on the basis of rational and objective considerations (Petter, 1989; Travis, Arenander & DuBois, 2004). Erickson describes in this regard to an episode of his family life. His three-year-old son had fallen down the stairs; he broke his lip and one tooth dug into his lower jaw. The child was bleeding profusely, and he was crying out in pain and fear. Erickson got near his son and, while the latter had momentarily stopped crying in order to breathe, said in a affable but firm voice, "It hurts, I know it hurts terribly." The child understood that his father recognized his pain. Then Erickson added, "And it will keep hurting."

It is never emphasized enough that one of the most important things in pediatric psychology is to talk to the pediatric patient in a sympathetic and understanding way. He should always feel that we grasped his situation and we know perfectly that he is suffering. Erickson kept talking to his son, "I know you would like the pain to stop." By saying so, he recognized the child's urgent need that the pain stop. Only at this point, Erickson said to the child with a certain confidence, knowing that only then the information could be accepted: "Maybe in a couple of minutes it won't hurt so much." This sort of direct suggestion perfectly harmonizes with the patient needs, and it can therefore be easily accepted.

A central point of this therapy is represented by the understanding of the rational meaning of the injuries, of the pain, and of the physical damage.

This had implied the acknowledgment of what was important for the child who—as a consequence—cooperated in the treatment of the traumatic event (Erickson, 1978). The example just described is a direct suggestion and a hypnosis technique.

The work on the patient started with the first sentence addressed to him. It became more obvious when the child began to pay attention to whatever was happening around him, during the medical treatment of his problem.

Never was he lied to and never was he given false information in conflict with the reality and with his understanding capability. In situations such as the one described, the patient has a strong and urgent need of seeing somebody taking care of him. The acknowledgment of such a need, along with the promptness in acting on the cause of the need, constitutes a very effective suggestion. It indeed helps the therapist in gaining the patient's complete cooperation, to adopt the adequate therapy.

As far as the "going through the body," clinical hypnosis and the relaxation techniques (for example, the Jacobsonian ones) are concerned, they can surely help the child in a variety of situations in which it could be necessary for some kind of relaxation. They are also indicated in specific situations, however. They can indeed represent a therapy even in acute and chronic pain disorders.

Children's palliative care encompasses the clinical, psychological, ethical, and spiritual aspects of care for children with life-threatening and life-limiting conditions. Children affected by these conditions have unique and multiple care needs that are very different from those of adults. Whereas in some countries child-specific palliative care services and practices have been in place for a number of years, in many others the recognition of needs and the development of dedicated pediatric palliative care services are still at an early stage.

3. DISTRACTION, RELAXATION, AND HYPNOSIS TECHNIQUES FOR CHILDREN

To ensure the best pain control, support has to be offered right from the first intrusive procedure in order to avoid anticipatory anxiety. Respiration, relaxation, visualization, desensibilization through the "switch technique" and the "magic glove," distraction and involvement, and muscular relaxation all have the common aim of focusing the child's mind and attention away from body perception of pain connected to the procedure. Different methods are utilized depending on the child's age and the level of consciousness required for the procedure:

    A. Distraction Techniques
    B. Relaxation Techniques
    C. Clinical Hypnosis Techniques

A. Distraction Techniques

A few simple techniques can make a difference in a child's hospital experience. Considering areas such as distraction, environment, positioning, and language may help a child have a positive hospital experience. Giving patients something else to focus on is especially effective. Age-appropriate distraction facilitates coping, helps manage pain, decreases the use of pharmacological methods, and builds trust between the staff and patient (Sharar et al., 2008).

Using Play Therapy in Pediatric Palliative Care: Listening to the Story and Caring for the Body

Parents and caregivers of dying children are generally the primary decision-makers in the child's care and can find the transition from active to palliative care particularly difficult. Nurses who understand the parents' perspective can better support them.

To be greatly comprehensive, palliative care for children must address more than pain control and symptom management (Van Breemen, 2009). Holistic care also encompasses attention to the child's relationships, hopes, fears, and wishes. Children reveal their hopes and fears through play. By being attuned to symbols and themes in play, nurses can better interpret the child's journey. Nurses can facilitate communication and connection between parents and children.

The Technique of Play by Play in Pain Procedures

Increase a child's understanding by explaining each step of the painful procedure and what to expect and telling him a story within a story. A story within a story, is a literary device or conceit in which one story is told during the action of another story (the procedures). Stories within stories can be of these types:

1. The inner story is told completely in the real world and could be extracted and told separately
2. Only fragments of it exist in the real world
3. None of the text of the inner story exists in the real world

THE TREASURE BOX. A box with small gifts or toys can be given to the child during or after their procedures. It is a behavioral intervention (the Treasure Chest) that employs the behavior modification techniques of self-monitoring and positive reinforcement to increase adherence to therapy in children (Cass, Talavera, Gresham, Moser & Joy, 2005).

THE PINWHEELS (ORIGAMI). Pinwheel (origami) is a type of traditional origami form that can be used as a toy pinwheel, as a base for more complicated models, or as a component of modular origami.

THE MAGIC BLANKET. We can give "magic powers" to a blanket for relaxation, comfort, and protection.

THE MAGIC WAND. For children, the plastic "wands" with shiny stars inside can be used for diversion

The Choices. Let the child have choices if any are possible, such as pop-up books. Reading and using the pop-ups can allow mind stimulation and distraction and may divert the child and alleviate some anticipatory pain. Be permissive regarding when pain will go away.

THE BLOWING BUBBLES. Blowing bubbles relaxes children by slowing and deepening the breath. Helping children experience fun, engaging activities is important. Not only does it keep them happy, creating positive bonds between the child and the family, it also encourages healthy development. In the early years, providing a variety of stimulations actually encourages the development of the brain. No wonder bubble blowers are one of the world's oldest and most popular toys. Children have to blow out air repeatedly during the injection, or procedures, as if they are blowing bubbles.

A simple distraction technique can be effective in helping children cope with the pain. The use of such a technique to relieve the pain and distress associated with even a brief painful procedure should be encouraged (French MD, Painter & Coury, 1994).

Counting

Have the school-age child count during a difficult part of the treatment or procedures:

> . . . Allow yourself to feel passive and indifferent . . .
> Counting each breath slowly from 10 to 1 . . .
> With each count feel yourself more and more relaxed . . .
> With each exhale allow the tension to leave your body . . .

The Use of Virtual Reality for Pain Control

Virtual reality is a relatively new technology that enables individuals to immerse themselves in a virtual world. This multisensory technology has been used in a variety of fields and most recently has been applied clinically as a method of distraction for pain management during medical procedures. Investigators have posited that virtual reality creates a nonpharmacological form of analgesia by changing the activity of the body's intricate pain modulation system (Mahrer & Gold, 2009).

Pain management in cancer patients is primarily achieved by potent pharmacological analgesics (e.g., opioids) but is necessarily complemented by nonpharmacological techniques, including distraction or hypnosis. Immersive virtual reality provides a particularly intense form of cognitive distraction during such brief, painful procedures and has undergone preliminary study by several research groups treating burn patients over the past decade.

Immersive virtual reality is logistically feasible, safe, and effective in ameliorating the pain and anxiety experienced in various settings of pain. Furthermore, the technique appears applicable to a wide age range of patients and may be particularly well-adapted for use in children (Sharar et al., 2008).

Emotions are often object related. It is yet an open question whether emotions and the associated perceptual contents that they refer to are processed by different parts of the brain or whether the brain regions that mediate emotions are also involved in the processing of the associated content they refer to. Using fMRI, it was demonstrated that simply combining music (rich in emotion but poor in information about the concrete world) with neutral films (poor in emotionality but rich in real-world details) yields increased activity in the hippocampus and lateral prefrontal regions. The finding that these regions, the heart of the emotional brain, respond increasingly to an emotional stimulus when they are associated with realistic scenes supports a fundamental role for concrete real-world content in emotional processing (Eldar, Ganor, Admon, Bleich & Hendler, 2007).

Mindfulness: Look Around You

Mindfulness is the here-and-now approach to living that makes daily life richer and more meaningful. It is approaching life like a child, without passing judgment on what occurs. Mindfulness means focusing on one activity at a time, so forget multitasking! Staying in the present tense can help promote relaxation and provide a buffer against anxiety and depression.

Practice it by focusing on your immediate surroundings. If you are outdoors, enjoy the shape and colors of flowers, hear a bird's call, or consider a tree. In the mall, look at the details of a dress in the window, examine a piece of jewelry and focus on how it is made, or window-shop for furniture, checking out every detail of pattern and style. As long as you can keep your mind focused on something in the present, stress will take a back seat. Attentional and emotional states alter the way we perceive pain. Recent findings suggest that the mechanisms underlying these two forms of pain modulation are at least partially separable. This concept is supported by the observation that attention and emotions differentially alter the sensory and affective dimensions of pain perception and apparently implicate different brain circuits (Villemure & Schweinhardt, 2010).

The Distancing From Pain

. . . Moving self away from pain, for example, imagine going to a favorite place
. . . Moving pain away from self, for example, imagine putting the discomfort in a balloon and watching it float away.
. . . Transferring it to another part of the body, for example, put all the discomfort in the little finger of the right hand.

Music

Music helps to soothe or distract, especially when the child picks the music. Music can calm the heartbeat and soothe the mind. So, when the going gets rough, take a musical stress detour by aligning your heartbeat with the slow tempo of a relaxing song.

Language and music, two of the most unique human cognitive abilities, are combined in song, rendering it an ecological model for comparing speech and music cognition. Variations in musical features affect word processing in sung language. Implications of the interactions between words and melody are discussed in light of evidence for shared neural processing resources between the phonological or semantic aspects of language and the melodic or harmonic aspects of music (Gordon et al., 2008).

Singing (Play Songs and Lullabies)

A child who has not gone too far in fear or anxiety may be soothed with singing or being sung to. Preverbal infants are conditioned to the different emotional messages contained in play songs and lullabies. However, it is unclear which performance properties of singing underlie infants' perception of the communicative intent of infant-directed singing. The overall pitch of a song is communicative to infants, and the affective nature of music can affect infants' pitch preferences (Tsang & Conrad, 2010). Lullabies promote new awareness, adaptation, and expression. A music therapist can enable the lulling through providing opportunities for music-contextualized "restorative resounding," expressed psychobiologically, verbally, musically, and metaphorically (O'Callaghan, 2008).

Pawuk and Schumacher introduced music therapy in hospice and palliative care. An eight-year-old boy with cancer wrote songs and records for a CD for his family. This demonstrates the role that music therapy plays in attending to the physical, emotional, and spiritual needs of hospice and palliative care patients and families while respecting their dignity and celebrating their lives (Pawuk et al., 2010).

The Diversional Talk

Talking about the weather, your last vacation, the child's family, an so on, with a comforting, rhythmic voice, can be calming.

Show Some Love, Give Your Patient a Fast Hug, at Least Once a Day

Induce the relaxation response by cuddling your pet, giving or receiving an unexpected hug with a friend or family member, snuggling with your spouse, or talking to a friend about the good things in your lives. When you do, you will be reducing your stress levels (Vincent, 2005). Social interaction helps your brain think better, encouraging you to see new solutions to situations that once seemed impossible. Physical contact, like petting your dog or cat or soft toys, may actually help lower blood pressure and decrease stress hormones.

Massage and Self-Massage

Massage is a very good way to release tension on the muscles. Exercise and massages are great ways to relax and can be very helpful in relieving pain and tension from muscles. Soft tissue massage is currently used in palliative care for the relief of anxiety and pain. Patients in palliative care can received soft tissue massage (hand or foot) every day. Soft tissue massage appears to be an appreciated source of support to dying patients in palliative care. The method is easy to comprehend and relatively short (20 minutes) which may imply that it is a suitable complement in nursing care for the patient (Cronfalk, Strang, Ternestedt & Friedrichsen, 2009).

Providing gentle massage to children is one of the great joys a massage therapist and a child can experience. Children respond very differently to touch and are often willing and excited recipients. Typically, they like to engage more actively than adults when receiving massage and a variety of different techniques can be used to enhance their massage experience. Surprisingly, pediatric massage is a field that has been given very little attention until now.

Powell, Cheshire, and Swaby (2010) studied children's experiences of their participation in a training and support program involving massage. This study reports on a research project that aimed to extrapolate the value of the Training and Support Programme, involving massage among children with cerebral palsy. Results showed that children enjoyed the relaxing aspects of massage and reported a number of improvements in their health, such as improved muscle relaxation, mobility and bowel movements and reduced pain.

Pediatric massage is a natural extension of working with the whole family in chronic pain relief and in cancer pain. At the University of Minnesota School of Nursing, massage therapy was studied for children with cancer. This pilot study aimed to determine the feasibility of providing massage to children with cancer to reduce symptoms in children and anxiety in parents. Changes in relaxation (heart and respiratory rates, blood pressure, and salivary cortisol level) and symptoms (pain, nausea, anxiety, and fatigue) were assessed in children. Anxiety and fatigue were measured in parents. Massage was more effective than quiet time was at reducing heart rate in children, anxiety in children less than fourteen years of age, and parent anxiety (Post-White et al., 2010). Pediatric massage differs from infant massage and includes massage for toddlers, preschool and school-age children, and adolescents and young adults.

There is some evidence to support the use of massage therapy to improve quality of life for people living with HIV/AIDS, particularly in combination with other stress-management modalities (Hillier, Louw, Morris, Uwimana & Statham, 2010).

Children at each stage of growth and development have different physical, emotional, and psychological needs. One of the pleasures of massaging children is that practitioners become attuned to providing what is needed at each life stage, and the relationship between the massage therapist and child evolves over time. Physiologically, children's bodies differ from adult bodies in significant ways. In children, the nervous system develops progressively and is somewhat predictive by age. For this reason, massage therapists working with children need to practice ongoing communication so they can best understand the sensations that children are feeling. Open communication is a key element of massaging children.

Light, calming strokes and feather touch create physical and emotional patterns of deep relaxation. Deepening and slowing of the breath and relaxed blood flow to the hands and feet are greatly desired.

A SIMPLE MASSAGE OR SELF-MASSAGE TECHNIQUE

Place both hands on your shoulders and neck . . .
Squeeze with your fingers and palms . . .
Rub sweet, keeping shoulders relaxed . . .
Wrap one hand around the other forearm . . .
Squeeze the muscles with thumb and fingers . . .
Move up and down from your elbow to fingertips and back again . . .
Repeat with other arm

For massage on children you can use simple, moderate-pressure strokes to the child's head and neck, arms, torso, legs, and back. Dividing time between these areas, say 4 minutes each, will address the full body and is enough to get the desired effect. Most children do fine fully clothed. A comfortable bed or chair in a quiet room is best. For parents seeking skilled bodywork for their kids, the massage is a great choice, done for about 20 to 30 minutes at a time.

In the process of maturing from infancy to adolescence, significant emotional and psychological development takes place. At each stage of growth and development, there are important considerations for massage therapists.

Verbal and nonverbal communication significantly affect whether children and adolescents feel safe and enjoy the massage. In approaching children and adolescents, friendly body language is important. For very young children, maintaining close proximity to the parent can minimize tension. When possible, clearly establishing a positive relationship with the parent can help the child to relax.

Many health-care professionals have long known the benefits of massage therapy for their pediatric patients. Massage has been shown to be beneficial to children with chronic pain. We highly recommend massage therapy for newborns, sick children, those with chronic disease, and those at end of life. Massage is an effective therapy for treatment of somatic pain of subhealth without adverse reactions and it should be generalized to application (Pang et al., 2010).

Soothing Touch

Rhythmic touch alleviates loneliness and fear and promotes relaxation in infants and children. The role of infant touch during early mother-infant interactions is very important. The way in which infant touch is organized with gaze and affect changes with the interactive context and underscores the important regulatory, exploratory, and communicative roles of touch during early socioemotional development (Moszkowski, Stack & Chiarella, 2009).

Distraction with the Magic Glove

For children age three to ten, the Magic Glove can be a simple distraction technique or a hypnotic technique if there is a deeper trance. According to Leora Kuttner, it can be used for blood draws, injections, and procedures. It may also be used on different areas of the body and presented as a magic patch, hat, sock, and so on. For a simple distraction technique, begin by explaining to the children that are in awake state that you will be teaching them a "special way" to help them change how much they feel. You can say that "you may feel something, but it will not bother you" or "I can help you change how your arm feels." It's important to avoid saying, "you won't feel any pain." Explain to the caregivers that you are teaching the children a strategy to help them use their mind to minimize their level of pain.

Begin by "testing" each arm prior to the placement of the Magic Glove. Apply equal pressure with the tip of a pencil to test each arm. Ask the child where you can press on each arm. Tell the child that you will press gently on each arm and full sensation should be felt. Reinforce the point that there is full sensation now and there will be less feeling after the Magic Glove is on. Ask the child to rate the feeling: a little, a lot, or not at all. This is not a pain assessment, just a feeling assessment. Ask the patient to put the hand or arm into yours to relax. You might say, "Relax into my hand or arm."

You may ask the child, "Where would you like the glove to begin and end?" Focus your touch on that area, making sure that you include the site of the needle insertion. Take the Magic Glove out of your pocket and stroke gently upward over designated area. Do this four to six times. Include the fingers as well. Enhance sensory focus on the glove by talking about it (Kuttner, 1991, 1996).

Positioning

Hold the younger child in any position that is most comforting and supportive to him or her.

Take an Attitude Break

Thirty seconds is enough time to shift your heart's rhythm from stressed to relaxed. The way to do that is to engage your heart and your mind in positive thinking. Start by envisioning anything that triggers a positive feeling, a vision of your parents or friends, the image of your pet, a memento from a vacation, whatever it is, conjuring up the thought will help slow breathing, relax tense muscles, and put a smile on your face. Creating a positive emotional attitude can also calm and steady your heart rhythm, contributing to feelings of relaxation and peace.

B. Relaxation Techniques

Children are not immune to stress and pain; it is an inevitable part of existence for everyone. Given the right tools, however, children can learn to effectively manage pain's suffering.

The Deep Breathing

Deep breathing is very useful for any person. Your child can learn to take a breath hold it and then release it; this slows breath, blood pressure, and heart rate and will feel healthier. Conversely, becoming aware of our breathing and learning to slow down and deepen each breath allows us to feel more relaxed. Becoming aware of our breathing is a simple strategy.

> Breathing involves taking a moderately deep breath in through nose and, pausing only briefly, letting the air out slowly through your nose . . .
> The slow gentle exhale is the key to sigh breathing . . .
> Be sure to lengthen your outward breath . . .
> Now, as you breathe out let go . . . relax your muscles of your face . . . your jaw and your shoulders . . .
> Let go of tension in your chest and stomach . . .
> Let your arms and legs relax . . .
> As your breath out feel a wave of relaxation, flow from the top of your head and all the way down to your feet. . . . As you continue to breathe in this manner for at least 10 to 20 cycles, direct your attention outside yourself . . .
> And deeper . . . and deeper . . . you relax your body . . . and your mind.

Breathe Deeply

Feeling stressed evokes tense, shallow breathing, while calm is associated with relaxed breathing. So to turn tension into relaxation, change the way you breathe.

> Let out a big sigh . . . dropping your chest . . . and exhaling through gently pursed lips . . . Now imagine your low belly . . . or center . . . as a deep . . . powerful place . . .
> Feel your breath coming and going as your mind stays focused there . . .
> Inhale . . . feeling your entire belly . . . sides and lower back expand
> Exhale . . . eeling peace and relaxation
> Repeat ten times, relaxing more fully each time.

The Progressive Muscles Relaxation

PMR is a technique of stress management developed by American physician Edmund Jacobson in the early 1920s. Jacobson argued that since muscular tension accompanies anxiety, one can reduce anxiety by learning how to relax the muscular tension. Jacobson trained his patients to voluntarily relax certain muscles in their body in order to reduce anxiety symptoms. PMR involves alternately tensing and relaxing the muscles.

A child, practicing it like play, may start by sitting or lying down in a comfortable spot and taking some deep breaths, and then he or she will proceed to tense, then relax, groups of muscles in a prescribed sequence (one such sequence is starting with the hands and moving up to the arms, shoulders, neck, and head and then down the torso and legs to the feet). You are going to focus on different muscles of the body and relax them in a progressive way. For example, you can focus on your arms, stretch them, hold them, and then release them at the same time that you release your breath.

The Progressive Muscle Relaxation of Jacobson in Children

- Assume a comfortable position. Your entire body, including your head, should be supported.
- We will try to pay attention to the feelings of muscular relaxation and tension.
- When you tense a particular muscle group, do so vigorously without straining, for 7 to 10 seconds.
- Concentrate on what is happening. Feel the buildup of tension in each particular muscle group. It is often helpful to visualize the particular muscle group being tensed.
- When you release the muscles, do so abruptly, and then relax, enjoying the sudden feeling of limpness.
- Allow the relaxation to develop for at least 15 to 20 seconds before going on to the next group of muscles.

Now tense forcefully all the muscles in your body. All the muscles will now become tight and tense.
Now tense forcefully the following muscles:
- legs: tense energetically . . . suddenly let go . . . relax and breathe
- gluteus: tense energetically . . . suddenly let go . . . relax and breathe
- abdominal: tense energetically . . . suddenly let go . . . relax and breathe
- back: tense energetically . . . suddenly let go . . . relax and breathe
- chest: tense energetically . . . suddenly let go . . . relax and breathe
- neck: tense energetically . . . suddenly let go . . . relax and breathe

- forehead: tense energetically . . . suddenly let go . . . relax and breathe
- shoulders: tense energetically . . . suddenly let go . . . relax and breathe

Now let go of all the tension and relax your body completely . . .
Feel the immediate well-being sensation . . .
Mentally scan your body for any residual tension . . .
If a particular area remains tense . . . repeat one or two tense-relax cycles for that group of muscles . . . Now imagine a wave of relaxation slowly spreading throughout your body . . . gradually penetrating every muscle group . . . and relax your body.

The immediate effects of PMR, include all the benefits of the relaxation mind-body response. The long-term effects of regular practice of PMR include

- A decrease in generalized anxiety
- A decrease in anticipatory anxiety related to procedures
- Reduction in the frequency and duration of panic attacks in chronic pain
- Improved ability to face pain situations through graded exposure
- An increased sense of control over moods
- Increased self-esteem

There are no contraindications for PMR. The effect of the tension-relaxation sequence is to cause deeper relaxation than would be achieved by simply attempting to relax.

Visualization, Metaphors, and Imagery

Visualization, metaphors, and imagery are very useful ways to relax children. The children should imagine beautiful places, with peace, and happiness and with people that they love.

Several lines of evidence suggest that mental motor imagery is subserved by the same cognitive operations and brain structures that underlie action. Additionally, motor imagery is informed by the anticipated sensory consequences of action, including pain (Coslett, Medina, Kliot & Burkey, 2010).

Imagery is an important aspect of teaching children any symbolic language. Before the age of 6, a child must have a rich imagination to master this relationship between symbols. Imagination helps us to create. By previsualizing things, it can then be transferred to paper, to the action in the physical world to create. Imagination creates the whole universe, and it is essential in the evolution of humans.

Another important aspect of imagination is that it allows the psyche to experience things safely. The psyche does not know the difference if something is real or imagined. Mythic play and visualization give a safe container to act out negative feelings, fears or aggressions, and desires that human's experience. We need to visualize things that give us pleasure to evoke that feeling within and satisfy ourselves. Bringing imagination to a child's world is one of the most important things we can do. We can easily explore and develop the vastness of a child's inner world through storytelling and also guided relaxations using imagery.

Allow children to create their own images that are appealing to them. What do they like? What makes them happy? Allow them to imagine people they love. You can create guided visualizations by starting one off on a journey, beginning with a place, such as a forest, outer space, a boat sailing to an island. Have them imagine it in detail. What sounds, smells, and sights do they experience? You can add characters, such as an animal guide, a fairy, a person who greets them. What happens next? Have them reach a special place. What is it? A bubbling pot, a magic door, a secret well? What comes out of it? What message is there for them? What image, object, animal is there just for them? Have them return, saying goodbye, returning with a magical object that was found, having a feeling of safety, comfort, joy, pain relief or relaxation.

Audiorecorded Guided Imagery

Audiorecorded guided imagery is a home-based, guided imagery treatment protocol, using audio and video recordings; it is easy for health-care professionals and patients to use, is inexpensive, and is applicable to a wide range of health-care settings. Guided imagery treatment plus medical care is superior to standard medical care only for the treatment of pain (van Tilburg et al., 2009).

C. Clinical Hypnosis Techniques for Children

Hypnosis and Self-Hypnosis in Children

Hypnosis is an altered state of consciousness. Some people describe hypnosis as a normal state of focused attention. They say they feel very relaxed and calm. During hypnosis, the mind is more open to suggestion than usual (Brugnoli, 1974). Hypnosis is a natural mental state. For example, children are often in a state of self-hypnosis when they are playing imaginary games. Children are open to suggestion while in a hypnotic state; they can learn to change their thoughts, feelings, behavior, and attitudes. Children can take these changes that happen during hypnosis and use them for self-improvement in their usual state of consciousness. Hypnosis can be used to help reduce anxiety, control pain, control the perception of discomfort during medical procedures, and lessen discomfort of physical symptoms.

There is broad agreement that a phenomenon we call hypnosis exists (Sutcher H., 2008). With children, the world revolves around them until experience helps expand that world. Because they are the center, everything is where they are.

When children are experiencing unrelenting stress or are worried, whether or not they are conscious of it, there are warning signs for those who have the eyes to see.

The imagination of children is very keen until parents, teachers, and others interfere. In many schools, the style of teaching in the classroom can tend to rule out the playful and imaginative, once children pass the second or third grade. When adults consider daydreaming worthless, when they call attention to its "cuteness," and associate imagination with lying, or otherwise imply ridicule and disbelief, the child gradually lets it weaken.

The doorway between the conscious and the unconscious mind is the imagination. For children, it is relatively easy to reach at the deepest levels in much less time than required by a good many adults. Stories, adventures, visualization, imaginative games, role-playing, magic, puppets, and costumes work most effectively with children. Any tools that stimulate the imagination should be at the hypnotherapist's disposal.

Hypnosis is an example of dissociation, whereby areas of an individual's behavioral control separate from ordinary awareness. Hypnosis would remove some control from the conscious mind, and the individual would respond with autonomic, reflexive behavior. Weitzenhoffer describes hypnosis via this theory as "dissociation of awareness from the majority of sensory and even strictly neural events taking place."

When a child is hypnotized, it might be that his or her imagination is dissociated and sends the imagined content back to the sensory cortex, resulting in dreams or visualizations, or that some senses are dissociated, resulting in hypnotic anesthesia. According to recent evidence, neurophysiological processes coupled to pain are closely related to the mechanisms of consciousness. This evidence is in accordance with findings that changes in states of consciousness during hypnosis strongly affect conscious perception and experience of pain and markedly influence brain functions. Past research indicates that painful experience may induce dissociated state, and information about the experience may be stored or processed unconsciously.

Reported findings suggest common neurophysiological mechanisms of pain and dissociation and point to a hypothesis of dissociation as a defense mechanism against psychological and physical pain that substantially influences functions of consciousness. The hypothesis is also supported by findings that information can be represented in the mind or brain without the subject's awareness. The findings of unconsciously present information suggest possible binding between conscious contents and self-functions that constitute self-representational dimensions of consciousness. The self-representation means that certain inner states of one's own body are interpreted as mental and somatic identity, whereas other bodily signals, currently not accessible to the dominant interpreter's access, are dissociated and may be defined as subliminal self-representations (Bob, 2008).

Techniques of Indirect or Direct Suggestions

THE INDIRECT SUGGESTIONS. The specific use of any word is important in indirect suggestions:

> "That hand" rather than "your hand"
> "Pretend for a while that . . .
> doesn't belong to you, think of it as a part of a sculpture or toy. . . ."

We can consider hypnosis delivered through immersive virtual reality (Patterson, Wiechman, Jensen & Sharar, 2006).

THE DIRECT SUGGESTIONS FOR ANALGESIA AND ANESTHESIA IN CHILDREN

> Request for numbness
> Re-create positive anesthetic experience
> "Imagine painting a numbing medicine on . . ."
> "Imagine putting an anesthetic into . . ."

DIRECT SUGGESTIONS: THE MAGIC GLOVE (IN HYPNOSIS STATE) FOR CHILDREN AGE 3 TO 10. In the hypnotic technique, we use a deeper relaxation state and trance than we did in the distraction technique. Hypnoanalgesia using The Magic Glove dramatically reduces the child's pain and anxiety when a medical procedure is necessary.

1. Explain that you are going to apply the Magic Glove to protect his arm. "You will know what is going on but you won't be bothered. You'll feel some pressure, but it won't bother you."

2. You have to induce the child in a deep relaxation and hypnotic state.
3. Use firm strokes over the child's hand, over each finger, up over the wrist, up to the elbow and the upper arm.
4. Stroke firmly but gently, repeating that the glove is going to protect hum.
5. Test that the other hand has full sensation with a pencil tip and test the arm with the Magic Glove.
6. Confirm the difference with the child.
7. Now the medical procedure can be started.

When the procedure is finished, "remove the glove," wake up the child, and test that there is no longer a sensation difference.

Deep Hypnosis Techniques in Children

Going into a trance is a skill. For many things, ultra-deep trances are not necessary. If you are going to create anesthesia in pain therapy or have some need to create a deeper hypnotic phenomenon, having a deeper trance is helpful.

The technique for deep hypnosis should contain three types of suggestions: (1) Deepening suggestions, (2) Suggestions that each time the children are hypnotized, they more easily and quickly go into a much deeper and relaxing state of hypnosis, and (3) Suggestions that children enjoy hypnosis state.

1. DEEPENING SUGGESTIONS. The deepening suggestions that are easiest to use in this situation are suggestions that relate to breathing, escalators, elevators and counting. Here are some examples:

Breathing

. . . and each and every deep and natural breath you take allows you to deepen your relaxation . . .

Counting

. . . In a moment, I'm going to count from 10 down to 1 . . .
And in allowing each number to help your body grow more relaxed . . .
your mind go more relaxed . . .
so that certain thoughts just fade away . . .
like sand slipping through your fingers . . .
You can find that easy relaxation of mind and body . . .

because of these words . . . just happens now . . .
ten easily relaxing all over again . . .
. . . nine . . . then eight deeper still . . .
. . . feeling great seven . . . six . . . five . . . mind and body relaxed . . .
four . . . relaxing more . . . three then two . . .
your deepening grew at one . . . deep levels . . . going deeper . . .
That's right . . .

Elevators and Escalators

In a moment I'm going to ask you to imagine yourself at the top of an escalator.
I'm going to count down from ten to one . . . as I say the number ten in your
imagination, step onto the escalator . . .
Allow yourself to go deeper into relaxation with each number I say.
When I reach the number 1, step off the escalator into a state of relaxation deeper than you've ever felt before.
ten . . . step on the escalator and go much deeper . . .
nine . . . relaxing more and more with each number . . .
eight . . . allowing yourself to go deeper and deeper with each number . . .
seven . . . each number and each easy, natural breath you take helps you relax
more fully . . .
six . . . five . . . doing deeper into relaxation . . .
four . . . feeling relaxation flow and every area of your body . . .
three . . . two . . . allowing your body feel a wonderful . . . at the relaxation . . .
one . . . now more deeply relaxed than ever before . . .

2. GO MORE EASILY AND QUICKLY GO INTO A MUCH DEEPER AND RELAXING STATE OF HYPNOSIS

. . . And each time you relax yourself . . . you more easily and quickly go into a
much deeper state of hypnosis . . .
. . . And . . . because you are learning . . . really learning what hypnosis is . . .
the next time you are hypnotized you will easily and quickly . . .
effortlessly and wonderfully enter a deep and profoundly useful trance . . .

3. ENJOY GOING INTO THE HYPNOSIS STATE

. . . You enjoy going easily and effortlessly achieving deeper and deeper levels
of hypnosis . . .
In a nutshell, here it is . . .

Create the child deepening hypnosis state with visualizations. Create a
posthypnotic reinduction cue for your subject.

Hypnosis Technique of Visualization
For Older Children or Adolescents

Have the child imagine going to a favorite place, talking with someone special. Try creating a peaceful visualization or "dreamscape."

To start, have the child simply visualize anything that keeps his or her thoughts away from current tensions. It could be a favorite vacation spot, a fantasy island, or something "touchable," such as the feel of silk. The idea is to take the child's mind off her or his stress and replace it with an image that evokes a sense of calm. The more realistic the daydream, in terms of colors, sights, sounds, even touch and feel, the more relaxation he or she will experience.

This hypnosis technique lasts from 3 to 10 minutes.

> . . . As you listen to the words of your inner self . . . picture the images that are
> being described in your mind . . .
> . . . Be open to the relaxation . . . and peace . . .
> My body . . . in time passing by . . .
> is becoming more and more pleasantly calm . . .
> Even more pleasantly calm . . .
> and a feeling of great well-being . . .
> imagine now a beautiful natural place . . . my favorite place . . .
> my favorite place . . .
> and look at the sky . . . look at the sky . . .
> a beautiful blue sky, with a few white clouds . . .
> they move slowly, almost rocking . . .
> a beautiful blue sky, a light breeze that caresses my face . . .
> and the bright sun . . . that gives me new energy . . .
> energy of the body and of the mind . . .
> I find my favorite place . . . in my favorite place . . .
> with beautiful blue sky and white clouds slowly moving . . .
> as time passes . . . time passes . . . and everything inside me becomes serene . . .
> . . . and calm . . . Great calm . . .
> great tranquility . . . it becomes part of me . . . and the time goes by . . .
> I feel well . . . I feel well . . . I feel really well . . .
> and everything else does not bother me anymore . . .

For this exercise repeat the sentences slowly, calmly at least ten times.

Relaxation, Hypnosis, and Music Therapy in Children

In children we can use music with relaxation and hypnosis techniques. There are some types of soft music and classical music that can really help focus and relax the mind. Songs that are recognized by children add to the enjoyment of the music. Therapeutic music helps children fall asleep sooner and with greater peace of mind. Adding nature sounds to music and hypnosis makes the heart rate respond to a slower beat, which in turn relaxes the body and mind.

Children need words, music, and nature sounds to be calmed and relaxed. The nature sounds include ocean waves, birds, ducks, horses, cows, heartbeats, sea gulls, streams, and many more. This is not only for a child's enjoyment; an adult will feel the same peace.

Therapeutic music is a gift to the senses that reassures the child that everything will be alright. Visual objects around the room or about the crib can only serve the child while the eyes are open. Therapeutic music continues to soothe and reassures as the eyes close and peaceful rest sets in (van Tilburg et al., 2009).

Functional neuroimaging studies show that music-evoked emotions can modulate activity in virtually all limbic and paralimbic brain structures. These structures are crucially involved in the initiation, generation, detection, maintenance, regulation and termination of emotions that have survival value for the individual and the species. Therefore, at least some music-evoked emotions involve the very core of evolutionarily adaptive neuroaffective mechanisms (Koelsch, 2010).

The origins of using music in hypnosis are not easy to find, but there are a few hints. Before the general use of the record player in the twentieth century, the hypnotherapist was limited to visual induction methods or the use of the humble metronome. The metronome is still in use today by some practitioners for inductions. It is a repetitive, slow, monotonous stimulus that focuses the conscious mind, allowing the hypnotherapist to communicate directly to the subconscious. We can use the metronome in hypnosis or music, with the power and the rhythm of words. Rhythm is what makes music and hypnosis move and flow. Rhythm is made up of sounds, emotions, and silences.

Music is capable of evoking exceptionally strong emotions and of reliably affecting the mood of individuals. The functional imaging studies, conducted so far on the investigation of emotion with music basically showed involvement of limbic and paralimbic cerebral structures (such as the amygdala, hippocampus, parahippocampal gyrus, temporal poles, insula, ventral striatum, orbitofronal, as well as cingulate cortex) during the processing of music with emotional valence, such as pleasant places (Koelsch, 2005).

Hypnosis in children works well because there are fewer years of reinforcing imprints on one's mind. Children are more susceptible to hypnosis. They have the drive to discover, and they hunger for new experiences.

Children are usually easily relaxed and focused. In order for this to happen, it is necessary to do a connection with the child, to give him the possibility of communicating with the adult, as well as he could do with a friend of the same age (and even better). Never has he to feel judged or being asked to be different. He must feel accepted as he is, so a therapist will be able to interest him in learning the physical and mental training necessary to reach a partial state of calm. Through this step, he will have the chance to excel in any situation because he will be able to exert an extraordinary self-control.

Another crucial moment of the therapy is represented by the explanation to the child how calm is the most important characteristic of a strong man. The information should be enriched with simple but effective examples taken from real life. The therapist could take a basketball player as a model: a champion waits for the right moment before launching the ball, he does not lose control, and then he scores a basket. This arouses the child's curiosity and makes the child willing to start training as soon as possible. He will sense that in this way that through relaxation, he could empower his capabilities, and he will be able to feel his spaces. Creativity is fundamental for the cognitive and emotional development of any child. First of all, it increases the quality of his thoughts, and second it makes the child understand his fears. Therefore, it enables him to get through them (Biondi, 1984).

So even in the pediatric patient the conscious and unconscious relationship acquires a key role only if we deal with the patient as with a complete being capable of self-regulation. The pediatric patient is, in fact, provided with a system of "self-able" to integrate the various functions necessary for interacting with the different situations one has to face in life. It is important to add that the state of calm, reached through relaxation and hypnosis techniques, showed itself to be therapeutic and anxiolytic. It could eliminate fears, and it could provide support.

In the end, it should be considered that in pediatrics, relaxation and hypnosis techniques have several uses, but it is necessary to keep in mind a few key steps: (1) to establish immediately a good relationship with the child and (2) to maintain his motivation high in pain therapy (Ferioli, 1974). The benefits of the therapeutic effect of hypnosis techniques are especially significant when either there is an urgent need of a state of relaxation we are in front of chronic diseases. In this last situation, the therapist—through relaxation and/or hypnosis—will be able to intervene precociously without leaving unresolved problems, which could become more difficult to treat with time.

Greater attention to symptom and pain control and the overall well-being of children with advanced disease might ease their suffering. Recognition of this problem by the medical community should prompt efforts to improve both communications between parents and caregivers and the quality of life for children who are dying of cancer and their family (Pearson, 2010).

Children are not supposed to die. Parents expect to see their children grow and mature. Ultimately, parents expect to die and leave their children behind. This is the natural course of life events, the life cycle continuing as it should. The loss of a child is the loss of serenity. The theme of parental mourning has been a universal one throughout the centuries. In the literature on bereavement, writers repeat certain themes, thoughts, and reflections; they talk of the powerful and often conflicting emotions involved in "the pain of grief and the spiral of mourning."

Sociologists and psychologists describe parental grief as complex and multilayered and agree that the death of a child is an incredibly traumatic event, leaving parents with overwhelming emotional needs. They also agree that this grief must be acknowledged and felt in its intensity. Death is an experience that is common to all mankind, an experience that touches all members of the human family. Death transcends all cultures and beliefs; there are both commonality and individuality in the grief experience. When a loved one dies, each person reacts differently. A child's death, however, is such a wrenching event that all affected by it express sadness and dismay and are painfully shaken.

Moreover, those who seek to comfort grieving parents need to recognize and understand the complexities of the parents' emotions and should avoid relying on preconceived ideas about the way a couple is supposed to grieve if their child dies. Reactions of grieving parents may seem overly intense, self-absorbing, contradictory, or even puzzling. For bereaved parents, the death of a child is such an overwhelming event that their responses may often be baffling not only to others but also to themselves. It is important obtaining help from traditional support systems, such as family, friends, professionals, or church groups; undergoing professional counseling; joining a parent support group, or acquiring information on the type of death that occurred as well as about their own grief (Warland, O'Leary, McCutcheon & Williamson, 2010).

REFERENCES

Accardi, M. C., & Milling, L. S. (2009). The effectiveness of hypnosis for reducing procedure-related pain in children and adolescents: A comprehensive methodological review. *Journal of Behavioral Medicine, 32*(4), 328–339.

Allen, R., Newman, S. P., & Souhami, R. L. (1997). Anxiety and depression in adolescent cancer: Findings in patients and parents at the time of diagnosis. *European Journal of Cancer, 33*(8), 1250–1255.

American Society of Anesthesiologists Task Force on Chronic Pain Management, American Society of Regional Anesthesia and Pain Medicine. (2010). Practice guidelines for chronic pain management: An updated report by the American Society of Anesthesiologists Task Force on Chronic Pain Management and the American Society of Regional Anesthesia and Pain Medicine. *Anesthesiology, 112*(4), 810-833.

Andrews, K., & Fitzgerald, M. (1997). Barriers to optimal pain management in infants, children, and adolescents: Biological barriers to paediatric pain management. *Clinical Journal of Pain, 13*(2), 138–143.

Bandura, A. (1963). *Social learning and personality development.* New York: Holt, Rinehart & Winston.

Benedetti, G. (1969, April).The unconscious from the neuropsychological viewpoint [Review]. *Der Nervenarzt, 40*(4), 149–155.

Biondi, M. (1984). I 4 canali del rapporto mente-corpo: dalla psicofisiologia dell'emozione alla psicosomatica scientifica. *Med. Psic., 29,* 421–456.

Boudarene, M., Legros, J. J., & Timsit-Berthier, M. (2002). Study of the stress response: Role of anxiety, cortisol and DHEAs. *L'Encephale, 28*(2), 139–146.

Brugnoli, A. (2005). *Stati di coscienza modificati neurofisiologici.* Verona, Italy: La Grafica Editrice.

Collins, J. J., Grier, H. E., Kinney, H. C., & Berde, C. B. (1995). Control of severe pain in children with terminal malignancy. *The Journal of Pediatrics, 126*(4), 653–657.

Craig, K. D. (1992). The facial expression of pain: Better than a thousand words? *APS Journal, 1*(3), 153–162.

Dubois, A., Bringuier, S., Capdevilla, X., & Pry, R. (2008). Vocal and verbal expression of postoperative pain in preschoolers. *Pain Management Nursing, 9*(4), 160–165.

Durrmeyer, X., Vutskits, L., Anand, K. J., & Rimensberger, P. C. (2010). Use of analgesic and sedative drugs in the NICU: Integrating clinical trials and laboratory data. *Pediatric Research, 67,* 117-127.

Eccles, J. C. (1966, July14). The ionic mechanisms of excitatory and inhibitory synaptic action. *Annals of the New York Academy of Sciences, 137*(2), 473–494.

Erickson, M. H. (1978a). *La mia voce ti accompagnerà.* Rome, Italy: Casa Editrice Astrolabio.

Erickson, M. H. (1978b). *Le nuove vie dell'ipnosi.* Rome, Italy: Casa Editrice Astrolabio.

Ferioli, W. (1976). *Introduzione all'impiego dell'ipnosi in pediatria.* Verona, Italy: Istituto H. Bernheim.

Franck, L., Noble, G., & Liossi, C. (2010). Translating the tears: Parents' use of behavioural cues to detect pain in normally developing young children with everyday minor illnesses or injuries. *Child: Care, Health and Development, 36*(6), 895–904.

Heath, J. A., Clarke, N. E., Donath, S. M., McCarthy, M., Anderson, V. A., & Wolfe, J. (2010). Symptoms and suffering at the end of life in children with cancer: An Australian perspective. *The Medical Journal of Australia, 192*(2), 71–75.

Hernandez-Peon, R., & Hagbarth, K. E. (1955). Interaction between afferent and cortically induced reticular responses. *Journal of Neurophysiology, 18*(1), 44–55.

Hester, N. O., Foster, R., & Kristensen, K. (1990). Measurement of pain in children: Generalizability and validity of the pain ladder and the poker chip tool. In D. C. Tyler & E. J. Krane (Eds.), *Pediatric pain* (Vol. 15. Advances in Pain Research and Therapy, pp. 79–84). New York: Raven Press, Ltd.

Jensen, M., & Patterson, D. R. (2006, February). Hypnotic treatment of chronic pain. *Journal of Behavioral Medicine, 29*(1), 95–124.

Kuttner, L. (1991). Helpful strategies in working with pre-school children in pediatric practice. *Pediatric Annals, 20*(3), 120–127.

Kuttner, L. (1996). *A child in pain: A guide for parents.* Seattle, WA: Hartley & Marks Publishers, Inc.

Langer, J. (1973.) *Teorie dello sviluppo mentale.* Barbera, Italy: Giunti.

Latremoliere, A., & Woolf, C. J. (2009). Central sensitization: A generator of pain hypersensitivity by central neural plasticity. *Journal of Pain, 10*(9), 895–926.

Legrain, V., Van Damme, S., Eccleston, C., Davis, K. D., Seminowicz, D. A., & Crombez, G. (2009). A neurocognitive model of attention to pain: Behavioral and neuroimaging evidence. *Pain, 144*(3), 230–232.

Liossi, C., & Hatira, P. (2003). Clinical hypnosis in the alleviation of procedure-related pain in pediatric oncology patients. *The International Journal of Clinical and Experimental Hypnosis, 51,* 4–28.

Loizzo, A., Loizzo, S., & Capasso, A. (2009). Neurobiology of pain in children: An overview. *The Open Biochemistry Journal, 3,* 18–25.

McGrath, P. J., & Unruh, A. M. (1999). Does gender affect appraisal of pain and pain coping strategies? *Clinical Journal of Pain, 15*(1), 31–40.

Melzack, R., & Katz, J. (2001). The McGill Pain Questionnaire: Appraisal and current status. In D. C. Turk & R. Melzack (Eds.), *Handbook of pain assessment* (2nd ed., pp. 35–52). New York: Guilford Press.

Moruzzi, G. (1981). *Fisiologia della vita di relazione.* Torino, Italy: UTET.

O'Rourke, D. (2004, June). The measurement of pain in infants, children, and adolescents: From policy to practice. *Physical Therapy, 84,* 560–570. Available at physicaltherapyjournal.com

Petter, G. (1989). *Dall'infanzia alla preadolescenza.* Barbera, Italy: Giunti.

Pruessner, J. C., Dedovic, K., Pruessner, M., Lord, C., Buss, C., Collins, L., ..., & Lupien, S. J. (2010). Stress regulation in the central nervous system: Evidence from structural and functional neuroimaging studies in human populations. *Psychoneuroendocrinology, 35*(1), 179–191.

Richardson, J., Smith, J. E., McCall, G., & Pilkington, K. (2006). Hypnosis for procedure-related pain and distress in pediatric cancer patients: A systematic review of effectiveness and methodology related to hypnosis interventions. *Journal of Pain and Symptom Management, 31*(1), 70–84.

Silva, Y. P., Gomez, R. S., Máximo, T. A., & Silva, A. C. (2007). Pain evaluation in neonatology. *Revista Brasileira de Anestesiologia, 57,* 565–574.

Smart, K., & Doody, C. (2007). The clinical reasoning of pain by experienced musculoskeletal physiotherapists. *Manual Therapy, 12*(1), 40–49.

Stallard, P., Williams, L., Velleman, R., Lenton, S., McGrath, P. J., & Taylor, G. (2002, July). The development and evaluation of the pain indicator for communicatively impaired children (PICIC). *Pain, 98*(1–2), 145–149.

Strathearn, L., Li, J., Fonagy, P., & Montague, P. R. (2008). What's in a smile? Maternal brain responses to infant facial cues. *Pediatrics, 122*(1), 40–51.

Vincent, J. L. (2005). Give your patient a fast hug (at least) once a day. *Critical Care Medicine, 33*(6), 1225–1229.

Weisman, S. J., Bernstein, B., & Schechter, N. L. (1998). Consequences of inadequate analgesia during painful procedures in children. http://archpedi.jamanetwork .com/article.aspx?articleid=189261 *Archives of Pediatrics & Adolescent Medicine, 152*(2), 147–149.

SUGGESTED READINGS

Acute Pain Management Guideline Panel. (1992). Acute pain management: Operative or medical procedures and trauma. Clinical practice guideline. AHCPR Pub. No. 92-0032. Rockville, MD: Agency for Health Care Policy and Research, Public Health Service, U.S. Department of Health and Human Services.

Aldrich, S., & Eccleston, C. (2000). Making sense of everyday pain. *Social Science and Medicine, 50*(11), 1631–1641.

American Academy of Pediatrics. (2005). AAP Publications Retired and Reaffirmed. *Pediatrics, 115,* 1438.

American Academy of Pediatrics, Committee on Pediatric Emergency Medicine. (1995). Guidelines for pediatric emergency care facilities. *Pediatrics, 96*(3), 526–537.

American College of Emergency Physicians. (1995). Pediatric equipment guidelines. *Annals of Emergency Medicine, 25,* 307–309.

American College of Emergency Physicians. (1997). Emergency care guidelines. *Annals of Emergency Medicine, 29,* 564–571.

American Medical Association Commission on Emergency Medical Services. (1990). Pediatric Emergencies. An excerpt from "Guidelines for Categorization of Hospital Emergency Capabilities." *Pediatrics, 85,* 879–887.

Andrè, T. A., & de Ajuriaguerra, J. (1948). *L'axe corporel. Muscolature et innervation.* Masson.

Arntz, A., Dreessen, L., & Merckelbach, H. (1991). Attention, not anxiety, influences pain. *Behaviour Research and Therapy, 29,* 41–50.

Athey, J., Dean, J. M., Ball, J., Wiebe, R., & Melese-d'Hospital, I. (2001). Ability of hospitals to care for pediatric emergency patients. *Pediatric Emergency Care, 17*(3), 170–174.

Atlas, L. Y., Bolger, N., Lindquist, M. A., & Wager, T. D. (2010). Brain mediators of predictive cue effects on perceived pain. *Journal of Neuroscience, 30,* 12964–12977.

Axia, G. (1986). *La mente ecologica. La conoscenza dell'ambiente nel bambino.* Barbera, Italy: Ed. Giunti.

Bandura, A., Barbaranelli, C., Caprara, G. V., & Pastorelli, C. (2001). Self efficacy beliefs as shapers of children's aspirations and career trajectories. *Child Development, 72*(1), 187–206.

Bantick, S. J., Wise, R. G., Ploghaus, A., Clare, S., Smith, S. M., & Tracey, I. (2002). Imaging how attention modulates pain in humans using functional MRI. *Brain, 125*(2), 310–319.

Bell, R. F., Wisloff, T., Eccleston, C., & Kalso, E. (2006). Controlled clinical trials in cancer pain. How controlled should they be? A qualitative systematic review. *British Journal of Cancer, 94*(11), 1559–1567.

Beyer, J. E., McGrath, P. J., & Berde, C. B. (1990). Discordance between self-report and behavioral pain measures in children aged 3–7 years after surgery. *Journal of Pain and Symptom Management, 5*(6), 350–356.

Boichat, C., Keogh, E., & Eccleston, C. (2011). *Higher General Distress is Related to Quicker Disengagement From Threat: Differences Between Supraliminal and Subliminal Presentation.* Presented at the British Pain Society Annual Conference, June 21–24, 2011, Edinburgh.

Brainard, D. H. (1997). The Psychophysics Toolbox. *Spatial Vision, 10*, 433–436.

Brown, C. A., & Jones, A. K. P. (2008). A role for midcingulate cortex in the interruptive effects of pain anticipation on attention. *Clinical Neurophysiology, 119*, 2370.

Buhle, J. T., & Wager, T. D. (2010). Performance-dependent inhibition of pain by an executive working memory task. *Pain, 149*, 19–26.

Buhle, J. T., Stevens, B. L., Friedman, J. J., & Wager, T. D. (2012). Distraction and placebo: Two separate routes to pain control. *Psychological Science, 23*, 246–253.

Caes, L., Vervoort, T., Eccleston, C., & Goubert, L. (2012). Parents who catastrophize about their child's pain prioritize attempts to control pain. *Pain, 153*(8), 1695–1701.

California Emergency Medical Services Authority. (1994). *Administration, Personnel, and Policy Guidelines for the Care of Pediatric Patients in the Emergency Department.* EMSC Project, Final Report. Sacramento, CA: California Emergency Medical Services Authority.

Clinch, J., & Eccleston, C. (2009). Chronic musculoskeletal pain in children: Assessment and management. *Rheumatology, 48*(5), 466–474.

Clinch, J., Eccleston, C., Malleson, P. N., & Connell, H. (2002). Chronic pain in adolescents: Evaluation of inter-disciplinary cognitive behaviour therapy. *Arthritis & Rheumatism, 46*(9), S313–S313.

Coghill, R. C., Sang, C. N., Maisog, J. H., & Iadarola, M. J. (1999). Pain intensity processing within the human brain: A bilateral, distributed mechanism. *Journal of Neurophysiology, 82*, 1934–1943.

Cohen, L. L., Vowles, K. E., & Eccleston, C. (2010a). Parenting an adolescent with chronic pain: An investigation of how a taxonomy of adolescent functioning relates to parent distress. *Journal of Pediatric Psychology, 35*(7), 748–757.

Cohen, L. L., Vowles, K. E., & Eccleston, C. (2010b). The impact of adolescent chronic pain on functioning: Disentangling the complex role of anxiety. *Journal of Pain, 11*(11), 1039–1046.

Craig, A. D., Chen, K., Bandy, D., & Reiman, E. M. (2000). Thermosensory activation of insular cortex. *Nature Neuroscience, 3,* 184–190.

Crombez, G., Eccleston, C., Baeyens, F., van Houdenhove, B., & van den Broeck, A. (1999). Attention to chronic pain is dependent upon pain-related fear. *Journal of Psychosomatic Research, 47*(5), 403–410.

Crombez, G., Eccleston, C., De Vlieger, P., Van Damme, S., & De Clercq, A. (2008). Is it better to have controlled and lost than never to have controlled at all? An experimental investigation of control over pain. *Pain, 137*(3), 631–639.

Crombez, G., Eccleston, C., & Van Damme, S. (2004). Hypervigilance and attention to pain. In R. Schmidt & W. Willis (Eds.), *Encyclopaedic reference of pain* (Vol. 2, pp. 919–931). Berlin, Germany: Springer-Verlag.

Crombez, G., Eccleston, C., Van den Broeck, A., Goubert, L., & Van Houdenhove, B. (2004). Hypervigilance to pain in fibromyalgia: The mediating role of pain intensity and catastrophic thinking about pain. *The Clinical Journal of Pain, 20,* 98–102.

Crombez, G., Eccleston, C., Van den Broeck, A., Van Houdenhove, B., & Goubert, L. (2005). The effects of catastrophic thinking about pain on attentional interference by pain: No mediation of negative affectivity in healthy volunteers and in patients with low back pain. *Pain Research & Management, 7,* 31.

Crozier, F., & Hancock, L. E. (2012). Pediatric palliative care. *Pediatric Nursing, 38*(4), 198–203.

Dahlquist, L. M., Gil, K. M., Armstrong, F. D., Ginsberg, A., & Jones, B. (1985). Behavioral management of children's distress during chemotherapy. *Journal of Behavior Therapy and Experimental Psychiatry, 16*(4), 325–329.

De Benedetti, F. (1978). Adolescence and modern mass media. *Minerva Medica, 69*(46), 3198–3201.

De Sousa, R. (1987). *The rationality of emotion.* Cambridge, MA: MIT Press.

Di Stefano, G. (1973). *Lo sviluppo cognitivo.* Barbera, Italy: Giunti.

Duggan, G. B., Keogh, E., Davies, R., Mountain, G., McCullagh, P., & Eccleston, C. (2012). *Inclusive Design and Chronic Pain: Designing Technology to Support Self-Management.* Presented at the British Pain Society Annual Scientific Meeting, April 24–27, 2012, Liverpool.

Durch, J. S., & Lohr, K. N. (Eds.). (1993). *Institute of medicine report: Emergency medical services for children.* Washington, DC: National Academy Press.

Eccleston, C. (1994). Chronic pain and attention: A cognitive approach. *British Journal of Clinical Psychology, 33*(4), 535–547.

Eccleston, C. (1995). The attentional control of pain: Methodological and theoretical concerns. *Pain, 63,* 3–10.

Eccleston, C. (2005). Managing chronic pain in children: The challenge of delivering chronic care in a "modernising" healthcare system. *Archives of Disease in Childhood, 90*(4), 332–333.

Eccleston, C. (2008). Children with chronic widespread pain: Hunting the Snark. *Pain, 138*(3), 477–478.

Eccleston, C. (2010). Evidence based psychological interventions for chronic pain. In K. Stannard & E. Kalso (Eds.), *Evidence-based pain management* (pp. 59–67). Oxford: Wiley-Blackwell.

Eccleston, C. (2011a). *A Cognitive Motivational View of Living With Chronic Pain.* Presented at Frontiers of Pain, The Australian Pain Society 31st Annual Scientific Meeting, June 12–16, 2011, Darwin.

Eccleston, C. (2011b). A normal psychology of chronic pain. *Psychologist, 24*(6), 422–425.

Eccleston, C., & Clinch, J. (2007). Chronic pain and disability: Assessment and treatment in the community. *Pediatrics and Child Health, 12*(2), 117–120.

Eccleston, C., & Crombez, G. (1999). Pain demands attention: A cognitive-affective model of the interruptive function of pain. *Psychological Bulletin, 125*(3), 356–366.

Eccleston, C., & Crombez, G. (2005). Attention and pain: Merging behavioural and neuroscience investigations. *Pain, 113*(1-2), 7–8.

Eccleston, C., & Crombez, G. (2007). Worry and chronic pain: A misdirected problem solving model. *Pain, 132*(3), 233–236.

Eccleston, C., Crombez, G., Scotford, A., Clinch, J., & Connell, H. (2004). Adolescent chronic pain: Patterns and predictors of emotional distress in adolescents with chronic pain and their parents. *Pain, 108*(3), 221–229.

Eccleston, C., Jordan, A. L., & Crombez, G. (2006). The impact of chronic pain on adolescents: A review of previously used measures. *Journal of Pediatric Psychology, 31*(7), 684–697.

Eccleston, C., & Malleson, P. (2003). Managing chronic pain in children and adolescents. *British Medical Journal, 326,* 1408–1409.

Eccleston, C., Palermo, T. M., de C Williams, A. C., Lewandowski, A., Morley, S., Fisher, E., & Law, E. (2009). Psychological therapies for the management of chronic and recurrent pain in children and adolescents. *Cochrane Database Systematic Reviews* (2), CD003968.

Eccleston, C., Wastell, S., Crombez, G., & Jordan, A. (2008). Adolescent social development and chronic pain. *European Journal of Pain, 12*(6), 765–774.

Erickson, M. H., & Rossi, E. L. (1976). Two level communication and the microdynamics of trance and suggestion. *American Journal of Clinical Hypnosis, 18*(3), 153–171.

Erickson, M. H., & Rossi, E. L. (1980). *The nature of hypnosis and suggestion.* New York: Irvington.

Erickson, M. H., Rossi, E. L., & Rossi, S. (1976). *Hypnotic realities: The induction of clinical hypnosis and indirect forms of suggestion.* New York: Irvington.

Evarts, E. (1978). I meccanismi cerebrali durante il movimento. *Le Scienze, 83,* 113–119.

Ewin, D. (1986). The effect of hypnosis and mind set on burns. *Psychiatric Annals, 16,* 115-118.

Fontana, L. (1981). Gli obiettivi psicomotori. *Psicologia e Scuola. Giunti–Barbera 5,* 34–40.

Fourie, D. P. (1997, June). "Indirect" suggestion in hypnosis: theoretical and experimental issues. *Psychological Reports, 80*(3, Pt 2), 1255–1266.

Gauntlett-Gilbert, J., & Eccleston, C. (2007). Disability in adolescents with chronic pain: Patterns and predictors across different domains of functioning. *Pain, 131*(1–2), 132–141.

Geers, A. L., & Lassiter, G. D. (1999). Affective expectations and information gain: Evidence for assimilation and contrast effects in affective experience. *Journal of Experimental Social Psychology, 35,* 394–413.

Goubert, L., Crombez, G., Eccleston, C., & Devulder, J. (2004). Distraction from chronic pain during a pain-inducing activity is associated with greater post-activity pain. *Pain, 110*(1–2), 220–227.

Gross, J. J. (1998). The emerging field of emotion regulation: An integrative review. *Review of General Psychology, 2*(3), 271–299.

Henderson, E. M., Rosser, B. A., Keogh, E., & Eccleston, C. (2012). Internet sites offering adolescents help with headache, abdominal pain, and dysmenorrhoea: A description of content, quality, and peer interactions. *Journal of Pediatric Psychology, 37*(3), 262–271.

Hester, N. O., & Barcus, C. S. (1986). Assessment and management of pain in children. *Pediatric Nursing Update, 1,* 1–8.

Hetz, W., Kamp, H. D., Zimmermann, U., Von Bohlen, A., Wildt, L., & Schuettler, J. (1996). Stress hormones in accident patients studied before admission to hospital. *Journal of Accident & Emergency Medicine, 13*(4), 243–247.

Houde, R. W. (1982). Methods for measuring clinical pain in humans. *Acta Anaesthesiologica Scandinavica, 74*(Suppl), 25–29.

Huguet, A., Eccleston, C., Miro, J., & Gauntlett-Gilbert, J. (2009). Young people making sense of pain: Cognitive appraisal, function, and pain in 8–16 year old children. *European Journal of Pain, 13*(7), 751–759.

Islam, N., Harris, N., & Eccleston, C. (2006). Does technology have a role to play in assisting therapy in a care or home environment? A review of practical issues for health practitioners. *Quality in Aging and Older Adults, 7*(1), 49–56.

Jay, S. M., & Elliott, C. H. (1990). A stress inoculation program for parents whose children are undergoing painful medical procedures. *Journal of Consulting and Clinical Psychology, 58*(6), 799–804.

Jordan, A. L., Eccleston, C., McCracken, L. M., Connell, H., Clinch, J., Sourbut, C. A., & Sleed, M. (2004). Developing an inventory to assess the impact of chronic pain on the lives of adolescents. *Annals of the Rheumatic Diseases, 63*(Suppl 1), 431.

Jordan, A. L., Eccleston, C., & Osborn, M. (2007). Being a parent of the adolescent with complex chronic pain: An interpretative phenomenological analysis. *European Journal of Pain, 11*(1), 49–56.

Keltner, J. R., Furst, A., Fan, C., Redfern, R., Inglis B, Fields, H. L. (2006). Isolating the modulatory effect of expectation on pain transmission: A functional magnetic resonance imaging study. *Journal of Neuroscience, 26*(16), 4437–4443.

Koyama, T., McHaffie, J. G., Laurienti, P. J., & Coghill, R. C. (2005). The subjective experience of pain: Where expectations become reality. *Proceedings of the National Academy of Sciences of the United States of America, 102,* 12950–12955.

Kuttner, L. (1997) Pain management in children. *Child and Adolescent Psychiatric Clinics of North America, 6*(4), 783–796

Kuttner, L. (author). (1998). *No Fears, No Tears–13 Years Later* [videotape]. Available from Fanlight Productions, 4196 Washington Street, Suite 2, Boston MA 02131. Telephone: 800-937-4113; Fax: 617-469-3379.

Kuttner, L. (author). (1985). *No Fears, No Tears: Children With Cancer Coping With Pain* [videotape]. Available from Fanlight Productions, 4196 Washington Street, Suite 2, Boston MA 02131. Telephone: 800-937-4113; Fax: 617-469-3379.

Lazarus, R. S. (1993). Coping theory and research: Past, present, and future. *Psychosomatic Medicine, 55,* 234–247.

Leventhal, H., Brown, D., Shacham, S., & Engquist, G. (1979). Effects of preparatory information about sensations, threat of pain, and attention on cold pressor distress. *Journal of Personality and Social Psychology, 37,* 688–714.

Lorenz, R., Hauck, M., Paur, R. C., Nakamura, Y., Zimmermann, R., Bromm, B., & Engel, A. K. (2005). Cortical correlates of false expectations during pain intensity judgments–A possible manifestation of placebo/nocebo cognitions. *Brain, Behavior and Immunity, 19*(4), 283–295.

Marcoli, A. (2001a). *Il bambino arrabbiato.* Rome, Italy: Oscar Saggi Mondadori.

Marcoli, A. (2001b). *Il bambino nascosto.* Rome, Italy: Oscar Saggi Mondadori.

McCann, J., Wang, H., Zheng, H., & Eccleston, C. (2012). An interactive assessment system for children with chronic pain. In *Proceedings of the IEEE-EMBS International Conference on Biomedical and Health Informatics,* January 5–7, 2012, Hong Kong and Shenzen.

McCaul, K. D., & Haugtvedt, C. (1982). Attention, distraction, and cold-pressor pain. *Journal of Personality and Social Psychology, 43,* 154–162.

McCracken, L. M., Gauntlett-Gilbert, J., & Eccleston, C. (2010). Acceptance of pain in adolescents with chronic pain: Validation of an adapted assessment instrument and preliminary correlation analyses. *European Journal of Pain, 14*(3), 316–320.

McCracken, L. M., MacKichan, F., & Eccleston, C. (2007). Contextual cognitive-behavioral therapy for severely disabled chronic pain sufferers: Effectiveness and clinically significant change. *European Journal of Pain, 11*(3), 314–322.

McCullagh, P. J., Nugent, C. D., Zheng, H., Burns, W. P., Davies, R. J., Black, N. D., ..., & Mountain, G. A. (2010). Promoting behaviour change in long term conditions using a self-management platform. In P. Langdon, P. J. Clarkson & P. Robinson (Eds.), *Designing inclusive interactions* (pp. 229–238). London: Springer.

McGlashan, T. H., Evans, F. J., & Orne, M. T. (1969). The nature of hypnotic analgesia and placebo response to experimental pain. *Psychosomatic Medicine, 31,* 227–246.

McGrath, P., Walco, G., Turk, D., Dworkin, R., Brown, M., Davidson, K., ..., & Zeltzer, L. (2008). Core outcome domains and measures for pediatric acute and chronic/recurrent pain clinical trials: PedIMMPACT recommendations. *Journal of Pain, 9*(9), 771–783.

McQuay, H. J., Derry, S., Eccleston, C., Wiffen, P. J., & Andrew Moore, R. (2012). Evidence for analgesic effect in acute pain-50 years on. *Pain, 153*(7), 1364–1367.

Montgomery, G. H., DuHamel, K. N., & Redd, W. H. (2000). A meta-analysis of hypnotically induced analgesia: How effective is hypnosis? *International Journal of Clinical and Experimental Hypnosis, 48,* 138–153.

Mounce, C., Keogh, E., & Eccleston, C. (2007). *Can We Make Sense of the Various Pain-Related Anxiety and Emotion Measures? Evidence for a Tripartite Structure.* Presented at the British Pain Society Annual Conference, April 22, 2007, Glasgow.

Murphy, T. M. (1986). Treatment of chronic pain. In R. D. Miller (Ed.), *Anesthesia.* New York: Churchill Livingstone.

National Emergency Medical Services for Children Resource Alliance, Committee on Pediatric Equipment and Supplies for Emergency. (1998). Guidelines for pediatric equipment and supplies for emergency departments. *Annals of Emergency Medicine, 31,* 54–57.

Olness, K. (1996). *Hypnosis and hypnotherapy with children.* New York: Guilford Press.

Palermo, T. M., & Eccleston, C. (2009). Parents of children and adolescents with chronic pain. *Pain, 146*(1-2), 15–17.

Palermo, T. M., Eccleston, C., Lewandowski, A. S., de C Williams, A. C., & Morley, S. (2010). Randomized controlled trials of psychological therapies for management of chronic pain in children and adolescents: An updated meta-analytic review. *Pain, 148*(3), 387–397.

Patterson, D. R., & Jensen, M. P. (2003). Hypnosis and clinical pain. *Psychological Bulletin, 129,* 495–521.

Petrovic, P., Petersson, K. M., Ghatan, P. H., Stone-Elander, S., & Ingvar, M. (2000). Pain-related cerebral activation is altered by a distracting cognitive task. *Pain, 85,* 19–30.

Peyron, R., Frot, M., Schneider, F., Garcia-Larrea, L., Mertens, P., Barral, F. G., ..., & Mauguiére, F. (2002). Role of operculoinsular cortices in human pain processing: Converging evidence from PET, fMRI, dipole modeling, and intracerebral recordings of evoked potentials. *NeuroImage, 17*(3), 1336–1346.

Ploghaus, A., Tracey, I., Gati, J. S., Clare, S., Menon, R. S., Matthews, P. M., & Rawlins, J. N. (1999). Dissociating pain from its anticipation in the human brain. *Science, 284*(5422), 1979–1981.

Posner, M. I., Snyder, C. R., & Davidson, B. J. (1980). Attention and the detection of signals. *Journal of Experimental Psychology, 109,* 160–174.

Price, D. D., Milling, L. S., Kirsch, I., Duff, A., Montgomery, G. H., Nicholls, S. S. (1999). An analysis of factors that contribute to the magnitude of placebo analgesia in an experimental paradigm. *Pain, 83*(2), 147–156.

Prkachin, K. M. (2009). Assessing pain by facial expression: Facial expression as nexus. *Pain Research & Management, 14*(1), 53–58.

Raz, A. (2005). Attention and hypnosis: Neural substrates and genetic associations of two converging processes. *International Journal of Clinical and Experimental Hypnosis, 53,* 237–258.

Risdon, A., Eccleston, C., Crombez, G., & McCracken, L. (2003). How can we learn to live with pain? A Q-methodological analysis of the diverse understandings of acceptance of chronic pain. *Social Science and Medicine, 56*(2), 375–386.

Rosser, B. A., & Eccleston, C. (2011). Smartphone applications for pain management. *Journal of Telemedicine and Telecare, 17*(6), 308–312.

Rosser, B. A., Keogh, E., Eccleston, C., & Mountain, G. A. (2010). *SMART2: Development Towards A Technology-Based System for Self-Management off Chronic Pain.* Presented at the ISAP 13th World Congress on Pain, August 29–September 2, 2010, Montreal.

Seminowicz, D. A., & Davis, K. D. (2007). A re-examination of pain-cognition interactions: Implications for neuroimaging. *Pain, 130,* 8–13.

Shih, S., & Sterling, G. (2002). Measuring and modeling the trajectory of visual spatial attention. *Psychological Review, 109,* 260–305.

Sleed, M., Eccleston, C., Beecham, J., Knapp, M., & Jordan, A. (2005). The economic impact of chronic pain in adolescence: Methodological considerations and a preliminary costs-of-illness study. *Pain, 119*(1-3), 183–190.

Solomon, R. (1980). Emotions and choice. In A. Rorty (Ed.), *Explaining emotions* (pp. 251–281). Los Angeles: University of California Press.

Spiegel, D., Kraemer, H., & Carlson, R. (2001). Is the placebo powerless? [Letter]. *New England Journal of Medicine, 345,* 1276.

Sugarmann, L. I. (1996). Hypnosis in a primary care practice: Developing skills for the "new morbidities." *Journal of Developmental and Behavioral Pediatrics, 17*(5), 300–305.

Suls, J., & Fletcher, B. (1985). The relative efficacy of avoidant and nonavoidant coping strategies: A meta-analysis. *Health Psychology, 4,* 249–288.

Tintinalli, J. E. (1996). Emergency medicine. *Journal of the American Medical Association, 275*(23), 1804–1805.

Valente, S. M. (2006, February). Hypnosis for pain management. *Journal of Psychosocial Nursing and Mental Health Services, 44*(2), 22–30.

Valet, M., Sprenger, T., Boecker, H., Willoch, F., Rummeny, E., Conrad, B., & Tolle, T. R. (2004). Distraction modulates connectivity of the cingulo-frontal cortex and the midbrain during pain—an fMR1 analysis. *Pain, 109*(3), 399–408.

Van Damme, S., Crombez, G., & Eccleston, C. (2004). The anticipation of pain modulates spatial attention: Evidence for pain-specificity in high-pain catastrophizers. *Pain, 111*(3), 392–399.

Van Damme, S., Crombez, G., & Eccleston, C. (2008). Coping with pain: A motivational perspective. *Pain, 139*(1), 1–4.

Van Damme, S., Crombez, G., Eccleston, C., & Koster, E. H. W. (2006). Hypervigilance to learned pain signals: A componential analysis. *Journal of Pain, 7*(5), 346–357.

Van Damme, S., Crombez, G., Eccleston, C., & Roelefs, J. (2004). The role of hypervigilance in the experience of pain. In G. J. G. Asmundson, J. W. S. Vlaeyen, & G. Crombez (Eds.), *Understanding and treating the fear of pain* (pp. 71–90). Oxford: Oxford University Press.

Van Damme, S., Crombez, G., Goubert, L., & Eccleston, C. (2009). Current issues and new directions in psychology and health: The costs and benefits of self-regulation—A call for experimental research. *Psychology and Health, 24*(4), 367–371.

Van Damme, S., Crombez, G., Hermans, D., Koster, E. H. W., & Eccleston, C. (2006). The role of extinction and reinstatement in attentional bias to threat: A conditioning approach. *Behaviour Research and Therapy, 44*(11), 1555–1563.

Van Damme, S., Crombez, G., Wiech, K., Legrain, V., Peters, M. L., & Eccleston, C. (2009). Why become more general when we can be more specific? [Comment]. *Pain, 144*(3), 342–343.

Van Damme, S., Lorenz, J., Eccleston, C., Koster, E. H. W., De Clercq, A., & Crombez, G. (2004). Fear-conditioned cues of impending pain facilitate attentional engagement. *Neurophysiologie Clinique = Clinical Neurophysiology, 34*(1), 33–39.

Van Ryckeghem, D. M. L., Van Damme, S., Crombez, G., Eccleston, C., Verhoeven, K., & Legrain, V. (2011). The role of spatial attention in attentional control over pain: An experimental investigation. *Experimental Brain Research, 208*(2), 269–275.

Verhoeven, K., Crombez, G., Eccleston, C., Van Ryckeghem, D. M. L., Morley, S., & Van Damme, S. (2010). The role of motivation in distracting attention away from pain: An experimental study. *Pain, 149*(2), 229–234.

Verhoeven, K., Van Damme, S., Eccleston, C., Van Ryckeghem, D. M. L., Legrain, V., & Crombez, G. (2011). Distraction from pain and executive functioning: An experimental investigation of the role of inhibition, task switching and working memory. *European Journal of Pain, 15*(8), 866–873.

Wager, T. D., Rilling, J. K., Smith, E. E., Sokolik, A., Casey, K. L., Davidson, R. J., ..., & Cohen, J. D. (2004). Placebo-induced changes in fMRI in the anticipation and experience of pain. *Science, 303*(5661), 1162–1167.

Wager, T. D., Scott, D. J., & Zubieta, J. K. (2007). Placebo effects on human [micro]-opioid activity during pain. *Proceedings of the National Academy of Sciences of the United States of America, 104*, 11056–11061.

Wager, T. D., van Ast, V. A., Hughes, B. L., Davidson M. L., Lindquist M. A., & Ochsner, K. N. (2009). Brain mediators of cardiovascular responses to social threat, part II: Prefrontal-subcortical pathways and relationship with anxiety. *Neuroimage, 47*(3), 836–851.

Walsh, J., Eccleston, C., & Keogh, E. (2012). *A Review of Methods for Investigating Induced Emotive Body Posture Expressions: An Appraisal of Their Application to Pain Research.* Presented at the International Association for the Study of Pain (IASP) 14th World Congress on Pain, August 27–31, 2012, Milan.

Weiss, H. B., Mathers, L. J., Forjuoh, S. N., & Kinnane, J. M. (1997). *Child and adolescent emergency department visit data book.* Pittsburgh, PA: Center for Violence and Injury Control, Allegheny University of the Health Sciences.

Wiffen, P., & Eccleston, C. (2009). The Cochrane pain, palliative and supportive care group: An update. *Palliative Medicine, 23*(2), 179–180.

Willer, J. C., Bouhassira, D., & Le Bars, D. (1999). Neurophysiological bases of the counterirritation phenomenon: Diffuse control inhibitors induced by nociceptive stimulation. *Neurophysiologie Clinique = Clinical Neurophysiology, 29,* 379–400.

Williams, A., Pither, C., Richardson, P., Nicholas, M., Justins, D., Morley, S., ..., & Eccleston, C. (1996). The effects of cognitive-behavioural therapy in chronic pain. *Pain, 65*(2-3), 282–283.

Wilson, T. D., Lisle, D. J., Kraft, D., & Wetzel, C. G. (1989). Preferences as expectation-driven inferences: Effects of affective expectations on affective experience. *Journal of Personality and Social Psychology, 56*(4), 519–530.

Chapter IX

CONCLUSION: QUANTUM PHYSICS AND MODIFIED STATES OF CONSCIOUSNESS– THE MIND BEYOND MATTER

Which are the scientific and philosophic relationships between neuro-physiology of the brain and the modified states of consciousness? Can we explain them?

Jean-Emile Charon was a physicist, an engineer, and a nuclear scientist. In 1959, however, he moved into metaphysics (while continuing to do his nuclear research), trying to extend the ideas of Albert Einstein as he searched for a unified theory to encompass the description of all physical phenomena. Charon published the results of his metaphysical inquiries in a number of works that have been translated throughout the world.

In "L'Esprit cet inconnu," his masterwork, he shows us how the entire universe is happening in each electron of each atom in creation. He writes, "My research focuses on unitary theories–those which strive to unify observable laws, by demonstrating that they are singular parts of a more general law–valid for all phenomena-defined as unitary law. If such a law exists, then it should be valid and verifiable at all dimensional levels, because it analyses the smallest up to the largest–from elementary particles to the entire cosmos" (Charon, 2004).

To discover what the universe is made of and how it works is the challenge of particle physics. Quantum universe presents the quest to explain the universe in terms of quantum physics, which governs the behavior of the microscopic, subatomic world. It describes a revolution in particle physics and a quantum leap in our understanding of the mystery and beauty of the life and the universe.

> The development during the present century is characterized by two theoretical systems essentially independent of each other: the theory of relativity and the

quantum theory. The two systems do not directly contradict each other; but they seem little adapted to fusion into one unified theory. . . . Experiments on interference made with particle rays have given brilliant proof that the wave character of the phenomena of motion as assumed by the theory do, really, correspond to the facts. . . . de Broglie conceived an electron revolving about the atomic nucleus as being connected with a hypothetical wave train, and made intelligible to some extent the discrete character of Bohr's "permitted" paths by the stationary (standing) character of the corresponding waves. (Albert Einstein, 1940)

The Bohr-Einstein debates were a series of public disputes about quantum mechanics between Albert Einstein and Niels Bohr who were two of its founders. Their debates are remembered because of their importance to the philosophy of science. An account of the debates has been written by Bohr in an article titled "Discussions with Einstein on Epistemological Problems in Atomic Physics."

A careful analysis of the process of observation in atomic physics, has shown that the subatomic particles have no meaning as isolated entities, but can only be understood as interconnections. (Capra, 2000)

Roger Penrose (1989) presents the argument that human consciousness is nonalgorithmic and thus not capable of being modeled by a conventional Turing machine type of digital computer. Penrose hypothesizes that quantum mechanics, plays an essential role in the understanding of human consciousness. The collapse of the quantum wave function is seen as playing an important role in brain function.

"There is no one reality. Each of us lives in a separate universe. That's not speaking metaphorically. This is the hypothesis of the stark nature of reality suggested by recent developments in quantum physics. Reality in a dynamic universe is non-objective. Consciousness is the only reality." With those words, M. R. Franks, a life member of the Royal Astronomical Society of Canada, a member of that organization since high school, and also a law professor, begins his new book *The Universe and Multiple Reality*. What is multiple reality? What are the exact processes by which mind interacts with matter at the quantum level?

Some say the universe is made of information. David Chalmers' "dual aspect theory" says that such information has both a physical aspect and an experiential (qualia) aspect. This is similar to what William James had said and Bertrand Russell's neutral monism, in which an underlying entity gives rise to both physical and mental qualities.

The conventional view is that the neural correlate of consciousness is in networks of neurons connected by chemical synapses, axons to dendrites, which are serial, though you can have parallel lines of serial connections. Axonal depolarizations, or spikes, are relatively easy to record and are robust. Therefore, the view is that spikes are the currency of consciousness. The vast majority of actual processing, however, occurs in dendrites (numerous dendites per neuron). Electrophysiological correlates of consciousness (e.g., gamma EEG, coherent 40 Hz) are produced by dendrites, and dendrites are interconnected by gap junctions (forming what I call hyperneurons) that actually do account for gamma EEG/40 Hz. Consciousness occurs in dendrites (John Eccles, Karl Pribram, Stuart Hameroff, Roger Penrose).

A hyperneuron may include tens or hundreds of thousands of gap junction, connected neurons. The quantum state may extend through the gap junctions, so that quantum computations in the collection of microtubules within the many dendrites of a single hyperneuron at a particular time mediate consciousness.

Professor Carlo Rovelli, scientist and quantum gravity theorist, pointed out that the Wheeler-DeWitt equation does not mention space either, suggesting that both space and time might turn out to be artifacts of something deeper. "If we take general relativity seriously," he said, "we have to learn to do physics without time, without space, in the fundamental theory" (2006).

Recent discoveries in quantum physics (the study of the physics of subatomic particles) and in cosmology (the branch of astronomy and astrophysics that deals with the universe taken as a whole) shed new light on how mind interacts with matter and universe. These discoveries compel acceptance of the idea that there is far more than just one universe and that we constantly interact with many of these "hidden" universes.

Our brain inside our skull has no experience of the external world. The brain only responds to internal states like, pH, electrolytes, hormones, ionic exchanges across cell membranes, and electrical impulses. So, how does the brain see an external world? That question goes back at least thousands of years, and the Greeks said that the world outside is nothing but a representation in our head.

Then of course Descartes recognized the same thing–that the only thing about which he could be sure was that he is, that he is conscious. I think, therefore I am. So, we are not really sure the outside world is as we perceive it. Some people would say it is a construction, an illusion. Some people would say it is an accurate representation. It is kind of a mix of views, and then when you add quantum properties to it, it is really uncertain if the world we perceive is the actual world out there.

According to the scientist Stuart Hameroff, it is also possible that quantum information is transduced in the retina in the cilia between the inner and outer segments before the photon even gets to the rhodopsin in the very back of the eye. So it is possible that there is additional quantum information being extracted from photons as they enter your eye through the retina. They might somehow more directly convey the actual essential quality or properties of the rose and the redness of the rose. Of course this gets right to the hard problem of conscious experience: that we have an actual quality of redness, pain, grief, sorrow, joy, happiness, and all feelings that are conscious awareness.

Since the structure of space-time geometry, what emptiness is made of is kind of holographic by quantum processes our retina and brain are able to access and connect to the essential qualities of the rose so that we have it in our head. Because space-time is sort of holographic, we are able to access it via quantum processes inside our brain.

"Second is guidance by Platonic wisdom. Penrose also embedded Platonic values in spacetime geometry which can guide our actions, and be viewed as following the way of the Tao, or divine guidance, or whatever you want to call it. And finally, even conceivably the possibility of afterlife or consciousness outside of the body" (Hameroff, 2010).

Robert Jahn and Brenda Dunne will describe the research carried out over the past quarter century in their PEAR laboratory, housed in Princeton University's School of Engineering and Applied Science. The results of numerous carefully controlled experiments provide strong evidence that human consciousness can play a proactive role in the establishment of physical reality. Initially intended to address the potential vulnerability of sensitive engineering systems and processes, these findings carry much broader implications that bear on our view of ourselves, our relationship to others, and to the cosmos in which we exist.

I think more like a quantum Hindu or Buddhist, in that there is a universal proto-conscious mind, which we access, and can influence us.

1. THE HUMAN BEING AND THE RELATIONSHIP BETWEEN BODY, MIND AND SPIRIT

Hypnotic therapy, mindfulness, and the meditative stages consider human beings as a whole of mind body and spirit. I am very glad to introduce you this theory, elaborated with my father Angelico Brugnoli.

How can we clearly explain the relationship between mind-body and spirit and the connections among hypnosis, mindfulness, meditative stages, and the activation of spiritual awareness and higher consciousness?

The human being is constituted by

1. the physical being (body)
2. the psychic being (mind)
3. the spiritual being (spirit, soul, higher consciousness)

To understand this concept we can imagine a cube where the width and the length are the physical and psychic side and the height is the spiritual side. We need to consider the human being in a part that forms the human being in a three-dimensional way:

therefore we will be talking of three sides of the human being
    body
        mind
            spirit

These three different components are intersecting one another to shape our three-dimensional cube, and they are part of the same person or entity.

For the human being, therefore, we are mind-body and spirit, and God that can be called the unknown being.

1–**the physical side (the body)** includes everything in the three-dimensional form that exists in the universe and also the time is part of it, which we can call time coordinate (because it differs from area to area on the earth and in the cosmos). The really physicality of the universe side includes all the cosmos, all the universe, and this also allows the psychic side to be part of it. The time coordinate is part of the body or physic side but relates also to the psychic.

2–**the psychic side is the mind**, and it is related to the body, or physic side, by the time coordinate and by the activation of the different cerebral zones.

3–**the spiritual side (the spirit)**

The psychic universe is related to the spiritual universe, as the point (focus) is to the whole. Therefore, what differentiates the transaction from the psychic field to the spiritual one is that the coordinate of time is not important any more. Like the vision of the universe, which is composed by the electric, the electromagnetic, magnetic, and gravitational fields, which are considered as a whole, we can consider also the psychic field connected with the physical one and creating a whole unit.

Let us try to find a rational explanation in the relationship between mind-body and spirit.

We can find a comparison in physics considering, for instance, the speed of light as a universal constant.

We call the speed of light V^1 and in this case it is a known speed.

V^1 is understood as the speed of light, of 300.000 km/second.

V^0 represents the absolute quiet of all material; therefore, there is no physical side when the speed of light is equal to 0

Between V^0 and V^1 exists the entire physical field that we know, such as from the subatomic world to the atomic aggregation; consequently, the molecular one up to the chemical compositions of all the metals, and different chemical essences up to man (human being) as a physical being.

Between V^0 and V^1 exists the entire physical universe we know.

In this field, therefore, between V^0 and V^1 exists also the time, understood as a measure and as a coordinate; the time therefore is part of the space so called of the four dimensions, between V^0 and V^1 time is measurable.

To understand the physical concept of mind and spirit, we can imagine the mind and the spirit, as power of V^1.

Obviously in the power of V at two, three, and so on, also the concept of time will change up to when it will not be measurable any more, and then perhaps until it disappears.

Throughout the power of V^1 you could find a physical explanation for the psychic field and the spiritual one. You can explore more deeply the analysis in this field. It is easy to understand that going in exponential progression, Infinite power of V exists, and maybe in the future it will be possible to explain other forms of knowledge until:

the Unknown Spiritual Being = V^n

Around 1990, Rovelli and Smolin obtained an explicit basis of states of quantum geometry, which turned out to be labelled by Roger Penrose's spin networks, and showed that the geometry is quantized, that is, the (nongauge-invariant) quantum operators, representing area and volume, have a discrete spectrum. The quantum mind hypothesis proposes that classical mechanics cannot fully explain consciousness and suggests that quantum mechanical phenomena, such as quantum entanglement and superposition, may play an important part in the brain's function and could form the basis of an explanation of consciousness.

Next, we will investigate whether this quantum world, like the classical world, is really composed of separate, independently existing entities. In other words, is this new world of potentiality a "Many" or a "One"? Our neuropsychological consciousness, made not only of the matter of mind but also of awareness and spirit, is potentiality a "many" or a "one"? Our Higher Consciousness and our spirituality, is potentiality a "many" or a "one"?

I leave you the answer, my friends, with your next scientific researches.

REFERENCES

Capra, F. (2000). *The Tao of physics.* Boston: Shambhala Publications.

Chalmers, D. (1996). *The conscious mind.* Oxford: Oxford University Press.

Charon, J. E. (2004). *The spirit: That stranger inside us.* Califormula Publishing.

Penrose, R. (1989). *Shadows of the mind: A search for the missing science of consciousness.* Oxford, UK: Oxford University Press.

Rovelli, C. (2006, October 13). Graviton propagator from background-independent quantum gravity. *Physical Review Letters, 97*(15), 151301. Epub Oct 10.

SUGGESTED READINGS

Armstrong, D. M. (1978). Naturalism, materialism and first philosophy. *Philosophia, 8,* 261–276.

Atkinson, R. C., & Shiffrin, R. M. (1968). Human memory: A proposed system and its control processes. In K. W. Spence & J. T. Spence (Eds.), *The psychology of learning and motivation* (Vol. 2, pp. 89–195). New York: Academic Press.

Bennett, M. V., & Zukin, R. S. (2004, February 19). Electrical coupling and neuronal synchronization in the mammalian brain [Review]. *Neuron, 41*(4), 495–511.

Bickle, J. (2003). *Philosophy and neuroscience: A ruthlessly reductive account.* Norwell, MA: Kluwer Academic Press.

Blackmore, S. (2003). *Consciousness: An introduction.* London: Hodder & Stoughton.

Bower, B. (2007, September 15). Consciousness in the raw: The brain stem may orchestrate the basics of awareness [Online]. *Science News.*

Brugnoli, A. (2004). Stato di coscienza totalizzante, alla ricerca del profondo Se. Verona, Italy: La Grafica Editrice.

Brugnoli A. (2005). *Stati di coscienza modificati neurofisiologici.* Verona, Italy: La Grafica Editrice.

Brugnoli, A. (2005). *Stati di coscienza modificati neurofisiologici.* Verona, Italy: La Grafica Editrice.

Capra, F. (1996). *The web of life: A new scientific understanding of living systems.* New York: Anchor Books. Available at http://www.worldcat.org/oclc/37800841& referer=brief_results

Carruthers, P. (2000). *Phenomenal consciousness.* Cambridge: Cambridge University Press.

Chalmers, D. J. (1995). Facing up to the problem of consciousness. *Journal of Consciousness Studies, 2*(3), 200–219.

Churchland, P. (1986). *Neurophilosophy.* Cambridge, MA: MIT Press.

Cowan, N. (1995). *Attention and memory: An integrated framework.* New York: Oxford University Press.

Crick, F., & Koch, C. (1995a). Are we aware of neural activity in primary visual cortex? *Nature, 375,* 121–123

Crick, F., & Koch, C. (1995b). Cortical areas in visual awareness [Reply]. *Nature, 377,* 294–295.

Damasio, A. (1994). *Descartes' error: Emotions, reason, and the human brain.* New York: Avon Books.

De Zazzo, J., & Tully, T. (1995). Dissection of memory formation: From behavioural pharmacology to molecular genetics. *Trends in Neuroscience, 18,* 212–218.

Dennett, D. (1991). *Consciousness explained.* London: Penguin Books.

Dermietzel, R. (1998). Gap junction wiring: A "new" principle in cell-to-cell communication in the nervous system? *Brain Research Reviews, 26,* 176–183.

Desimone, R., & Duncan, J. (1995). Neural mechanisms of selective visual attention. *Annual Review of Neuroscience, 18,* 193–222.

Farthing, G. W. (1992). *The psychology of consciousness.* Englewood Cliffs, NJ: Prentice-Hall.

Fries, P., Schroder, J.-H., Roelfsema, P. R., Singer, W., & Engel, A. K. (2002). Oscillatory neuronal synchronization in primary visual cortex as a correlate of stimulus selection. *Journal of Neuroscience, 22,* 3739–3754.

Frost, S. E. (1989). *Basic teachings of the great philosophers.* New York: Anchor Books.

Fuster, J. M. (1997). *The prefrontal cortex: Anatomy, physiology, and neuropsychology of the frontal lobe* (2nd ed.). Philadelphia: Lippincott, Williams & Wilkins.

Galarreta, M., & Hestrin, S. (1999). A network of fast-spiking cells in the neocortex connected by electrical synapses. *Nature, 402,* 72–75.

Goldstein, J. (1983). *The experience of insight.* Boston: Shambhala.

Gombrich, R. F. (1988). *Theravāda Buddhism: A social history from ancient Benares to modern Colombo.* London: Routledge.

Hameroff, S. (2010, January). The "conscious pilot"–dendritic synchrony moves through the brain to mediate consciousness. *Journal of Biological Physics, 36*(1), 71–93.

Hameroff, S. R. (1987). Ultimate computing: Biomolecular consciousness and nano technology. Philadelphia: Elsevier Science Publishers. Available at http://www.quantumconsciousness.org/ultimatecomputing.html

Hameroff, S. R., & Watt, R. C. (1982). Information processing in microtubules. *Journal of Theoretical Biology, 98,* 549–561. Available at http://www.quantumconsciousness.org/documents/informationprocessing_hameroff_000.pdf

Hameroff, S. R. (2008). That's life!–The geometry of πelectron clouds. In D. Abbott, P. C. W. Davies & A. K. Pati (Eds.), *Quantum aspects of life* (pp. 403–426).

London: Imperial College Press. Retrieved Jan 21, 2010. Available at http://www.quantumconsciousness.org/documents/Hameroff_received-1-05-07.pdf

Hormuzdi, S. G., Filippov, M. A., Mitropoulou, G., Monyer, H., & Bruzzone, R. (2004). Electrical synapses: A dynamic signaling system that shapes the activity of neuronal networks. *Biochimica et Biophysica Acta, 1662,* 113–137.

Jackson, F. (1982). Epiphenomenal qualia. *Philosophical Quarterly, 32,* 127–136.

Kaiser, J., & Lutzenberger, W. (2003). Induced gamma-band activity and human brain function. *Neuroscientist, 9,* 475–484.

Knudsen, E. I. (2007). Fundamental components of attention. *Annual Review of Neuroscience, 30*(1), 57–78.

Lao Tzu. (1963). *Tao Te Ching.* London: Penguin Books.

Lazar, S. W., Bush, G., Gollub, R. L., Fricchione, G. L., Khalsa, G., & Benson, H. (2000). Functional brain mapping of the relaxation response and meditation. *NeuroReport, 11*(7), 1581–1585.

LeBeau, F. E. N., Traub, R. D., Monyer, H., Whittington, M. A., & Buhl, E. H. (2003). The role of electrical signaling via gap junctions in the generation of fast network oscillations. *Brain Research Bulletin, 62,* 3–13.

Lehmann, D., Grass, P., & Meier, B. (1995). Spontaneous conscious covert cognition states and brain electric spectral states in canonical correlations. *International Journal of Psychophysiology, 19,* 41–52.

Leroy, E. B. (1933). *Les visions du demi-sommeil.* Paris: Alcan.

Levine, J. (1983). Materialism and qualia: The explanatory gap. *Pacific Philosophical Quarterly, 64,* 354–361.

Marshall, W., Simon, C., Penrose, R., & Bouwmeester, D. (2003). Towards quantum superpositions of a mirror. *Physical Review Letters, 91*(13), 130401-1–130401-4.

McFarlane, T. J. (1995). Quantum mechanics and reality [Online]. Available at www.integralscience.org

Merker, B. (2007, September). Consciousness in the raw. *Science News Online.* Available at http://www.sciencenews.org/articles/20070915/bob9.asp

Mosca, A. (2000). A review essay on Antonio Damasio's *The Feeling of What Happens: Body and Emotion in the Making of Consciousness. PSYCHE, 6*(10).

Nagel, E. (1961) *The structure of science.* London: Routledge.

Penrose, R. (1989b). *The emperor's new mind: Concerning computers, minds and the laws of physics.* Oxford, UK: Oxford University Press.

Searle, J. (1992). *The rediscovery of the mind.* Cambridge, MA: MIT Press.

Searle, J. R. (1990). Consciousness, explanatory inversion and cognitive science. *Behavioral and Brain Sciences, 13,* 585–642.

Sellars, R. W. (1919). The epistemology of evolutionary naturalism. *Mind, 28*(112), 407–426.

Taylor, J. (2000, February). The enchanting subject of consciousness (or is it a black hole?). *PSYCHE, 6*(2).

Van Gulick, R. (2004). Higher-order global states (HOGS): An alternative higher-order model of consciousness. In R. J. Gennaro (Ed.), *Higher-order theories of consciousness: An anthology* (pp. 67–92). Amsterdam: John Benjamins B. V.

Vogels, T. P., Rajan, K., & Abbott, L. F. (2005). Neural network dynamics. *Annual Review of Neuroscience, 28,* 357–376.

INDEX